JRCALC Clinical Practice Supplementary Guidelines 2017

Edited for JRCALC and AACE by

Simon N Brown, Dhushy Kumar and Cathryn James

on behalf of NASMeD by

Julian Mark and medical director colleagues

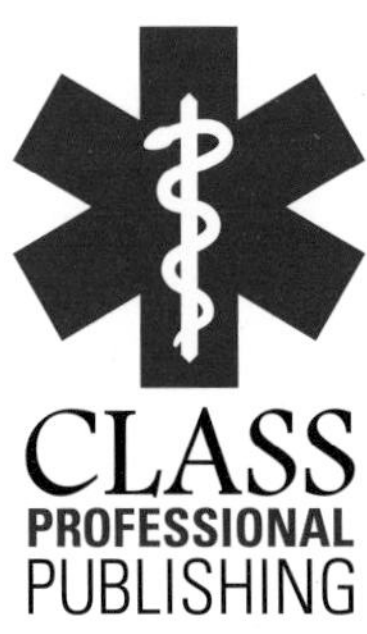

September 2017

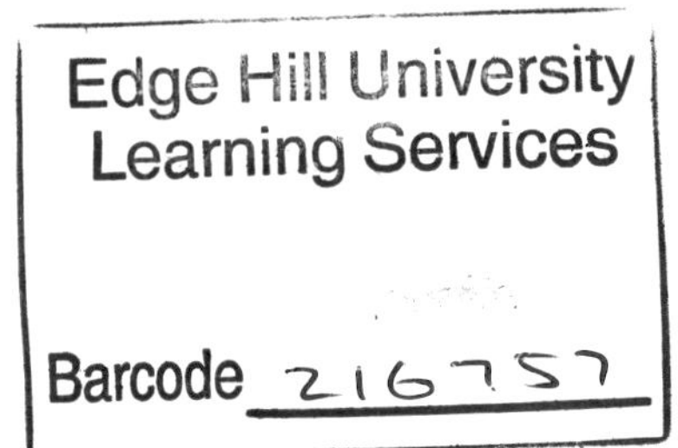

The information presented in this book is accurate and current to the best of the authors' knowledge. The authors and publisher, however, make no guarantee as to, and assume no responsibility for, the correctness, sufficiency or completeness of such information or recommendation.

Printing history

First edition published 2000, second edition 2004, third edition 2006

Fourth edition published 2013, reprinted 2014, 2015 (twice, Version 1.3)

The content for Reference Edition 1.3 and Pocket Book 1.2 was updated in January 2015.

2016 edition published 2016, reprinted 2016 (Version 1.5)

This supplement published 2017.

Reprinted 2017.

The authors and publisher welcome feedback from the users of this book.

Please contact the publisher:

Class Professional Publishing,

The Exchange, Express Park, Bristol Road, Bridgwater TA6 4RR

Telephone: 01278 427 800

Email: icpg@class.co.uk

Website: www.classprofessional.co.uk

Class Professional Publishing is an imprint of Class Publishing Ltd

A CIP catalogue record for this book is available from the British Library

This edition: JRCALC Clinical Practice Supplementary Guidelines 2017 ISBN 978 1 85959 654 8

ISSN 2514-6084

Also available: JRCALC Clinical Practice Supplementary Guidelines 2017 ISBN 978 1 85959 659 3 (ebook)

Clinical Practice Guidelines 2016 ISBN 978 1 85959 594 7 (print)

Clinical Practice Guidelines 2016 ISBN 978 1 85959 595 4 (ebook)

Designed and typeset by RefineCatch and DLXML Associates

Edited by Emma Milman and Heather Cushing

Line illustrations by David Woodroffe and Gary Holmes

Printed in Slovenia by arrangement with KINT Ljubljana

Contents

Disclaimer

The Association of Ambulance Chief Executives and the Joint Royal Colleges Ambulance Liaison Committee have made every effort to ensure that the information, tables, drawings and diagrams contained in these guidelines are accurate at the time of publication. However, the guidelines are advisory and have been developed to assist healthcare professionals, and patients, to make decisions about the management of the patient's health, including treatments. This advice is intended to support the decision making process and is not a substitute for sound clinical judgement. The guidelines cannot always contain all the information necessary for determining appropriate care and cannot address all individual situations; therefore, individuals using these guidelines must ensure they have the appropriate knowledge and skills to enable suitable interpretation.

JRCALC has referenced NICE in these guidelines. NICE guidance is prepared for the National Health Service in England, and is subject to regular review and may be updated or withdrawn. NICE has not checked the use of its content in these guidelines to confirm that it accurately reflects the NICE publications from which it is taken.

Users of these guidelines must always be aware that such innovations or alterations after the date of publication may not be incorporated in the content.

The Association of Ambulance Chief Executives and the Joint Royal Colleges Ambulance Liaison Committee do not guarantee, and accepts no legal liability of whatever nature arising from or connected to, the accuracy, reliability, currency or completeness of the content of these guidelines.

Although some modification of the guidelines may be required by individual ambulance services, and approved by the relevant local clinical committees, to ensure they respond to the health requirements of the local community, the majority of the guidance is universally applicable to NHS ambulance services. Modification of the guidelines may also occur when undertaking research sanctioned by a research ethics committee.

Whilst these guidelines cover a range of paramedic treatments available across the UK they will also provide a valuable tool for a range of care providers. Many of the assessment skills and general principles will remain the same. All clinical staff must practise within their level of training and competence.

Foreword

Welcome to the JRCALC Clinical Practice Supplementary Guidelines 2017, which complement the UK Ambulance Services Clinical Practice Guidelines 2016. You will find here some valuable minor amendments and updates, but most importantly, significant new guidance.

Sepsis has for too long been under recognised and under treated across the healthcare sector. Recent campaigns have raised awareness and the new guidance presented here includes practical steps ambulance clinicians can take to improve care.

Maternal and obstetric emergencies can often present challenges and concerns for pre-hospital clinicians. The completely revised and updated guidelines provide the detailed knowledge and practical information required for safe, effective practice and decision making.

Caring for an ageing population is of course a growing need, and the new section on falls in the older adult provides strategies for dealing with one of the common calls for pre-hospital clinicians.

All the guidance presented here by JRCALC supports thoughtful delivery of care by professionals rather than the following of flowcharts or protocols. Paramedics are developing their practice and we trust that these guidelines support that journey.

JRCALC would like to thank all those that contributed to this supplement, our committee members who acted as lead authors and the groups of expert and enthusiastic healthcare professionals who gave so willingly of their time. Emma Milman acted as the lead editor for Class Professional and Cathryn James of AACE provided expertise, knowledge and energy. Final thanks are due to the ambulance service medical directors (NASMeD), who requested this guidance and have supported its contents.

DHUSHY SURENDRA KUMAR

Chair, Joint Royal Colleges Ambulance Liaison Committee

SIMON N BROWN

Chair, JRCALC Guideline Development Groups

STEVE IRVING

Executive Officer, Association of Ambulance Chief Executives

Guideline Developers and Contributors

The authors and editors would like to thank everyone who has contributed to these 2017 supplementary guidelines. Many people have given freely and generously of their time to help draft, develop and improve the guidelines. In particular, we wish to acknowledge the work of the members of JRCALC and the National Ambulance Service Medical Directors group (NASMeD). Contributors have come from multidisciplinary groups and include healthcare professionals, educators and patients.

Editorial Leads

CATHRYN JAMES, *Clinical Support for NASMeD and JRCALC guidelines editor, AACE*

STEVE IRVING, *Executive Officer, AACE*

DHUSHY KUMAR, *Consultant in Critical Care, Prehospital Care and Anaesthesia, University Hospitals Coventry and Warwickshire, chair of JRCALC*

SIMON N BROWN, *GP and Assistant Medical Director, South Central Ambulance Service, JRCALC member, Royal College of GPs*

JULIAN MARK, *Executive Medical Director, Yorkshire Ambulance Service, chair of NASMeD*

Reference Groups:

OBSTETRICS AND GYNAECOLOGY

KIM HINSHAW, *Consultant Obstetrician and Gynaecologist, City Hospitals Sunderland, JRCALC Royal College of Obstetricians and Gynaecologists*

AMANDA MANSFIELD, *Consultant Midwife, London Ambulance Service, JRCALC The Royal College of Midwives*

SALLY ARNOLD-JONES, *Paramedic, Clinical Development Manager, South Western Ambulance Service*

ANNMARIE BRESLIN, *Midwife and Advanced Life Support Obstetrics faculty*

CLAIRE CAPITO, *Supervisor of Midwives, Support Midwife for London*

PROFESSOR TIM DRAYCOTT, *Consultant Obstetrician, Bristol. Representing PROMPT (PRactical Obstetric Multi-Professional Training) programme*

SIMON GRANT, *Consultant in Obstetrics and Fetal Medicine, North Bristol. Representing MOET (Managing Obstetric Emergencies and Trauma) programme*

CLAIRE HENDERSON, *Paramedic, London Ambulance Service*

SHARON JORDAN, *Midwife, Senior Labour Ward Coordinator*

MICHELLE KNIGHT, *Lead Midwife, Epsom and St Helier Hospital*

PROFESSOR PAUL LEWIS, OBE, *Emeritus Professor, Bournemouth University, Honorary Fellow of the Royal College of Midwives. Representing ALSO (Advanced Life Support in Obstetrics) UK programme*

DENICE MACE, *Senior Clinical Midwife, Sunderland. Representing POET (Prehospital Obstetric Emergency Training) programme*

STEPHANIE MICHAELIDES, *Midwife, Programme Leader, Middlesex University*

ROGER NEUBERG, *retired Consultant in Obstetrics and Gynaecology, Leicester. Representing ALSO (Advanced Life Support in Obstetrics) UK programme*

NICK SILLETT, *Advanced Paramedic Practitioner, London Ambulance Service*

JACQUI TOMKINS, *Chair of Independent Midwives UK*

AARTI ULLAL, *Consultant Obstetrician, City Hospitals Sunderland*

CATHY WINTER, *Research Midwife, Bristol. Representing PROMPT (PRactical Obstetric Multi-Professional Training) programme*

JONATHAN WYLLIE, *Professor of Neonatology and Paediatrics, Durham University, Consultant Neonatologist, James Cook University Hospital*

AIMEE YARRINGTON, *Paramedic and Midwife, West Midlands Ambulance Service*

FALLS IN OLDER ADULTS

ALISON WALKER, *Consultant in Emergency Medicine, Harrogate and District Hospital, JRCALC member*

MARK BAXTER, *Orthogeriatrician, University Hospital Southampton*

JAY BANERJEE, *Consultant in Emergency Medicine, University Hospitals of Leicester*

KEITH COLVER, *Paramedic, Clinical Governance Manager, Scottish Ambulance Service*

DAWNE GARRETT, *Professional Lead – Older People and Dementia Care, The Royal College of Nursing*

JOANNA GARRETT, *Paramedic, Clinical Development Officer, South Western Ambulance Service*

JAMES GOUGH, *Paramedic, Welsh Ambulance Service*

TIM JONES, *Advanced Paramedic Practitioner, Clinical Practice Lead, Welsh Ambulance Service*

ANN MURRAY, *Programme Lead, Falls Programme, Active and Independent Living Programme, Scottish Government*

IAN MURSELL, *Consultant Paramedic, East Midlands Ambulance Service*

DUNCAN ROBERTSON, *Consultant Paramedic, North West Ambulance Service*

VICKY KYPTA, *Specialist Paramedic, South East Coast Ambulance Service*

DANIEL HAWORTH, *Advanced Practice Paramedic and Pathway Development Manager, North East Ambulance Service*

JAQUI LINDRIDGE, *Consultant Paramedic, London Ambulance Service*

SAFEGUARDING

SARAH THOMPSON, *Nurse, Head of Safeguarding and Staying Well Service, Designated Officer for Allegations, South Western Ambulance Service*

NIKKI HARVEY, *Nurse and Head of Safeguarding, Welsh Ambulance Service*

SAM THOMPSON, *Forensic Paramedic, Kent Police and Senior Lecturer, St George's, University of London*

SIMON CHASE, *Paramedic, Safeguarding Lead and Freedom to Speak Up Guardian, East of England Ambulance Service*

JANE MITCHELL, *Paramedic and Safeguarding Lead, South East Coast Ambulance Service*

ALAN TAYLOR, *Paramedic and Head of Safeguarding, London Ambulance Service*

SEPSIS

DHUSHY KUMAR, *Consultant in Critical Care, Prehospital Care and Anaesthesia, University Hospitals Coventry and Warwickshire, chair of JRCALC*

BARRY MURPHY-JONES, *Paramedic, Clinical Watch Manager/Clinical Audit Facilitator, London Ambulance Service*

MIKE SMYTH, *Paramedic, NIHR Clinical Doctoral Research Fellow, University of Warwick*

JAMES WENMAN, *Consultant Paramedic, South Western Ambulance Service*

GRAHAM MCCLELLAND, *Research Paramedic, North East Ambulance Service*

SIMON STOCKLEY, GP, *The Royal College of General Practitioners, JRCALC member*

PAUL KELLY, *Paramedic, Scottish Ambulance Service*

MATTHEW INADA-KIM, *Consultant Acute Physician, Hampshire Hospitals, National Clinical Advisor Sepsis, Sepsis Lead for the National Patient Safety Collaborative*

TRACY NICHOLLS, *Paramedic, Head of Clinical Quality, East of England Ambulance Service*

TRAUMA

CHERYLENE CAMPS, *Paramedic, Duty Operations Manager, East Midlands Ambulance Service*

PROFESSOR SIR KEITH PORTER, *Professor of Clinical Traumatology, University Hospitals Birmingham, JRCALC member, Royal College of Surgeons Edinburgh*

COLVILLE LAIRD, *GP, JRCALC member, Royal College of Surgeons Edinburgh*

SIMON N BROWN, *GP and Assistant Medical Director, South Central Ambulance Service, JRCALC member and member of the Royal College of GPs*

PAIN MANAGEMENT

MARTIN PARKINSON, *Paramedic, Yorkshire Ambulance Service*

SHYAM BALASUBRAMANIAN, *Consultant in Pain Medicine and Anaesthesia, University Hospitals Coventry*

Contributors

RICHARD BERRY, *Specialist Paramedic, South Central Ambulance Service*
ALICE BRETON, *Education and Research Development Lead, Royal College of Surgeons Edinburgh*
MARK MILLINS, *Associate Director Paramedic Practice, Yorkshire Ambulance Service*
RICHARD PILBERY, *Research Paramedic, Yorkshire Ambulance Service*
KEVIN WEBB, *Paramedic, Clinical Effectiveness Manager, Welsh Ambulance Service*
JOHN WASS, *Professor, Endocrinologist, Oxford University Hospitals*
KATHERINE WHITE, *Chair, Addison's Disease Self Help Group*
MENAI OWEN-JONES, *Chief Executive Officer, The Pituary Foundation*
DAVE WHITMORE, *Paramedic and Clinical Advisor, London Ambulance Service*
IAN WILMER, *Advanced Paramedic Practitioner, London Ambulance Service*

Guideline Development Methodology

The methodology used by JRCALC (Joint Royal Colleges Ambulance Liaison Committee) to develop the UK Ambulance Services Clinical Practice Guidelines is designed to comply with the criteria used by the AGREE II (Appraisal of Guidelines for Research and Evaluation in Europe) instrument. This process is a leading academic tool to identify good quality guidelines: http://www.agreetrust.org/

The purpose of the AGREE II, is to provide a framework to:

- assess the quality of guidelines
- provide a methodological strategy for the development of guidelines
- inform what information and how information ought to be reported in guidelines.

By adopting these principles, guidelines are developed that support safe decision making and high quality patient care.

Guideline Selection

JRCALC, NASMeD (National Ambulance Service Medical Directors) and the ALPG (Ambulance Lead Paramedic Group) will advise on those clinical guidelines which need updating and those clinical conditions which need a new guideline developing. These are then prioritised and assessed with regard to urgency and risk. Clinical topics can be identified through a variety of means including the monitoring of serious incidents within individual UK Ambulance Service Trusts, preventing future death directives issued by coroners and national service reconfiguration e.g. the move to major trauma centres and networks. In addition JRCALC provide extensive clinical expertise and advice on potential new developments to ensure that the guidelines capture latest best practice and future innovations.

Feedback

Is welcome via

JRCALC@AACE.org

Editorial Independence

No external funding has been received for the development of these guidelines and no competing or conflicting interests have been declared by those involved in their development.

How to Use this Book

The UK Ambulance Services Clinical Practice Guidelines is a reference book with accompanying Pocket Book and iCPG companion app to assist ambulance clinicians and pre-hospital practitioners with information on the common conditions and injuries encountered on emergency calls. These resources give practical guidance on assessment and management, and detailed listings of drug routes and dosages.

This supplementary edition contains new and updated guidance to be used in conjunction with the 2016 edition of the UK Ambulance Services Clinical Practice Guidelines.

The content is divided into sections focussing on general guidance, medical conditions, trauma, maternity care and specific drug information. Where relevant, information on the treatment of children is provided separately.

Each guideline is organised to provide background information on the nature and incidence of each condition or circumstance to aid assessment and decision making, as well as specific and detailed information on the management of patients. Many of the guidelines are supplemented with algorithms for step-by-step direction.

Throughout the guidelines coloured text is used to refer the clinician to further relevant guidance; the colour relates to the section of the book within which the guidance falls:

General Guidance

Resuscitation

Medical

Trauma

Maternity Care

Drugs

Special Situations

The drugs section contains guidance on the drugs that can currently be administered by paramedics. The individual tables list dosage information by patient age for each preparation. The Page for Age section lists the routes and dosages for each drug appropriate to each age range.

The Pocket Book that accompanies the reference and supplementary editions provides clinicians with all the drugs tables and Page for Age data, as well as algorithms and tables for specific conditions and circumstances to assist in the assessment and management of patients.

The iCPG companion app holds exactly the same content as the reference, supplementary and pocket books in an easy-to-use, dynamic format that is accessible and practical for use in day-to-day practice. It updates in real time with best practice information. Visit www.icpg.co.uk for more information.

Update Analysis

The 2017 supplementary guidelines are published in addition to the UK Ambulance Service Clinical Practice Guidelines 2016.

Section 1

General Guidance	***Addition/update of guidance and rationale***
Pain Management in Adults	This guideline has been significantly updated. ● The 0–10 point verbal numerical scale in which 0 refers to no pain and 10 is the worst imaginable pain is recommended. ● For patients with communication difficulties and dementia, the Abbey Pain Scale is recommended. ● Clinical evaluation of chronic pain is covered. ● Ambulance clinicians should consider biopsychosocial factors. ● 'Balanced analgesia' with a multimodal pain plan is recommended by JRCALC in pre-hospital pain management and involves administration of analgesics with different mechanisms of action. ● An algorithm on the routes of administration according to pain severity is included. ● Pain measurements and re-assessments will help to monitor progress. ● New information is provided about Methoxyflurane (Penthrox).
Safeguarding Children	This guideline has been significantly updated in line with current legislation. ● Members of staff have a duty of care to report abuse or neglect. If the abuse is not reported, the victim may be at greater risk. ● Emotional abuse, sexual abuse, child sexual exploitation/abuse, physical abuse and neglect are discussed. ● Mandatory reporting of female genital mutilation (FGM) is included.
Sexual Assault	This guideline has been significantly updated. ● Sexual assault may be concurrent with other injuries that will need treating. ● The decision to report a sexual assault on an adult is entirely the decision of the victim. There is no statutory obligation for victims of sexual violence to report to police and many victims elect not to report to protect their safety, privacy or both. ● Where the victim requests police involvement, forensic awareness is essential. Within the limits of any immediate care needs, there is a responsibility to preserve evidence. ● Sexual Assault Referral Centres provide recent victims of sexual assault with immediate care and crisis support from specialist staff trained to allow patients to make informed decisions. ● Patients refusing referral to support services place a duty of care on clinicians to ensure their immediate safety. Encouraging patients to call a friend or relative for support is a priority. In these cases, patients should be given details of their nearest GUM clinic and rape crisis services.
Safeguarding Adults at Risk	This guideline has been significantly updated in line with current legislation. ● Ambulance clinicians are often the first professionals to make contact with adults at risk and may identify initial concerns regarding abuse. The role of the ambulance service is not to investigate suspicions but to ensure that any suspicion is passed, with the consent of the adult (where no consent, state why), to the appropriate agency (e.g. social care or the police) in line with locally agreed procedures. ● The six key principles underpinning the Care Act guidance are covered: empowerment, prevention, proportionality, protection, partnership and accountability. ● Types and signs of abuse are explained. ● Mandatory Reporting of FGM is included. ● The NHS, including the ambulance service, has a statutory responsibility to comply and engage with Prevent. Any member of staff identifying concerns that vulnerable people may be radicalised, should report to the safeguarding service, their Prevent lead or their line manager in the Trust.

Domestic Abuse	This is a new guideline. ● If staff suspect a crime has been committed resulting in harm to the patient, the police must be called. ● Listen closely to the patient for disclosure, and document this on the patient record. ● If possible, take the patient away from the scene. ● Treatment should avoid disturbing evidence where possible. ● Take into account any information that is disclosed by children. ● Never leave a child with an alleged perpetrator if transporting the patient to hospital. ● Accommodate patient wishes where possible.

Section 3a

Medical – Undifferentiated Complaints	***Addition/update of guidance and rationale***
Altered Level of Consciousness	Adrenal insufficiency (adrenal crisis) is added as a red flag condition that should be considered as a cause of altered level of consciousness.
Medical Emergencies in Adults – Overview	More detail is included about the management of patients with adrenal insufficiency (adrenal crisis). Emphasis is on its potentially life threatening nature, the risk of circulatory collapse, the need for early and prompt treatment and administration of hydrocortisone, fluids and rapid transport.
Sepsis	This is a completely new guideline. We purposely decided not to develop or include a sepsis screening algorithm or tool. JRCALC recommends using tools that have been agreed locally in your own organisation, or across a network or region, along with use of a NEWS score. We are aware of the development of NEWS2, and this guideline will be updated after it becomes available. The red, amber and green tables in the febrile illness in children guideline are slightly different from the more up-to-date tables in this new sepsis guideline. This will be addressed as part of a future update in the febrile illness in children guideline. ● Think 'could this be sepsis?' if a person presents with fever/feeling unwell with a NEWS greater than or equal to 5. ● Think 'could this be sepsis?' if a person looks unwell with a history of infection. ● NEWS does not diagnose sepsis – it simply identifies sick patients who need urgent senior medical review and intervention. ● Keep on scene times to a minimum – delaying transport may increase mortality. ● Provide a pre-alert and NEWS score to the receiving hospital – 'patient has suspected sepsis' – in line with local arrangements.

Section 3b

Medical – Specific Conditions	***Addition/update of guidance and rationale***
Asthma (Adults)	Reference to T piece nebuliser is removed.
Asthma (Children)	Reference to T piece nebuliser is removed.

Section 4

Trauma	*Addition/update of guidance and rationale*
	Four pieces of trauma guidance have been updated in line with NICE major trauma guidance. Emphasis on conveyance destination, major trauma centres and use of ATMIST is included.
Limb Trauma	• Emphasis on major trauma centres, use of ATMIST and antibiotics for open fractures. • Do not irrigate open fractures of the long bones, hindfoot or midfoot. • Management of amputations, partial amputations and degloving are covered.
Spinal Injury and Spinal Cord Injury	This guideline replaces the Neck and Back Trauma guideline • Immobilise the whole spine until it is positively cleared. • Immobilise the whole spine in all unconscious blunt trauma patients. • Falls are a frequent cause of SCI in the older person. Maintain a high index of suspicion in cases of older people who have had low energy falls. • If the cervical spine is immobilised, the thoracic and lumbar spine also needs immobilisation. • Asking a patient to self-extricate is acceptable, but is not clearing the cervical spine. • Standard immobilisation is by means of collar (unless contraindicated or counterproductive), head blocks, tape and scoop. • Longboard is solely used as an extrication device, and not for transporting patients to hospital. • Aspiration of vomit, pressure sores and raised intracranial pressure are major complications of immobilisation. • Red flag signs and symptoms of the medical emergency Cauda Equina Syndrome (CES) are covered. • A new immobilisation algorithm is presented.
Major Pelvic Trauma	• Always suspect a pelvic fracture in a blunt high-energy trauma. • Give tranexamic acid as soon as possible for active or suspected active bleeding from a pelvic fracture.
Thoracic Trauma	• $EtC0_2$ presents an immediate picture of the patient's condition. • Open chest wounds: seal the wound with a proprietary dressing with a valve, but if none are available use a three-sided dressing. • Open thoracostomy can be performed if an appropriately skilled practitioner is available.
Falls in Older Adults	This is a completely new guideline. • The term 'mechanical fall' is not an appropriate term to use when describing a fall. • Initial assessment should exclude the possibility of syncope. • A thorough and careful physical examination is required along with a high index of suspicion, to exclude common but easily missed injuries. • Some older people who fall may prefer to be managed in the community or at home, and where possible this should be supported, particularly where family/carers can also provide support. • All older people who have fallen resulting in an ambulance call/attendance, but are then managed at home, should be offered referral pathways as per local guidelines. • Ambulance clinicians have a role to play in talking with people who are at risk of falling, or who have fallen, to try and prevent further falls.

Update Analysis

Section 5

<table>
<tr><th>Maternity Care</th><th>Addition/update of guidance and rationale</th></tr>
<tr><td></td><td>The full section has been updated and significantly revised, helpful visual photographs and new algorithms are included. Maternal resuscitation and newborn life support are now included in the maternity care sections; previously, these were in the resuscitation section of the book. Trauma in pregnancy has also been moved from the trauma section to the maternity care section.</td></tr>
<tr><td>Maternity Care (including Obstetric Emergencies Overview)</td><td>This replaces the Obstetrics and Gynaecology Emergencies Overview guideline.
● Human Factors, MBRRACE-UK, communication, information sharing and consent are covered.
● A new section on special cases, including concealment, denial and unknown pregnancy is added.
● FGM is discussed.
● The appropriate destination to convey mother and baby is discussed.
● A new pre-hospital maternity emergency management for normal birth algorithm is provided.</td></tr>
<tr><td>Birth Imminent: Normal Birth and Birth Complications</td><td>● New algorithms on management of eclampsia, cord prolapse, post-partum haemorrhage, breech birth and shoulder dystocia are included.
● Tranexamic acid can be administered for PPH.
● For a woman experiencing an abnormal labour or birth, transfer immediately to the nearest obstetric unit.
This includes:
– severe vaginal bleeding
– preterm or multiple births
– prolapsed umbilical cord
– continuous severe abdominal/epigastric pain
– maternal convulsions (eclampsia)
– presentation of the baby other than the head (e.g. arm or leg or buttocks)
– shoulder dystocia.
● If the woman presents with an obvious medical or traumatic condition that puts her life in imminent danger, transfer to the nearest ED with an obstetric unit.
● The period of gestation is important in informing the appropriate course of action, including the most appropriate location for conveyance, namely an ED, an early pregnancy unit or an obstetric unit.
● In the event of an obstetric emergency, detailing the exact emergency via a pre-alert call will assist the ED or maternity unit to summon the appropriate staff.
● Maintaining normothermia in the newborn is critical while on scene and during conveyance. The optimum body temperature of the baby should be between 36.5 and 37.5 degrees.
● The use of specific internal manoeuvres may be appropriate where a registered paramedic has received additional training to undertake them.</td></tr>
</table>

Care of the Newborn	This guideline has been updated. • All babies should initially be kept warm. Skin-to-skin contact is an effective measure in keeping babies warm, and early feeding is key. • A newborn baby will need to be transferred to hospital for the following reasons: – any baby that required resuscitation – perinatal hypoxia (APGAR score below 5). – meconium staining or aspiration – baby of a diabetic mother – small for dates/growth-restricted baby – prematurity (gestation <37 weeks) or a term baby >37 with respiratory distress syndrome/ abnormal – breathing pattern – major congenital abnormalities, even if the baby appears well at birth – red flags suggesting a high risk of early onset neonatal bacterial infection – safeguarding concerns known to the ambulance service or communicated by the maternity unit. • Perinatal hypoxia, hypothermia, hypoglycaemia, neonatal jaundice, preterm delivery, congenital abnormalities and early onset neonatal sepsis are covered.
Haemorrhage During Pregnancy (including Miscarriage and Ectopic Pregnancy)	• A new algorithm on haemorrhage during pregnancy is included. • Haemorrhage during pregnancy is broadly divided into two categories, occurring in early and late pregnancy. • Haemorrhage may be revealed (evident vaginal blood loss) or concealed (little or no obvious loss). • Practical guidance for management of pregnancy loss and fetal tissue in early pregnancy is included. • Pregnant women may appear well even when a large amount of blood has been lost (tachycardia may not appear until 30% of circulating volume as symptoms of hypovolaemic shock occur very late, by which stage the woman is critically ill). • Obtain venous access with large bore cannulae (16G). • In the presence of a confirmed miscarriage, intramuscular administration of Syntometrine should be considered.
Pregnancy-induced Hypertension (including Eclampsia)	IV magnesium sulphate can be administered by paramedics for eclamptic convulsions if available to you. This would need to be given under a PGD: Patient Group Direction. Magnesium sulphate is not currently included in the JRCALC drugs section, but a review of the whole drugs section will take place next year, reviewing additional drugs that may be in common use.
Vaginal Bleeding: Gynaecological Causes	• More detail on the types and causes of vaginal bleeding is included. • Reference is made to the sexual assault guideline. • Photos to aid the assessment of blood loss are included. • Following gynaecological surgical interventions, heavy, ongoing vaginal bleeding commencing 7–14 days post procedure may indicate underlying infection.
Maternal Resuscitation	• A team approach to prehospital resuscitation, definitions of maternal deaths and reversible causes of maternal collapse are covered. • DO NOT withhold or terminate maternal resuscitation. • ALWAYS manage pregnant women in cardiac arrest at greater than 20 weeks' gestation with manual displacement of the uterus to the maternal left. • If resuscitation attempts fail to achieve ROSC within 5 minutes of the cardiac arrest, undertake a TIME CRITICAL transfer to the nearest ED with an obstetric unit attached. • Place an early pre-alert to enable the ED team to summon the maternity team, as an immediate peri-mortem caesarean section (resuscitative hysterotomy) may be performed.

Newborn Life Support	• Do not place the baby in a plastic bag or polythene wrapping as there is a lack of pre-hospital evidence demonstrating the role of these in the prevention of newborn hypothermia in either significantly preterm (<32 weeks) or term infants. • New photographs are provided.
Trauma in Pregnancy	• All trauma is significant. • If the pregnant woman is found in cardiac arrest or develops cardiac/respiratory arrest en-route, commence advanced life support and pre-alert the nearest ED with an obstetric unit. • Resuscitation of the woman may facilitate resuscitation of the fetus. • Due to the physiological changes in pregnancy, signs of shock may be slow to appear following trauma, hypotension being an extremely late indication of volume loss. Signs of hypovolaemia during pregnancy are likely to indicate a 35% (class III) blood loss and must be treated aggressively. • If sexual assault or domestic violence is suspected, consideration must be given to potential safeguarding issues and provision made to ensure safety is maintained.

Section 6

Drugs	***Addition/update of guidance***
Drugs Overview	• Paediatric drug doses are based on a child's weight, on a milligram per kilogram basis. • When a child's weight is known, it is better to administer according to their weight rather than their age. • When a child is clearly larger or smaller than would be expected for their age (their parents/carers will often be aware of this), an 'older' or 'younger' Page for Age chart should be selected for that child, dependent on the chart that most closely reflects their actual weight.
Atropine	Bradycardia following Return of Spontaneous Circulation (ROSC) is added as an indication for atropine.
Diazepam	• The doses have been amended and simplified. • Confusion over 'large' and 'small' doses has been removed. • Smaller rectal doses for patients 70 years and over are outlined. • The full dose should be given so that convulsion recurrence is much less likely. • The adult convulsions guideline is currently undergoing review, and recent evidence on the medicines management of convulsions will be sought, reviewed and considered.
Entonox	• Nitrous oxide may have a deleterious effect if used in patients with an air-containing closed space since nitrous oxide diffuses into such a space with a resulting increase in pressure. • Intraocular injection of gas within the past four weeks is added as a contra-indication.
Hydrocortisone	• More emphasis on the need to administer for patients in adrenal crisis, in line with changes to altered level of consciousness and medical emergencies updates. • Actions has been added: Glucocorticoid drug that restores blood pressure, blood sugar, cardiac synchronicity and volume. High levels are important to survive haemorrhagic shock. Therapeutic actions include suppression of inflammation and immune response. • Contra-indications have been simplified. • If in doubt it is better to give hydrocortisone.
Misoprostol	• Administer subligually unless the patient is unable to maintain their airway. • The vaginal route is not appropriate in post-partum haemorrhage or for miscarriage, but rectal route may be considered when appropriate (e.g. impaired consciousness).

Naloxone Hydrochloride (Narcan)	The indication to give Naloxone to reverse respiratory and central nervous system depression in a neonate following maternal opioid use during labour has been removed. There is little evidence to support its use in neonates. If Naloxone is given to neonates born to opioid addicted mothers there are concerns that it may produce withdrawal effects. Emphasis should be on effective drying and stimulation of the baby, systematic airway management with bag valve-mask ventilation and maintaining newborn temperature between 36.50C to 37.50C. Where these interventions do not achieve established respiratory effort the newborn should be rapidly conveyed to the nearest Emergency Department with an Obstetric Unit attached. The pre-alert should detail the neonatal emergency. The newborn should be conveyed, where necessary, ahead of the mother.
Oxygen	● Decompression illness added to the high levels of supplemental oxygen for adults with critical illnesses table. ● Patients over 50 years of age who are long-term smokers with a history of exertional breathlessness and no other known cause of breathlessness should be treated as having COPD. ● Target saturation for patients with paraquat or bleomycin poisoning are 85–88%.
Paracetamol	● Dosage tables have been amended. ● Consideration is given to patients that weigh under 50kg. ● Tablets may be broken in half. ● Paracetamol is not recommended for patients with cardiac chest pain. ● Intravenous doses from birth are included. ● A new caution is added to reduce the risk of paracetamol overdose.
0.9% Sodium Chloride	● Changes to fluid regimes in trauma and sepsis are included. ● Seek advice to exceed maximum dose of fluid boluses in trauma in children.
Tranexamic Acid	● Women suffering from post-partum haemorrhage (PPH) is added as an indication. Use TXA alongside uterotonic drugs (drugs that stimulate the uterus to contract) such as syntometrine and misoprostol.
Intravascular Fluid Therapy (Adults)	● This guideline is updated alongside the sepsis guideline.

List of Abbreviations

The glossary of terms listed below is designed to assist reading ease and is **NOT** provided as a list of short-hand terms. The Joint Royal Colleges Ambulance Liaison Committee reminds the user that abbreviations are not to be used in any clinical documentation.

Term	
AAA	Abdominal Aortic Aneurysm
ABCDE	**A** – Airway
	B – Breathing
	C – Circulation
	D – Disability
	E – Exposure and environment
AC	Alternating Current
ACPO	Association of Chief Police Officers
ACS	Acute Coronary Syndrome
ADHD	Attention Deficit Hyperactivity Disorder
ADRT	Advance Decision to Refuse Treatment
AED	Automated External Defibrillation
AHF	Acute Heart Failure
ALoC	Altered level of consciousness
ALS	Advanced Life Support
AMH	Adult Mental Health Services
AMHP	Approved Mental Health Professional
APC	Antero-Posterior Compression
APGAR	**A** – Apperance
	P – Pulse rate
	G – Grimace or response to stimulation
	A – Activity or muscle tone
	R – Respiration
ARDS	Acute Respiratory Distress Syndrome
ATMIST	**A** – Age
	T – Time of incident
	M – Mechanism
	I – Injuries
	S – Signs and symptoms
	T – Treatment given / immediate needs
ATP	Anti-Tachycardia Pacing
AV	Atrioventricular
AVPU	**A** – Alert
	V – Responds to voice
	P – Responds to pain
	U – Unresponsive
bd	Twice daily
BG	Blood Glucose
BIA	Best Interest Assessors
BLS	Basic Life Support
BM	Stick Measures blood sugar
BP	Blood Pressure
bpm	Beats per minute
BR	Breech

Term	
BSA	Body Surface Area
BTS	British Thoracic Society
BVM	Bag-Valve-Mask
<C>ABCDE	**<C>** – Catastrophic haemorrhage
	A – Airway
	B – Breathing
	C – Circulation
	D – Disability
	E – Exposure and environment
CAMHS	Child and Adolescent Mental Health Services
CBRNE	Chemical, Biological, Radiological, Nuclear and Explosive
CBT	Cognitive Behavioural Therapy
CCS	Central Cord Syndrome
CD	Controlled Drug
CES	Cauda Equina Syndrome
CEW	Controlled Electrical Weapon
CHD	Coronary Heart Disease
CHF	Congestive Heart Failure
CMHT	Community Mental Health Team
CMI	Combined Mechanical Injury
CNS	Central Nervous System
CO	Carbon monoxide
CO_2	Carbon dioxide
COP	Code of Practice
COPD	Chronic Obstructive Pulmonary Disease
CPAP	Continuous Positive Airway Pressure
CPN	Community Psychiatric Nurse
CPP	Cerebral Perfusion Pressure
CPR	Cardiopulmonary Resuscitation
CRT	Capillary Refill Test
CRT	Cardiac Resynchronisation Therapy
CSA	Child Sexual Abuse
CSE	Child Sexual Exploitation
CSE	Convulsive (tonic-clonic) status epilepticus
CT	Computerised Tomography
CVA	Cerebo Vascular Accident
DC	Direct Current
DIC	Disseminated Intravascular Coagulation
DKA	Diabetic Ketoacidosis
DM	Diabetes Mellitus

List of Abbreviations

Term	
DNA	Deoxyribonucleic Acid
DNACPR	Do Not Attempt Cardio-Pulmonary Resuscitation
DoLS	Deprivation of Liberty Safeguards
DPA	Data Protection Act
DVT	Deep Vein Thrombosis
E	Ecstasy
EC	Enteric Coated
ECG	Electrocardiograph
ED	Emergency Department
EDD	Estimated Date of Delivery
EMS	Emergency Medical Services
EOC	Emergency Operations Centre
ERC	European Resuscitation Council
ET	Endotracheal
ETA	Expected Time of Arrival
EtCO2	Exhaled (end-tidal) carbon dioxide
FAST	**F** – Face **A** – Arms **S** – Speech **T** – Test
FBAO	Foreign Body Airway Obstruction
FC	Febrile Convulsions
FEV	Forced Expiratory Volume
FLACC	**F** – Face **L** – Legs **A** – Activity **C** – Cry **C** – Consolability
FII	Fabricated or Induced Illness
FGM	Female Genital Mutilation
FVC	Forced Vital Capacity
g	Grams
GBS	Group B Strep Infection
GCS	Glasgow Coma Scale
GI	Gastrointestinal
GP	General Practitioner
GTN	Glyceryl Trinitrate
HART	Hazardous Area Response Team
HCP	Healthcare Professional
HIV	Human Immunodeficiency Virus
HR	Heart Rate
HSE	Health and Safety Executive
HVS	Hyperventilation Syndrome
IBS	Irritable Bowel Syndrome
ICD	International Classification of Diseases
ICD	Implantable Cardioverter Defibrillator

Term	
ICE	Infant Cooling Evaluation
ICP	Intracranial Pressure
IGIV	Immunoglobulin Intravenous
IHD	Ischemic Heart Disease
IM	Intramuscular
IMCA	Independent Mental Capacity Advocates
IO	Intraosseous
IPAP	**I** – Intent **P** – Plans **A** – Actions **P** – Protection
IQ	Intelligence Quotient
ISVA	Independent Sexual Violence Adviser
ITU	Intensive Care Unit
IV	Intravenous
IVC	Inferior Vena Cava
J	Joule
JRCALC	Joint Royal Colleges Ambulance Liaison Committee
JVP	Jugular Venous Pressure
kg	Kilogram
kPa	Kilopascal
kV	Kilovolt
LBBB	Left Bundle Branch Block
LC	Lateral Compression
LMA	Laryngeal Mask Airway
LMP	Last Menstrual Period
LOC	Level of Consciousness
LPA	Lasting Power of Attorney
LSD	Lysergic Acid Diethylamide
LVF	Left Ventricular Failure
MAOI	Monoamine Oxidase Inhibitor antidepressant
MAPPA	Multi-Agency Public Protection Arrangements
MAP	Mean Arterial Pressure
MBRRACE	Mothers and Babies: Reducing Risk through Audits and Confidential Enquiries
MCA	Mental Capacity Act
mcg	Microgram
MDMA	Methylene Dioxymethamphetamine
MECC	Making Every Contact Count
mg	Milligram
MH	Mental Health
MHA	Mental Health Act
MHSOP	Mental Health Services for Older People
MI	Myocardial Infarction

List of Abbreviations

Term	
MINAP	Myocardial Ischaemia National Audit Project
ml	Millilitre
mmHG	Millimetres of Mercury
mmol	Millimoles
mmol/l	Millimoles per Litre
MOI	Mechanisms of Injury
MSC	**M** – Motor **S** – Sensation **C** – Circulation
msec	Millisecond
NARU	National Ambulance Resilience Unit
Neb	Nebulisation
NEET	Not in Education, Employment or Training
NEWS	National Early Warning Score
NG	Nasogastric
NHS	National Health Service
NICE	National Institute for Health and Care Excellence
NiPPV	Non-invasive Positive Pressure Ventilation
NLS	Newborn Life Support
NPIS	National Poisons Information Service
NSAID	Non-Steroidal Anti-inflammatory Drug
NSTEMI	Non-ST Segment Elevation Myocardial Infarction
O_2	Oxygen
OOH	Out of Hours
OPA	Oropharyngeal Airway
ORS	Oral Rehydration Salt
P	Parity
PaO2	Partial pressure of oxygen
PCO_2	Measure of the Partial Pressure of Carbon dioxide
PE	Pulmonary Embolism
PEaRL	Pupils Equal and Reacting to Light
PEA	Pulseless Electrical Activity
PEF	Peak Expiratory Flow
PEFR	Peak Expiratory Flow Rate
PHTLS	Pre-hospital Trauma Life Support
PIH	Pregnancy Induced Hypertension
POM	Prescription Only Medicine
PPCI	Primary Percutaneous Coronary Intervention
PPE	Personal Protective Equipment
PPH	Post-Partum Haemorrhage
pr	Per Rectum
PreSep	Prehospital Early Sepsis Detection
PRESS	Prehospital Recognition of Severe Sepsis

Term	
PSM	Patient Specific Medication
prn	When required medication
PV	Per Vaginam
RAID	Rapid Assessment, Interface and Discharge
RCT	Randomised Controlled Trial
ROLE	Recognition Of Life Extinct
ROSC	Return of Spontaneous Circulation
RR	Respiratory Rate
RSV	Respiratory Syncytial Virus
RTC	Road Traffic Collision
RVF	Right Ventricular Failure
RVP	Rendezvous Point(s)
SAD	Supraglottic Airway Device
SARC	Sexual Assault Referral Centre
SaO2	Oxygen Saturation Of Arterial Blood
SBAR	**S** – Situation **B** – Background **A** – Assessment **R** – Recommendation
SBI	Serious Bacterial Infection
SBP	Systolic Blood Pressure
SC	Subcutaneous
SCENE	**S** – Safety **C** – Cause including MOI **E** – Environment **N** – Number of patients **E** – Extra resources needed
SCI	Spinal Cord Injury
SOCRATES	**S** – Site **O** – Onset **C** – Character **R** – Raditation **A** – Associated symptoms **T** – Time **E** – Exacerbation **S** – Severity
SORT	Special Operations Response Team
SpO2	Oxygen Saturation Measured With Pulse Oximeter
SSRIs	Selective Serotonin Re-Uptake Inhibitors
STEMI	ST Segment Elevation Myocardial Infarction
STI	Sexually transmitted infections
SUDEP	Sudden Unexpected Death in Epilepsy
SUDI	Sudden Unexpected Death in Infants
SUDICA	Sudden Unexpected Death in Infants, Children and Adolescents

List of Abbreviations

Term	
SVT	Supraventricular Tachycardia
TARN	Trauma Audit Research Network
TBI	Traumatic Brain injury
TBSA	Total Body Surface Area
TEP	Tracheoesophageal Puncture
TIA	Transient Ischaemic Attack
TLoC	Transient loss of conciousness
TOBY	Total Body Hypothermia for Neonatal Encephalopathy

Term	
URTI	Upper Respiratory Tract Infection
UTI	Urinary Tract Infection
VF	Ventricular Fibrillation
VS	Vertical Shear
VT	Ventricular Tachycardia
VTE	Venous Thromboembolism
WHO	World Health Organisation

1

General Guidance

Pain Management in Adults

1. Introduction

- Relief of pain is one of the most important clinical outcomes in paramedic practice. Often, pain is the chief complaint that has resulted in seeking assistance. Apart from the humanitarian dimension, managing pain has several clinical benefits. Analgesia should be swiftly initiated as soon as clinically possible after arriving on scene. There is no reason to delay pain relief because of uncertainty with the definitive diagnosis. It does not affect later diagnostic efficacy, but may potentially aid in arriving at a prompt diagnosis, as patients are more cooperative when comfortable. Intense pain can modify the nervous system leading to chronic persistent pain – a troublesome long-term problem with huge health and socioeconomic impact.
- Barriers to effective pain management include:
  - patient factors (general condition, communication, cooperation)
  - knowledge and experience of the clinician
  - environment and available resources.

2. Assessment

- Pain is a complex and dynamic experience and all clinicians should place the requirements and needs of the individual at the forefront of all assessments. Ideally, multidisciplinary assessment ascertains the most appropriate and efficient course of treatment in both acute and chronic pain conditions, but limited resources in the pre-hospital environment can make comprehensive assessment a challenging task.
- The pain experience of individuals is influenced by bio-psycho-social factors, such as:
  - the nature of any underlying medical condition
  - age, gender, genetics
  - prior pain experience, culture, beliefs
  - environment and social conditions.

2.1 Measuring Pain

- Although different scoring systems are used to gauge the intensity of pain, patients' experiences cannot be objectively validated in the same way as other vital signs. JRCALC recommend the 0–10-point verbal numerical scale in which 0 refers to no pain and 10 is the worst imaginable pain. In most pre-hospital situations, this score is suitable to assess severity of pain and the response to treatment. As there is inter-individual variability, the trend in the scores is more important than the absolute value in assessing efficacy of treatment. Apart from initial assessment and scoring, subsequent periodical measurement after each intervention is a recommended practice. However, no pain assessment tool is set in stone and the patient's needs should always be considered above the findings of the assessment tool.
- Scoring can be difficult in patients with dementia, cognitive impairment, altered level of consciousness or communication difficulties. In these scenarios, pain is assessed through behavioural cues. Remember: no behaviour is unique to pain; behaviour is unique to individuals.[1]
- The prevalence of persistent pain in older adults is high, with the main causes originating as a result of degenerative changes. In both sexes, incidence of arthritis increases with age. Both osteoarthritis and osteoporosis are more common in women. Due to unmet healthcare needs, other concurrent medical conditions or poor compliance with medications, managing pain in older adults is often suboptimal. This has adverse effects on mood, sleep and activity. Ageing-related alteration to pharmacokinetics, pharmacodynamics and polypharmacy also contribute to poorly controlled pain. Older adults may not complain or effectively communicate their needs. In addition, they may also be living with dementia. The process of assessing older adults should be the same as for younger people, utilising numerical or pictorial pain assessment scales. Where there is suspected dementia, the Abbey Pain Scale is used to measure pain (refer to Figure 1.1).

The Abbey Pain Scale

For measurement of pain in people who cannot verbalise.

How to use scale: While observing the patient, score questions 1 to 6.

Q1. Vocalisation
e.g. whimpering, groaning, crying
Absent 0 ***Mild 1*** ***Moderate 2*** ***Severe 3*** — Q1 ☐

Q2. Facial expression
e.g. looking tense, frowning, grimacing, looking frightened
Absent 0 ***Mild 1*** ***Moderate 2*** ***Severe 3*** — Q2 ☐

Q3. Change in body language
e.g. fidgeting, rocking, guarding part of body withdrawn
Absent 0 ***Mild 1*** ***Moderate 2*** ***Severe 3*** — Q3 ☐

Q4. Behavioural change
e.g. increased confusion, refusing to eat, alteration in usual patterns
Absent 0 ***Mild 1*** ***Moderate 2*** ***Severe 3*** — Q4 ☐

Q5. Physiological change
e.g. temperature, pulse or blood pressure outside normal limits, perspiring, flushing or pallor
Absent 0 ***Mild 1*** ***Moderate 2*** ***Severe 3*** — Q5 ☐

Q6. Physical changes
e.g. skin tears, pressure areas, arthritis, contractures, previous injuries
Absent 0 ***Mild 1*** ***Moderate 2*** ***Severe 3*** — Q6 ☐

Add scores for Q1 to Q6 and record here → Total pain score ☐

Now tick the box that matches the Total Pain Score →

0–2 No pain	3–7 Mild	8–13 Moderate	14+ Severe

Finally, tick the box which matches the type of pain →

Chronic	Acute	Acute on chronic

Abbey J, De Bellis A, Piller N, Esterman A, Gilles L, Parker D, Lowcay B. The Abbey Pain Scale.
Funded by the JH & JD Gunn Medical Research Foundation 1998–2002.
(This document may be reproduced with this reference retained.)

Figure 1.1 – The Abbey Pain Scale.

2.2 Clinical Evaluation of Acute Pain

- Assessment and treatment of acute pain has to be immediate with minimal interruption to other aspects of the patient's life. Poorly managed acute pain can result in certain changes in the nervous system, commonly described as 'plasticity', which predispose to development of chronic pain. Knowledge of exacerbating and relieving factors can complement pain management.
- A commonly used mnemonic in acute pain assessment is SOCRATES:
  - **Site** (e.g. calf pain due to deep venous thrombosis; associated chest pain may be due to pulmonary embolism).
  - **Onset** (acute onset or progressive worsening of an underlying condition).
  - **Character** (aching pain with movements can be musculoskeletal; burning pain, pins and needles can be neuropathic).
  - **Radiation** (back pain radiating to legs can be due to nerve root irritation; chest pain with radiation to the left arm can be due to angina).
  - **Associated symptoms** (fever, chills, nausea may be due to infectious cause).
  - **Time**/duration.
  - **Exacerbation** and relieving factors (pain with movement may be musculoskeletal, pain associated with bowel and bladder disturbance may be due to abdominal problems).
  - **Severity** (scoring tools to assess baseline intensity and monitor progress).
- All patients with pain should have at least two pain scores taken, the first one before the treatment and the subsequent measurements after the treatment is commenced. Scoring and systematic assessment increases awareness of pain management, reveals previously unrecognised pain and improves analgesic administration.

2.3 Clinical Evaluation of Chronic Pain

- Chronic pain is not prolonged acute pain. The experience of pain is influenced by 'bio-psycho-social' factors, such as medical condition, mood, sleep, beliefs and behavior, cultural and social factors.
- Patients with chronic pain may have heightened sensitivity of the nervous system and are prone to develop exacerbation episodes necessitating a call for urgent help.
- The fundamental principles of assessing these patients are the same as described above, but consideration should be given to psychological and social factors. The challenges for paramedics include seeing these patients for the first time and hence difficulty in obtaining a global picture, and limited resources/time to conduct a comprehensive assessment. This may result in disbelief of the patient's report of pain. Without precise knowledge of patient's background medical history, malingering may be suspected and this impression may negatively affect the quality of care. A safer approach is to seek and accept the patient's self report of their pain.

Examples of questions to assess patients with chronic pain

- How would you rate your pain on a 0 to 10 scale at the **present**, where 0 is 'no pain' and 10 is 'worst imaginable pain'?
- In the past six months, how intense was your **worst** pain, rated on a 0 to 10 scale?
- In the past six months, on **average**, how intense was your pain, rated on a 0 to 10 scale?
- In the past six months, how much has the pain interfered with your daily activities, rated on a 0 to 10 scale where 0 is 'no interference' and 10 is 'unable to carry on any activities'?
- In the past six months, how much has the pain changed your ability to take part in recreational, social and family activities where 0 is 'no change' and 10 is 'extreme change'?
- In the past six months, how much has the pain changed your ability to do housework where 0 is 'no change' and 10 is 'extreme change'?
- About how many days in the past six months have you been kept from your usual activities (work, school or housework) because of pain?

3. Management

- Whenever possible, treat the cause (for example, glyceryl trinitrate sublingual spray for angina and oxygen for sickle cell crisis). When the cause is not readily treatable or if it is not apparent, then other analgesic interventions are necessary.
- The pain relief options are:
  - psychological (e.g. reassurance, distraction)
  - physical (e.g. dressing burns wound, splinting fracture)
  - pharmacological (e.g. paracetamol, NSAID, morphine).
- 'Balanced analgesia' with a multimodal pain plan is recommended by JRCALC in pre-hospital pain management and involves administration of analgesics with different mechanisms of action. The synergistic effects should improve effectiveness while limiting the side effects. An example is the combination of paracetamol and morphine. Studies show that the dose of morphine can be reduced by 40–50% when administered alongside paracetamol or ibuprofen. This complementary effect not only offers a more effective pain solution for the patient, but will also improve safety when paramedics administer morphine. Often, a combination of pharmacological and non-pharmacological methods may be necessary, for example, Entonox, morphine or ketamine may be required to enable the application of a splint for fractures.

Pain Management in Adults

- Treatment of acute pain may not follow the WHO analgesic ladder as closely as in other elective clinical scenarios. Initially, effective pain control is facilitated with stronger opioids and, wherever appropriate, local anaesthetic techniques. Entonox can be judiciously used for a short period until the other analgesics have had time to take effect. Once controlled, enteral options, such as regular oral opioid analgesics (codeine) and then simple analgesics (paracetamol, NSAID) are introduced.
- Any pain relief must be accompanied by careful explanation of the patient's condition and the pain relief methods being used. Understanding the basic sites of action of different analgesics will aid in choosing the optimal combinations.

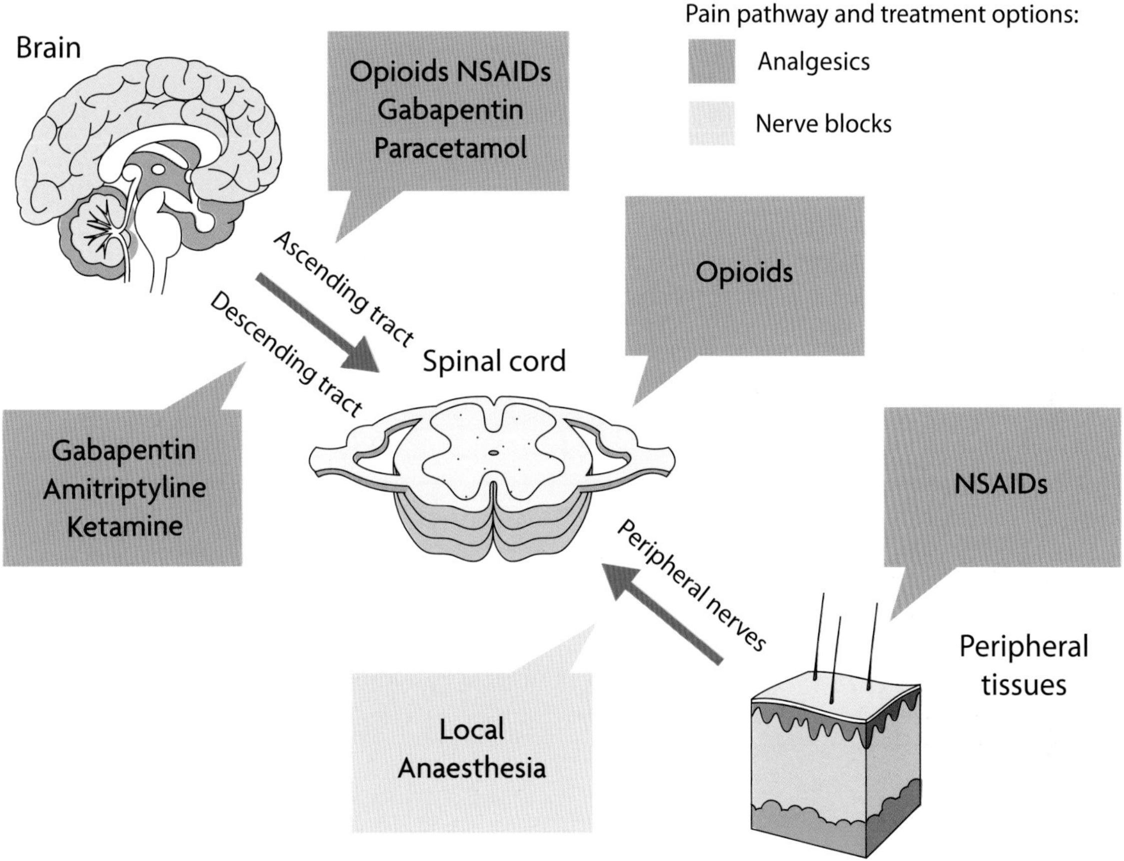

Figure 1.2 – Pain pathway and treatment options.

3.1 Choice of Analgesics

Refer to Figure 1.3.

- Simple analgesics:
  - paracetamol, non-steroidal anti-inflammatory drugs (NSAID), e.g. ibuprofen, Diclofenac, Naproxen.
- Opioids:
  - codeine, morphine.
- Miscellaneous:
  - Entonox, Methoxyflurane, ketamine, local anaesthetic blocks.

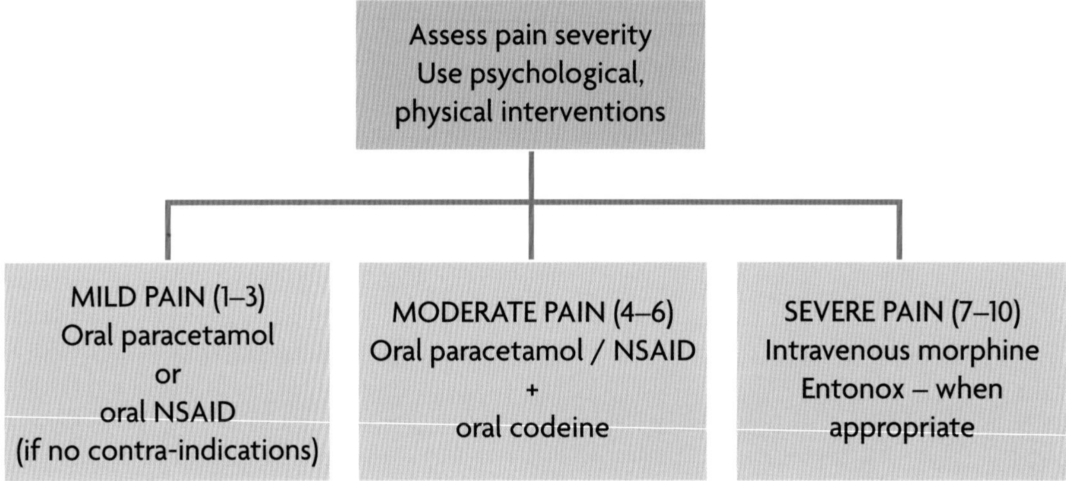

Figure 1.3 – Choice of analgesics.

3.2 Routes of Administration

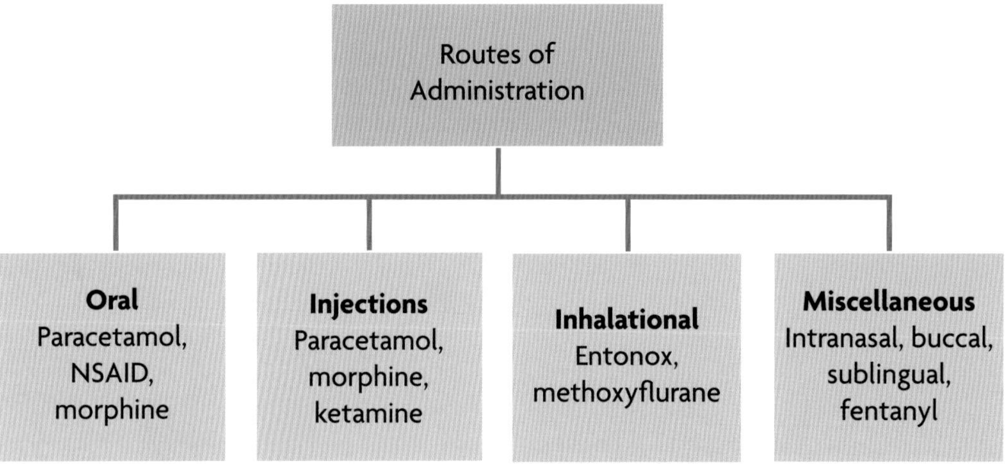

Figure 1.4 – Routes of administration.

- The oral route is mostly sufficient for mild to moderate pain. In severe pain, the intravenous route has the advantage of rapid onset and the dose can be titrated against analgesic effect. In a subgroup of patients, such as those suffering from sickle cell disease or requiring end of life care, intramuscular or subcutaneous injections are appropriate and local Trust guidelines should be followed. In specific circumstances, the intraosseous route may be considered.
- In vulnerable adults or needle-phobic adults, where venepuncture may be required in a non-urgent situation, tetracaine 4% gel/amethocaine can be applied to the skin overlying a suitable vein and the area covered with an occlusive dressing. Such an application takes about 30–40 minutes to work.
- The intranasal route of offering pain relief has many advantages over the traditional routes. It overcomes the cannulation barrier associated with the administration of opioid analgesia that has been shown to be a major problem in the young, the elderly, the shocked patient and the cognitively impaired. Studies looking at pain management in children have found that the intranasal route offers a kinder and less intrusive mechanism for drug delivery while at the same time offering the same level of analgesia as the intravenous route.
- Inhalational analgesia is particularly useful when venous access is not readily secured or when there is a need for immediate relief of severe pain. It can be used as the first analgesic while other pain relief is instituted, or in conjunction with other medications until satisfactory control is achieved. Inhalational analgesia is only for short-term use.

3.3 Chronic Pain[2, 3]

- These patients are commonly on pain medications, such as gabapentin, pregabalin, amitriptyline, duloxetine, and a significant dose of opioids. Unlike acute pain management, complete resolution of symptoms can be challenging in 'acute on chronic' pain management. Understanding the complexity of chronic pain helps in handling the situation. Ensuring compliance to the prescribed chronic pain medications can help to avoid adding more medicines. Patients may be on a significant dose of opioids such as morphine, oxycodone, fentanyl or buprenorphine patches. Recent evidence throws light on the limitations of using stronger opioids in chronic pain management.

- If patients require intravenous morphine or inhalation of Entonox to help break the pain-spasm cycle and enable assessment, it is prudent to reiterate that this is only a short-term intervention for temporary relief; long-term exposure to opioids or Entonox can be potentially harmful. If the patient is found with intense muscle spasm and mobilising is difficult, slow intravenous injection of diazepam (into a large vein at a rate of not more than 5 mg/minute) up to a maximum dose of 10 mg can help relieve the spasm.
- In general, the treatment plan for patients with chronic pain runs closely alongside the principle of 'start low and go slow' with regards to the analgesics. If clinical assessment did not identify any fresh cause for exacerbation of pain, reassurance, compliance with prescribed medicines, simple non-pharmacological interventions, such as a TENS machine, may minimise the need for transportation to the emergency department and instead facilitate elective review with the general practitioner or the pain clinic.
- Modern medicine has heavily relied on the 'biomedical model', where clinicians regarded diseases as derangement in normal body structure and function that can be fixed with a drug or a procedure. We now recognise that the brain does not work in isolation, especially in pain. When managing chronic illnesses, the major shortcoming is lack of emphasis placed on the person as a whole. The bio-psycho-social model encompasses all the three important facets that influence pain experience, i.e. biological, psychological and social factors (refer to Table 1.1).

Table 1.1 – THE BIO-PSYCHO-SOCIAL MODEL

Biological

Concerns itself with the biological aspects of the illness and is usually managed within the biomedical model. Although alleviating pain with good analgesics is still the main aim, it is equally important that clinicians do not reduce the problem of pain to simply labeling it as a broken or dysfunctional part of the body in isolation and apply a specific treatment for that cause.

Psychological

Explores the emotional aspect of the person and behaviour, or indeed the change in the behaviour that accompanies pain. Commonly, patients with persistent pain also have mental health issues such as anxiety and depression, either as a cause or as an association. Timely recognition of mental health difficulties and facilitating appropriate psychological support can avoid escalation into other complex long-term problems.

Social

Pain-related beliefs and behaviour could have social repercussions at home, work and in the wider society. Patients will rationalise what is happening to them within a social model, which will have impacts on their relationships, family, employment etc. In chronic pain, a social constructionist approach will help to develop a holistic treatment plan.

Table 1.2 – NON-PHARMACOLOGICAL METHODS OF PAIN RELIEF

• **Physical**	• Cooling of burns can reduce the pain. Burns should not be cooled for longer than 20 minutes total time and care should be taken with large burns to avoid hypothermia. • Splintage and immobilisation of fractures provides pain relief as well as minimising ongoing tissue damage, bleeding and other complications. • Warm blankets can help to keep the patient comfortable and avoid hypothermia.
• **Psychological**	• Fear and anxiety worsen pain; reassurance and explanation can go a long way towards alleviation of pain. • Distraction makes pain easier to tolerate; simple conversation is the simplest form of distraction.

Table 1.3 – PHARMACOLOGICAL METHODS OF PAIN RELIEF (refer to specific drug protocols)

• **Oral analgesia**	• Paracetamol and ibuprofen may be used in isolation or together for the management of mild to moderate pain when used in appropriate dosages. It is important to assess the presence of contra-indications to all drugs, including simple analgesics. Non-steroidal anti-inflammatory drugs are responsible for large numbers of adverse events, because of their gastrointestinal and renal side effects and their effects on asthmatics. Some ambulance services may also choose to add a paracetamol/codeine combination and/or other opioid-based oral analgesics to their formulary. • Oral morphine is useful for less severe pain but has the disadvantage of delayed onset, some unpredictability of absorption and having to be given in a set dose. It has the advantage of avoiding the need for intravenous access. It is widely used for patients with mild/moderate pain from injuries such as fractures.
• **Parenteral analgesia (intravenous, intramuscular, subcutaneous, intraosseous)**	• Morphine is approved for administration by paramedics. Intravenous morphine is a potent analgesic to manage acute pain, but has significant side effects. For satisfactory relief, in presentations such as severe musculoskeletal pain, co-administration of intravenous paracetamol should be considered. This will improve effectiveness while keeping the dose of morphine to a minimum. As with other opioids, effects of morphine are reversed with the opioid-antagonist, naloxone. The person administering opioids should have the expertise and resources for maintaining airway, breathing and circulation, and have ready access to naloxone. Decisions to reverse the opioid's effect using naloxone should be made cautiously as this will return the patient to their pre-treatment pain level. Another common unpleasant side effect of opioids is nausea and vomiting, which may require administration of an antiemetic, such as ondansetron. • Intramuscular and subcutaneous injections are offered in special circumstances, such as patients with sickle cell disease or end-of-life care pathways as per pre-agreed local Trust guidelines. Occasionally, when the only available vascular access is the intraosseous route and the patient is in severe pain, intraosseous morphine can safely be administered with good effect.
• **Inhalational analgesia**	• Entonox (50% nitrous oxide, 50% oxygen) is a good analgesic for adults who are able to self-administer and who can rapidly be taught to operate the demand valve. It is fast acting but has a very short half-life, so the analgesic effect wears off rapidly when inhalation is stopped. It can be used as the first analgesic while other pain relief is instituted. It can also be used as part of a balanced analgesic approach, particularly during painful procedures such as splint application and patient movement. It is safest to avoid its use in situations such as head injuries (as it can raise intracranial pressure) and pneumothorax (or any other condition where air is trapped in the body).

Table 1.4 – METHODS THAT REQUIRE APPROPRIATELY TRAINED PRACTITIONERS

• **Ketamine analgesia**	• Ketamine is a NMDA receptor antagonist with some action on opioid receptors. Depending upon the dose, it can produce analgesia, sedation or anaesthesia. It is particularly useful in serious trauma because it is less likely to significantly depress blood pressure or respiration compared to other agents. Ketamine is also useful in entrapments, where a person can be extricated with combined analgesic and sedative effects. • When used in moderate to higher dosages, adults may experience unpleasant side effects, such as hallucinations and agitation. Ketamine produces salivation so careful airway management is important, although unnecessary interference should be avoided as laryngospasm may occasionally occur. Concurrent use of atropine may minimise excessive salivation.
• **Methoxyflurane (Penthrox)**	• Methoxyflurane is an inhaled analgesic designed for self-administration. It can be used as a non-opioid alternative to morphine or in conjunction with morphine for very severe pain. Evidence has shown that methoxyflurane works well when combined with morphine and, therefore, morphine administration is encouraged at the earliest possible opportunity (as with Entonox) to work alongside methoxyflurane as part of a multi-modal approach to pain management.[4] If methoxyflurane treatment has been initiated prior to the arrival of clinicians on scene, this should be continued providing the treatment is helping to manage pain and the clinician is confident in using methoxyflurane. It is particularly useful when venepuncture cannot be achieved or when there is a need for immediate relief of severe pain. It also has advantage over Entonox in patients with chest injuries/ pneumothorax. • Methoxyflurane is presented in 3 ml doses, which will provide analgesia for approximately 30 minutes. At analgesic doses, a maximum dose of 6 ml per day is considered safe.
• **Intranasal opioids (e.g. Fentanyl)**	• Evidence of its effectiveness in the emergency department has highlighted the potential of intranasal Fentanyl for helping paramedics treat severe pain where venous access is compromised. Studies have shown that intranasal Fentanyl compares with the analgesic standard set by intravenous administration. Also, due to the lack of significant histamine release with Fentanyl, the risk of hypotension is less; this is especially useful in trauma situations. The combined lung surface area of around 50–75 m^2 offers a large capillary-rich environment for absorption. In addition, the duration of action of 30 minutes offers greater control for the clinician. Intranasal Fentanyl at a dose of 1.5 mcg/kg, to a maximum of 100 mcg divided evenly between nares, appears to be a safe and effective analgesic in the pre-hospital management of acute severe pain and may be an attractive alternative to both oral and intravenous opiates.
• **Local anaesthetic techniques**	• There is limited room for regional nerve blocks because of the environment and the need to transport the patient to hospital in a timely manner. However, they can be effective in certain circumstances of severe pain and do not induce drowsiness or disorientation. Examples include femoral nerve/ fascia iliaca block for lower limb injuries such as a fractured femur. Clinicians undertaking regional analgesia techniques must be suitably trained, and should be able to manage local anaesthetic toxicity.

KEY POINTS

Pain Management in Adults

- **Timely management of pain has clinical benefits.**
- **Pain relief does not affect later diagnosis.**
- **Multimodal analgesia is effective and has to be tailored to both patient and practitioner variables.**
- **Pain measurements and re-assessments will help to monitor progress.**

Further Reading

Further important information and evidence in support of this guideline can be found in the Bibliography.[5, 6, 7, 8]

Bibliography

1 Alzheimer's Australia. *Pain and Dementia*. Available from: https://www.fightdementia.org.au/files/helpsheets/Helpsheet-DementiaQandA16-PainAndDementia_english.pdf, 2011.

2 Von Korff M, Ormel J, Keefe FJ, Dworkin SF. Grading the severity of chronic pain. *Pain* 1992, 50: 133–149.

3 Scottish Intercollegiate Guidelines Network. *Management of Chronic Pain* (SIGN 136). Edinburgh: SIGN, 2013

4 Bendall JC, Simpson PM, Middleton PM. Effectiveness of prehospital morphine, fentanyl, and methoxyflurane in pediatric patients. *Prehospital Emergency Care* 2011, 15(2).

5 Lo JC, Kaye DA. Benzodiazepines and muscle relaxants. *Essentials of Pharmacology for Anesthesia, Pain Medicine, and Critical Care*. New York: Springer, 2015: 167–178.

6 National Institute for Health and Care Excellence. *Diazepam*. Available from: https://bnf.nice.org.uk/drug/diazepam.html.

7 Lord B, Deveson M. Assessment and management of chronic pain in adults: implications for paramedics. *Journal of Paramedic Practice* 2011, 3(4): 166–172.

8 Pak SC, Micalos PS, Maria SJ, Lord B. Nonpharmacological interventions for pain management in paramedicine and the emergency setting: a review of the literature. *Evidence-Based Complementary and Alternative Medicine* 2015 (2015).

Safeguarding Children

1. Introduction

- Safeguarding is everyone's responsibility and a statutory duty under the Children Act.[1] Ambulance clinicians must be aware of the signs, symptoms and indicators of abuse and neglect that constitute harm. This applies to staff who have direct contact, either face-to-face or on the telephone.
- Throughout this section, reference to a child equates to someone who is not yet 18 years of age.
- Members of staff in an ambulance trust have a **duty of care to report abuse or neglect**. If the abuse is not reported, the victim may be at greater risk. They may also feel discouraged from disclosing again, as they may feel they were not believed. This may put other people at risk.
- All partners who work with children, including local authorities, police, the health service, courts, professionals, the private and voluntary sectors and individual members of local communities, share the responsibility for safeguarding and promoting the welfare of children and young people. It is vital that all partners are aware of, and appreciate, the role that each of them plays in this area.[2]
- Healthcare professionals have a statutory duty to report, while social care and the police have statutory authority to investigate allegations or suspicions of child abuse.
- Ambulance clinicians are often the first professionals on scene and, therefore, may identify initial concerns regarding a child's welfare and alert social care, the police, the GP, or other appropriate health professional, in line with locally agreed procedures. Accurate recording of events/actions may be crucial to subsequent enquiries.
- The role of the ambulance service is not to investigate suspicions but to ensure that any suspicion is passed to the appropriate agency (e.g. social care or the police). Ambulance clinicians need to be aware of child abuse issues and the aim of this guideline is to:
  - ensure all staff are aware of, and can recognise, cases of suspected child abuse or children at risk of significant harm, and provide guidance enabling operational and control staff to assess and report cases of suspected child abuse
  - where appropriate, ensure that all staff involved in a case of suspected abuse are aware of the possible outcome and of any subsequent actions.
- Further information on local procedures can be obtained from the safeguarding services within individual ambulance trusts.

2. Significant Harm

- All children have the right:
  - to be protected from significant harm/ill-treatment
  - to be protected from impairment of their health[a] and development
  - to grow up in circumstances consistent with the provision of safe and effective care.
- The maltreatment of children, physically, emotionally, sexually or through neglect, can have a major impact on their health, well-being and development.
- There are no absolute criteria on which to rely when judging what constitutes significant harm. In some cases, a single traumatic event may constitute significant harm, but more generally it is a compilation of significant events, both acute and long-standing, which interrupt, change or damage the child's physical and psychological development. Considerations include:
  - the degree and extent of physical harm
  - the duration and frequency of abuse and neglect
  - the extent of premeditation
  - the degree of threat, coercion, sadism and bizarre or unusual elements.
- In order to understand and identify significant harm, consider:
  - the nature of harm, in terms of maltreatment or failure to provide adequate care
  - the impact on the child's health and development
  - the child's development within the context of the family and wider environment
  - any special needs, such as a medical condition, communication impairment or disability, that may affect the child's development and care within the family and the capacity of parents/carers to meet adequately the child's needs.
- Consideration is needed towards other siblings and/or vulnerable people living in the household/establishment.
- Abuse and neglect are forms of maltreatment, and children may suffer as a result of a deliberate act or failure on the part of a parent, legal guardian or carer to act to prevent harm (descriptions of abuse and neglect are detailed in Table 1.5).
- Children can be abused in any care or community setting, and abuse can be perpetrated by those known to them or by a stranger.

a Health means physical or mental health.

Table 1.5 – EXAMPLES OF TYPES OF ABUSE AND NEGLECT

Emotional abuse

The persistent emotional maltreatment of a child so as to cause severe and persistent adverse effects on the child's emotional development, which may:

- involve conveying to the child(ren) that they are worthless or unloved, inadequate, or valued only insofar as they meet the needs of another person
- involve not giving the child opportunities to express their views, deliberately silencing them or 'making fun' of what they say or how they communicate
- feature age or developmentally inappropriate expectations being imposed on children (e.g. interactions that are beyond the child's developmental capability), as well as overprotection and limitation of exploration and learning, or preventing the child from participating in normal social interaction
- involve seeing or hearing the ill-treatment of another
- involve serious bullying (including cyberbullying), causing children frequently to feel frightened or in danger, or the exploitation or corruption of children.

Some level of emotional abuse is involved in all types of maltreatment of a child, though it may occur alone.

Emotional abuse alone can be difficult to recognise as the child may be physically well cared-for and the home in good condition. Some common factors that may indicate emotional abuse are:

- if the child is constantly denigrated/humiliated before others
- if the child is constantly given the impression that the parents are disappointed in them
- if the child is blamed for things that go wrong or is told they may be unloved/sent away
- if the parent does not offer any love or attention (e.g. leaves them alone for a long time)
- if the child is obsessive about cleanliness, tidiness etc.
- if the parent has unrealistic expectations of the child (e.g. educational achievement/toilet training)
- if the child is either bullying others or being bullied themselves
- if there is an atmosphere of domestic abuse, adults or parents with mental health problems or a history of drug or alcohol abuse (toxic trio)
- if there is evidence of self-harm, intentional overdose or the excessive use of alcohol on the part of either the parent(s) or child
- unusual behaviour of the parents/carers towards the child(ren) in an emergency situation (e.g. are they comforting a distressed child? What is the interaction like between the child and care giver?).

Sexual abuse

Sexual abuse involves forcing or enticing a child or young person to take part in sexual activities. Both girls and boys of all age groups are at risk.

The sexual abuse of a child is often planned and chronic. A large proportion of sexually abused children have no physical signs, and it is therefore necessary to be alert to behavioural and emotional factors that may indicate abuse.

The activities may involve physical contact, including assault by penetration (e.g. rape or oral sex) or non-penetrative acts, such as masturbation, kissing, rubbing and touching outside of clothing. They may include non-contact activities, such as involving children in looking at, or in the production of, sexual images, watching sexual activities, encouraging children to behave in sexually inappropriate ways, or grooming a child in preparation for abuse (including via the internet).

Men, women and children perpetrate sexual abuse. However, most abuse is perpetrated by someone known to the child.

Child sexual exploitation/abuse (CSE/CSA)

Sexual exploitation/abuse of children and young people under 18 can involve gangs or individuals. It is defined when children and young people receive something (such as food, accommodation, drugs, alcohol, cigarettes, affection, gifts or money) as a result of performing, and/or others performing on them, sexual acts. It can occur through direct contact or the use of the internet or mobile phones. Perpetrators have power over the child(ren) because of their age, gender, intellect, physical strength and/or resources. Both girls and boys of all age groups are at risk.

There are four models used to describe CSE:

1. **Peer on peer exploitation**: outlines instances when children are sexually exploited by their own peers who could be known to them at school, through mutual friends or in the neighbourhood.
2. **Boyfriend model**: targets children by posing as boyfriends and showers the child(ren) with attention, which results in them becoming infatuated. The perpetrator then initiates a sexual relationship with the child, who is then expected to return it as 'proof of their love', or they are told they owe money for the gifts, and sexual activities are a way of paying back.
3. **Party model**: organised by groups who lure young people by offering drinks, drugs and car rides often for free and an introduction to an exciting environment. This often results in incriminating evidence being obtained at the party, such as photos or videos of sexual acts, that is then used to exploit through fear.
4. **Exploitation through befriending and grooming**: befriending directly by the perpetrator, either in person, or online, or through other children or young people.

Table 1.5 – EXAMPLES OF TYPES OF ABUSE AND NEGLECT *continued*

Children who are most vulnerable and at higher risk of CSE/CSA are:

- missing or runaway children
- children in care
- those with experience of sexual abuse or violence in the home
- neglected
- homeless/sofa surfing
- misusing substances
- children with mental health issues
- those with a learning disability
- not in education, employment or training (NEET).

Physical abuse

Physical abuse may involve hitting, shaking, throwing, poisoning, burning (including cigarette burns or scalding), suffocating, use of restraint, spitting, force feeding or otherwise causing physical harm. Physical harm may also be caused when a parent or carer fabricates the symptoms of, or deliberately induces, ill-health; this situation is commonly described as 'fabricated or induced illness' (FII).

Neglect

Neglect is the persistent failure to meet a child's basic physical and/or psychological needs, and is likely to result in the serious impairment of the child's health or development. Neglect may occur during pregnancy as a result of maternal substance abuse.

A neglected or abused infant may show signs of poor attachment. They may lack the sense of security to explore, and appear unhappy and whining. There may be little sign of attachment behaviour, and the child may move aimlessly around a room or creep quietly into corners.

Signs of potential neglect include:

- poor weight gain
- failure to use prescribed medication or medication withheld by parent/carer
- severe nappy rash
- tooth decay
- failure to immunise
- poor hygiene and dirty clothes
- obesity
- poor growth
- delayed development
- failure to attend appointments
- delayed presentation
- poor physical condition
- child not at school
- child not registered with a GP
- clothes not consistent with the climate.

2.1 Children in Need

- Children are defined as being 'in need' when:
  - they are unlikely to reach or maintain a satisfactory level of health or development
  - their health and development will be significantly impaired without the provision of services (section 17 (10) of the Children Act 1989) [1]
  - they have a disability.
- Local authorities have a duty to safeguard and promote the welfare of children in need.

3. Recognition of Abuse

Ambulance clinicians may receive information or make observations that suggest that a child has been abused or is at risk of harm, for example:

- the nature of the illness/injury
- the account given for the illness/injury may be inconsistent with what is observed, this is known as 'disguised compliance'
- observation of hazards in the home (e.g. alcohol or drug paraphernalia, home conditions such as lack of bedding)
- child(ren) has/have been locked in a room
- signs of distress shown by other children in the home
- observations regarding the condition of other children or adults in the household (e.g. an environment where domestic abuse has taken place). In the case of domestic dispute between adults, the presence of children in the household creates a need to notify even if the child(ren) was/were not injured
- parents or carers who seek medical care from a number of sources.

3.1 Non-accidental/Deliberate Injury

- When assessing an injury in any child, you should be aware of the possibility of the injury being non-accidental/deliberate and you should consider this possibility in every case, even if you promptly dismiss the idea.
- For an injury to be accidental it should have a clear, credible and acceptable history and the findings should be consistent with the history and with the development and abilities of the child.

3.2 Suspicion of Abuse

Suspicions should be raised by:

- any injury in a non-mobile (non-independent) baby
- accidents/injuries in unusual places (e.g. the buttocks, trunk, inner thighs)
- extensive injuries or signs of both recent and old injuries

- small deep burns in unusual places
- repeated burns and scalds
- 'glove and stocking' burns
- poor state of clothing, cleanliness and/or nutrition
- delayed reporting of the injury
- inappropriate sexual knowledge for the child's age
- overt sexual approaches to other children or adults
- fear of particular people or situations (e.g. bath time or bedtime)
- drug and alcohol abuse
- suicide attempts and self-injury
- running away and fire-setting
- environmental factors and family situations (e.g. domestic abuse, drug or alcohol abuse, learning disabilities that effects parents, carers and/or child).

The following symptoms should give cause for concern and further assessment:

- soreness, discharge or unexplained bleeding in the genital area (including anal area and severe nappy rash)
- chronic vaginal/anal infections
- bruising, grazes or bites to the genital/anal or breast area
- sexually transmitted infections
- pregnancy, especially when the identity of the father is vague or if it is a concealed or denied pregnancy.

When assessing an injured child, you should use your clinical knowledge regarding what level of accidental injury would be appropriate for their stage of development. Although stages of development vary (e.g. children may crawl or walk at different ages), injuries can broadly be divided between mobile and non-mobile children.

4. Non-mobile (Non-independent) Babies

- Babies aged under 1 year are the most vulnerable group of children as they cannot speak for themselves and are dependent on their parents/carers. Any injury in a non-mobile baby requires review by a clinician. If there is any doubt, the clinician should speak with the on-call paediatrician in the acute trust and/or the child should be conveyed.
- Healthy babies do not bruise or break their bones easily. They do not bruise themselves with their fists or toys, bruise themselves by lying against the bars of a cot, or acquire bruises on the legs when they are held for a nappy change. When in an environment, checks can be made for safety equipment, such as stair gates etc.
- Bruising on the ears, face, neck, trunk and buttocks is particularly suspicious. A torn frenulum (behind the upper lip) is rarely accidental in babies, and bleeding from the mouth of a baby should always be regarded as suspicious.

4.1 Fractures

- Fractures may not be obvious on observation and the baby may present only with crying on handling. Often a fracture will not be diagnosed until an X-ray is performed. Fractures in babies are seldom caused by 'rough handling' or putting their legs through the bars of the cot. Babies rarely fracture their skull after a fall from a bed or a chair. Fractures in non-mobile infants should be assessed by an experienced paediatrician to exclude non-accidental injury (refer to Table 1.6 for types of fractures).
- Children's bones tend to bend rather than break and require considerable force to damage them. There are various kinds of fractures (refer to Table 1.6), depending on the direction and strength of the force that caused them.
- Unless there is an obvious bony deformity, bone injuries may not be apparent on initial clinical assessment. A clear history and appreciation of the mechanism of injury are crucial parts of the initial assessment and must be clearly documented.

Table 1.6 – TYPES OF BONE FRACTURES

Greenstick

The bones bend rather than break. This is a very common accidental injury in children.

Transverse

The break goes across the bone and occurs when there is a direct blow or a direct force on the end of the bone (e.g. a fall on the hand may break the forearm bones or the distal humerus).

Spiral or oblique

A fracture line that goes right around the bone or obliquely across it is due to a twisting force, which may be a feature in non-accidental injuries.

Metaphyseal

Occur at the extreme ends of the bone and are usually only confirmed radiologically. These are caused by a strong twisting force.

Skull

These must be consistent with the history and explanation given. Complex (branched), depressed or fractures at the back of the skull are suspect of abuse.

Rib

These do not occur accidentally, except in a severe crushing injury. Any other cause is highly suspicious of non-accidental injury.

4.2 Shaking Injuries

- When small babies are shaken violently their head and limb movements cannot be controlled, causing brain damage and haemorrhage within the skull. This can also be caused by being thrown.
- Finger bruising on the chest may indicate that a baby has been held tightly and shaken. These babies usually

present with collapse or respiratory problems and the diagnosis is only made on further detailed assessment.

5. Mobile Babies and Toddlers

5.1 Bruising

- It is normal for toddlers to have accidental bruises on the shins, elbows and forehead. Bruises in unusual areas such as the back, upper arms and abdomen do not tend to occur accidentally. Defensive wounds commonly occur on the forearm, upper arm, back of the legs, hands or feet. You may see clusters of bruises on the upper arm, outside of the thigh or on the body. You may see bruises with dots of blood under the skin. A bruised scalp and swollen eyes may suggest that hair has been pulled violently.
- Bruising caused by a hand slap leaves a characteristic pattern of 'stripes' representing the imprint of fingers. Forceful gripping leaves small round bruises corresponding to the position of the fingertips. 'Tramline' bruising is caused by a belt or stick, and shows as lines of bruising with a white patch in between.

5.2 Burns and Scalds

- Burns and scalds can result from hot liquids, hot objects, flames, chemicals or electricity.
- Burns are caused by the application to the skin of dry heat, and the depth of the burn will depend on the temperature of the object and the length of time it is in contact with the skin.
- Abusive burns are frequently small and deep, and may show the outline of the object (e.g. the soleplate of an iron), whereas accidental burns rarely do so because the child will pull away in response to pain.
- Cigarette burns are not common. They are round, deep and have a red flare around a flat brown crust. These burns usually leave a scar.
- Scalds are caused by steam or hot liquids. Accidental scalds may be extensive but show splash marks unlike the sharp edges of damage done when the child is dunked in hot water (although splash marks may also feature in a non-accidental burn indicating that the child had tried to escape hot water). The glove and stocking pattern of burns on the arms and legs is typical of non-accidental injury. The head, face, neck, shoulders and front of the chest are the areas affected when a child pulls over a kettle accidentally.

5.3 Bite Marks

Bites result in small bruises forming part or all of a circle. They are usually oval or circular in shape. There may be visible wounds, indentations or bruising from individual teeth.

5.4 Deliberate Poisoning and Attempted Suffocation

These are very difficult to assess and may need a period of close observation in hospital. Deliberate poisoning, such as might be found in a child in whom illness is fabricated or induced by carers with parenting responsibilities (fictitious or induced illness), may be suspected when a child has repeated puzzling illnesses, usually of sudden onset. The signs include unusual drowsiness, apnoeic attacks, vomiting, diarrhoea and fits. There may be respiratory problems due to suffocation.

6. Older Children and Adolescents

- If the injury is accidental, older children will give a very clear and detailed account of how it happened. The detail will be missing if they have been told what to say.
- Overdosing and other self-harm injuries must be taken seriously in this age group, as they may indicate sexual or other abuse (such as exploitation).

6.1 Parental Factors

Parental unavailability for whatever reason increases the risk to the child of all forms of abuse, especially neglect and emotional abuse. Specific consideration of the effects of the parent's problem on the children must be made, whatever the circumstances of presentation. Sources of stress within families may have a negative impact on a child's health, development or well-being, either directly or because they affect the capacity of parents to respond to their child's needs. Sources of stress may include social exclusion, domestic abuse, unstable mental illness of a parent or carer, or drug and alcohol misuse. Parents who appear overanxious about their child when there is no sign of illness or injury may be signalling their inability to cope.

Parental factors that might have a negative impact on parenting capacity include:

- learning difficulties
- mental health problems
- substance abuse
- domestic abuse
- chronic ill health
- physical disability
- unemployment or poverty
- homelessness/frequent moves
- social isolation
- young, unsupported parents
- parents with poor role models of their own
- lack of, or poor, education
- criminality
- unwanted or unplanned pregnancy.

7. Special Circumstances

7.1 Individuals Who Pose a Risk to Children

- Once an individual has been sentenced and identified as presenting a risk of harm to children, agencies have a responsibility to work collaboratively to monitor and manage the risk of harm to others.
- Where an offender is given a community sentence, Offender Managers or Youth Offending Team workers will monitor the individual's risk of harm to others and their behaviour, and liaise with partner agencies as appropriate.
- Multi-Agency Public Protection Arrangements (MAPPA) should be in place to enable agencies to work together within a statutory framework for managing risk of harm to the public.
- There are certain work forces that are exempt from the Rehabilitation of Offenders Act 1974. Patient-facing roles within the ambulance service are part of this. Safer recruitment checks will be undertaken including an enhanced DBS (Disclosure and Barring Service).

7.2 Disabled Children

Abuse may be difficult to separate from symptoms of disability (e.g. increase in seizures in a child with epilepsy if anticonvulsants are withheld). Induced and fabricated illness may be even more difficult to recognise because the child may have coexistent diagnoses.

Important points to remember about abuse of disabled children are:

- It may be more common than abuse of non-disabled children, but evidence for this is poor.
- It may be under-reported.
- Children may have difficulty communicating their abuse.
- Abuse may compound pre-existing disability, or be the cause of the disability.
- All forms of abuse are seen, including neglect and sexual abuse.
- It is easy to fail to recognise abuse in disabled children by making too many allowances for the disability as a cause of problems.
- Be aware that professionals can be drawn into collusion with families; this is a term known as 'disguised compliance'.

These children are at risk of achieving poor outcomes. Ambulance clinicians need to be aware of the role they can play in recognition of these children, identifying their particular needs and preventing significant harm. In the current multicultural society of the United Kingdom, it is important to recognise that there may be children and families in need of skilled interpreters, and that differences may exist in child-rearing practices in minority groups.

7.3 Special Circumstances for Consideration

- **Children and young people living away from home** – many looked-after children and young people that live independently have been abused or neglected prior to going into care. This is a particular group where assessment may be made more difficult, because of pre-existing symptoms and behaviour. There should be a low threshold in seeking advice from experienced professionals in these circumstances (e.g. designated/named professional).
- **Asylum-seeking children or refugees, both with families and unaccompanied** – the importance of having skilled interpreters in assessment of these children cannot be over-emphasised. The children's behaviour on entering the country may already have been influenced by previous experience. It is important to remember their general health needs and that families will need help in accessing services. It is also important to refer children who are victims of human trafficking.
- **Children with maladjusted parent(s)/carers** (see also **Parental Factors**) – these include children of substance-misusing parents/carers, children living with domestic abuse, children whose parents/carers have chronic mental or physical health problems, children whose parents/carers have a learning disability, children with a parent/carer in prison, children living in flexi-families. Effects on the child/ren can be profound and include fearfulness, withdrawal, anxious behaviour, lack of self-confidence and social skills, difficulties in forming relationships, sleep disturbance, non-attendance at school, aggression, bullying, post-traumatic stress disorder, behaviour suggestive of ADHD.

The following children may also have unmet health needs (low immunisation levels, poor dental health and either poor or non-attendance at clinic appointments).

- **Children in the armed forces** – extra strains are placed upon the families engendered by frequent moves, frequent changes of school, separation of parents by the nature of the job, and separation from immediate support from family and friends.
- **Children of travelling families** – are subjected to the same problems because of frequent moves. They may also suffer from poor health, poor access to primary healthcare and vaccinations, in addition to poor living conditions.
- **Runaway children and exploitation** – many runaway children may already have been the subject of abuse and are at risk of exploitation. They are also at risk of child trafficking for sexual exploitation.
- **Children as young carers** – neglect and emotional abuse may be part of the difficulties of taking on parental responsibilities and a caring role at a young age. Young carers lose out on normal childhood experiences and should be considered at higher risk of abuse whether intentional or unintentional (e.g. school attendance, peer groups).

8. Mandatory Reporting of Female Genital Mutilation (FGM)

On 31st October 2015 the FGM Act introduced a mandatory reporting duty that requires health and social care professionals as well as teachers to report known cases of FGM in those under 18 years of age to the police.

FGM is child abuse and the current procedure is set out below:

- **Children and vulnerable adults** – if any child (under 18) or vulnerable adult has symptoms or signs of FGM, or if there is good reason to suspect they are at risk of FGM on consideration of their family history or other relevant factors, they **must** be referred using existing safeguarding procedures as with all instances of child abuse. This will involve referral to police and social care in the usual way.
- In all cases where staff are unsure of their actions, they should seek the advice of the Trust Safeguarding Service.

9. Assessment and Management

If physical, sexual, or emotional abuse or neglect is suspected, follow local procedures; information can be obtained from the named professional for safeguarding within individual ambulance Trusts. Ambulance clinicians may obtain contact information from ambulance control.

9.1 If the Child is the Patient

- The first priority is the health and safety of the child. Ambulance clinicians should follow the usual **ABCDE** and **<C>ABCDE** assessment (refer to **Medical Emergencies in Children (Overview)** and **Trauma Emergencies Overview (Children)**). Children with significant injury should be transferred to further care without delay.
- Where a child is thought to be at immediate risk, they should be referred to the police as an emergency by contacting ambulance control for a 999 response.

In all circumstances:

- Limit questions to those of routine history taking, asking questions only in relation to the injury or for clarification of what is being said. It is important to stop questioning when suspicions are clarified. Unnecessary questioning or probing may affect the credibility of subsequent evidence.
- Accept the explanations given and do not make any suggestions to the child as to how an injury or incident may have happened.
- Care must be taken not to directly accuse parents or carers of abuse as this may result in a refusal to transfer to further care and place the child at further risk. Always work in partnership with parents or carers as far as possible, and inform them of concerns and the need to share these with the statutory agencies, unless to do so would put the child or others at greater risk of harm. Professional curiosity and judgement is crucial as to what information should be shared with parents.
- Any allegation of abuse made by a child is an important indicator and should always be taken seriously – it is important to listen to the 'voice of the child' and what they are saying. Do not ask probing questions. Consider what is a 'safe space' for them to talk.
- Adult responses can influence how able a child feels to reveal the full extent of the abuse. Listen and react appropriately to instil confidence. It is important to note that children may only tell a small part of their experience initially.
- It is important to make an accurate record of events and actions. Write down exactly what the child says. Their first language may not be English and care must be taken not to use family members or carers as interpreters in cases of suspected abuse. Take note of any inconsistency in history and any delay in calling for assistance.
- On arrival at hospital inform the receiving staff and the most senior member of nursing staff on duty of any concerns or suspicions. When reporting suspected abuse, the emphasis must be on shared professional responsibility and immediate communication.
- Complete safeguarding documentation/report as per local procedures; complete in private if possible. Follow local/Trust protocols/guidelines.
- Ambulance clinicians must report suspected child abuse to the relevant statutory bodies (e.g. social care and the police), but they do not have a statutory duty to investigate it.
- Where a practitioner feels that their concerns have not been taken up (commonly known as professional challenge), they have a duty to escalate their concerns to a higher level by discussing this with their line manager, a more experienced colleague or named/designated doctor or nurse.

9.2 If the Child is Not the Patient

- If the circumstances are suspicious, the ambulance clinician(s) should consider the implications of leaving the child.
- If the child is accompanying another person (e.g. a parent/carer) who is being conveyed, the ambulance clinician(s) should inform ED staff of their concerns and remember to report through their own safeguarding services as required.
- If no one is transferred to hospital, follow local/Trust protocols/guidelines and inform them of the incident/concerns at the earliest opportunity.
- Complete safeguarding documentation/report as per local procedures; complete in private if possible. Follow local/Trust protocols/guidelines.

9.3 Allegations Against Ambulance Clinicians

- An allegation made by a child against an ambulance clinician is no different from an allegation made against any other healthcare professional, and the appropriate procedures should be followed, that is a referral to social care or the police. In other words, a child protection inquiry must follow such allegations.

Safeguarding Children

- No staff, regardless of their position, volunteer, commissioned service or person associated with delivering services on behalf of an NHS Trust, must act in any way that constitutes any of the following:
  - Behaviour that harms, or may harm, a child, young person or adult.
  - Behaviour that results in a criminal offence against, or related to, a child, young person or adult.
  - Behaviour towards a child, young person or adult that indicates s/he is unsuitable to work in a position of trust.
- The member of staff who is alleged to have abused the child must report the allegation to his line manager/named professional, who should follow employment procedures, that is a possible restriction of practice or suspension while investigations are conducted. There should be close liaison between the police carrying out the investigation and the line manager/named professional, who should be guided by the police as to how much information about the inquiry should be relayed to the member of staff. There will also need to be a support system in place for the member of staff.

KEY POINTS

Safeguarding children

- **The safety and welfare of the child is paramount.**
- **There is a duty to report concerns. Staff should not investigate suspicions themselves.**
- **Be aware of any special circumstances that the child is in which may increase the risk of abuse.**
- **Police should be involved where there may be an immediate risk to the child.**
- **Staff should document the circumstances giving rise to their concern as soon as possible.**

Further Reading

Further important information and evidence in support of this guideline can be found in the Bibliography.[3, 4, 5, 6, 7, 8, 9, 10, 11, 12, 13, 14, 15, 16, 17, 1819]

Other useful resources include:

Barnado's – http://www.barnados.org.uk/

Child Exploitation and Online Protection Centre – http://www.ceop.gov.uk

Childline – http://www.childline.org.uk/

Children's Legal Centre – http://www.childrenslegalcentre.com

DCSF – http://www.dcsf.gov.uk/

Every Child Matters – http://www.everychildmatters.co.uk/

Kidscape – http://www.kidscape.org.uk

National Service Framework for Children, Young People and Maternity Services – https://www.gov.uk/government/publications/national-service-framework-children-young-people-and-maternity-services

NSPCC – http://www.nspcc.org.uk

Family Lives – http://www.familylives.org.uk/

Samaritans – http://www.samaritans.org.uk

Think You Know – http://www.thinkuknow.co.uk/

Victim Support – http://www.victimsupport.org.uk

Victoria Climbié Enquiry – https://www.gov.uk/government/uploads/system/uploads/attachment_data/file/273183/5730.pdf

Bibliography

1 Department of Health. *The Children Act 1989*. London: HMSO, 1989. Available from: https://www.gov.uk/government/uploads/system/uploads/attachment_data/file/441643/Children_Act_Guidance_2015.pdf.

2 Department for Children, Schools and Families. *Working Together to Safeguard Children: A guide to interagency working to safeguard and promote the welfare of children*. London: HMSO, 2015. Available from: https://www.gov.uk/government/uploads/system/uploads/attachment_data/file/419595/Working_Together_to_Safeguard_Children.pdf.

3 National Institute for Health and Clinical Excellence. *When to Suspect Child Maltreatment* (CG89). London: NICE, 2009. Available from: https://www.nice.org.uk/guidance/cg89.

4 Department of Children, Schools and Families. *Safeguarding Disabled Children – Practice guidance*. London: HMSO, 2009. Available from: https://www.gov.uk/government/uploads/system/uploads/attachment_data/file/190544/00374-2009DOM-EN.pdf.

5 Department of Health. *The Data Protection Act 1998*. London: HMSO, 1998. Available from: http://www.legislation.gov.uk/ukpga/1998/29/contents.

6 Department of Health. *Responding to Domestic Abuse: A handbook for health professionals*. London: HMSO, 2005.

7 Department of Health. *Women's Mental Health: Into the mainstream*. London: HMSO, 2002.

8 Department of Health. *Improving Safety, Reducing Harm – Children, young people and domestic violence*. London: HMSO, 2009.

9 Home Office. *Adoption and Children Act 2002*. London: HMSO, 2002. Available from: http://www.legislation.gov.uk/ukpga/2002/38/contents.

10 Home Office. *Female Genital Mutilation Act 2003*. London: HMSO, 2003. Available from: http://www.legislation.gov.uk/ukpga/2003/31/pdfs/ukpga_20030031_en.pdf.

11 Krug E, Dahlberg L, Mercy J, Zwi A. Lozano R. *World Report on Violence and Health*. Geneva: World Health Organisation, 2002.

12 O'Keefe M. Predictors of child abuse in martially violent homes. *Journal of Interpersonal Violence* 1995, 10: 3–25.

13 Royal College of Paediatrics and Child Health. *Safeguarding Children and Young People: Roles and competences for health care staff*. Available from: http://www.rcpch.ac.uk/sites/default/files/asset_library/Education%20Department/Safeguarding/Safeguarding%20Children%20and%20Young%20people%202010G.pdf. 2010.

14 Scottish Parliament. *Prohibition of Female Genital Mutilation (Scotland) Act 2005*. Edinburgh: HMSO, 2005. Available from: http://www.refworld.org/pdfid/47d159902.pdf.

15 Sullivan PM, Knutson JF. Maltreatment and Disabilities: A population-based epidemiological study. *Child Abuse and Neglect* 2000, 24(10): 1257–1273.

16 Taskforce on the Health Aspects of Violence Against Women and Children Improving Safety. *Responding to Violence Against Women and Children – the role of the NHS*. Available from: http://www.fflm.ac.uk/wp-content/uploads/documentstore/1268669895.pdf, 2010.

17 Walby S, Allen J. *Domestic Violence, Sexual Assault and Stalking: Findings from the British Crime Survey*. Home Office Research Study 276. Available from: http://womensaidorkney.org.uk/wp-content/uploads/2014/08/Home-office-research.pdf, 2004.

18 WHO/UNICEF/UNFPA. *Female Genital Mutilation: A joint statement*. Geneva: WHO. Available from: http://apps.who.int/iris/bitstream/10665/41903/1/9241561866.pdf, 1997.

19 World Health Organization. *Eliminating Female Genital Mutilation: An interagency statement*. Geneva: WHO. Available from: http://www.un.org/womenwatch/daw/csw/csw52/statements_missions/Interagency_Statement_on_Eliminating_FGM.pdf, 2008.

1. Introduction

- Sexual assault is extremely distressing, causing a broad spectrum of psychological, emotional and physical effects on patients. They may be agitated or hysterical, in shock or disbelief, or calm and extremely controlled. Clinicians should understand there is no 'normal' response and have no expectation of the patient exhibiting a prescribed pattern of behaviour.[1]
- It may be appropriate for the patient to be accompanied by another person. The patient may be anxious when left alone with a person of the same sex as the assailant. On the other hand, they may be reassured by the presence of a professional person. The wishes of the patient must be considered and attempts made to reassure them and make them feel safe.
- The patient has just experienced a major psychological and potentially physical trauma, often committed by someone they believed in and trusted. The clinician must not only manage their physical, medical and psychological needs, but must absolutely act as the patient's advocate, facilitating their wishes wherever possible.
- Patients experiencing sexual assault may believe they are responsible for the assault and need reassuring that they are victims and what has happened was not their fault.[2]
- A sensitive and kind approach by those providing an initial response is known to be beneficial in facilitating recovery and decreasing long-term use of health services post rape. In contrast, health professionals inexperienced in dealing with survivors, who use insensitive language, subscribe to rape myths and stereotypes, who are judgemental, inconsiderate or critical, are known to increase the risk of revictimising the survivor, delaying recovery, sometimes forever.[3]
- Importantly, victims of sexual violence must be treated with respect and dignity irrespective of either the victim's or the clinician's social status, race, religion, culture, sexual orientation, lifestyle, sex or occupation.[1]
- It is not the role of the clinician to determine if the assault has occurred; that is the job of the courts. Instead they must provide a sensitive, non-judgemental, holistic approach that is neither moralistic nor opinionated. Victims who blame themselves, or fear being blamed or doubted, are less likely to report sexual assault. Recovery may also be hampered by the blame or disbelief of others, whether real or perceived. Body language, gestures and facial expressions all contribute to conveying an atmosphere of believing the patient's account, which is known to be critical to recovery.[4]
- The intimate nature of sexual assault, combined with the inevitable feelings of guilt and shame these patients experience, complicates their care. During the assault, they may have seen, experienced and been forced to do things that are outside their normal moral or ethical code. They may believe it to be unspeakable.
- Many victims cite fear of not being believed as a reason for not reporting sexual assault and recovery may be hindered when others disbelieve or blame the patient for the assault. Validation of the patient's feelings is thus critical to recovery.[3] Body language, gestures and facial expressions all contribute to conveying an atmosphere of believing the patient's account.

2. Disclosure to Police

- Some patients will refuse care or transfer to hospital because they believe police may be informed without their consent and fear perceived catastrophic consequences. Historically reporting without patient consent has been common practice amongst both control room and operational staff of all levels.
- The decision to report a sexual assault on an adult is entirely the decision of the victim. There is no statutory obligation for victims of sexual violence to report to police and many victims elect not to report to protect their safety, privacy or both.[5]
- Similarly, no statutory obligation mandates the reporting by healthcare professionals of cases involving rape or sexual assault.[5] Where the patient is an adult with full capacity to consent, and is not classed as 'vulnerable', there is no requirement for clinicians to breach confidentiality and report to police without consent. Control room staff should not routinely inform police and request their attendance unless this is the specific wish of the patient, and no attempt to persuade or coerce the patient to agree to police attendance should be made by anyone involved in their care pathway at any time.[6,7]
- The only exception to this would be where disclosing the information is necessary to prevent a serious crime or serious harm to others. Generally, if the ambulance service is involved, the serious crime has already occurred. Unless there are reasonable grounds to assume there is imminent risk to either the patient or the public, the patient's decision, as an autonomous adult, should be fully respected.[8]
- Where it is perceived there is a clear and present immediate danger to the patient or others if disclosure to police is not made, and that risk is greater than the possible consequences to the patient of disclosure, then it would be appropriate to breach that confidentiality.

3. Forensic Requirements

- Where the victim requests police involvement, forensic awareness is essential. Within the limits of any immediate care needs, there is a responsibility to preserve evidence. Where police are on scene and injuries do not require emergent care, the police will normally take responsibility for the patient.[9]
- While awaiting police arrival patients should be kept within the environment in which they present, unless this is unsafe or increasing the patients distress; if so, they can be moved to the ambulance, seated on a

clean sheet and wherever possible discouraged from any activities that jeopardise collection of evidence. This will include cutting, removing or changing clothing, eating or drinking, passing urine or opening bowels or washing.[9]

- Where the patient cannot be dissuaded from the natural need to clean themselves, they should be encouraged to place any tissues or towels along with any bloodstained clothes into paper (not plastic) bags, which do not destroy biological evidence.[9]
- Where patients are transported to hospital and police action is requested, all blankets, sheets, towels and associated paraphernalia should be passed to police for forensic retrieval.[9]

Additional forensic information:

- Where patients have not presented for immediate care following rape, clinicians should be aware of how long forensic material may be preserved within the patient. The approximate times after contact for which evidentially relevant material has been identified – the 'forensic window' - is detailed in Table 1.7.
- Differences exist between pre- and post-pubescent patients; this is because the vaginal area is hostile to semen in pre-pubescent patient.

Table 1.7 – PRESERVATION OF FORENSIC MATERIAL[9]

Type of Incident	Type of Sample	Forensic Window
Digital penetration	Vulval, vaginal, peri-anal and anal swabs	Up to 12 hours
Oral penetration	Mouth swabs and oral rinse	Up to 48 hours – even where the patient has eaten, drunk or brushed their teeth
Anal penetration	Peri-anal, perineal, internal anal and rectal swabs Penile swabs	Up to 72 hours
Vaginal penetration	Vulval, vaginal and endocervical swabs	Pre-pubescent: Up to 72 hours Post-pubescent: Up to 120 hours

4. Care Pathways

As primary caregiver and advocate, clinicians should inform the patient of their options without judgement, bias or coercion. Any physical examination should allow identification of life threatening injuries and those requiring emergent care only. Genital areas should only be exposed and examined if there is evidence of bleeding requiring immediate treatment.

Allow the patient space and as much choice about options for their treatment as possible. Options for the care of sexual assault victims may be summarised as:

- **Accident and Emergency**:
  - if the victim has injuries requiring emergent care
  - if the level of distress makes it impossible for the patient to consent or coherently express their wishes.
- **Police**:
  - only where the patient gives express and informed consent as discussed above.
- **Sexual Assault Referral Centres (SARC)**:
  - SARCs provide recent victims of sexual assault with immediate care and crisis support from specialist staff trained to allow patients to make informed decisions. They also provide access to acute physical assessment with testing for STIs, provision of post-infection prophylaxis and emergency contraception.[10]
  - SARCs also facilitate access to the criminal justice system. Forensic retrieval may be undertaken regardless of whether the patient reports to police or not. Where the patient decides not to report, forensic samples may be stored, allowing patients time to consider their options until after the immediate 'crisis period'.[10]
  - SARCs provide direct access to Independent Sexual Violence Advisers (ISVAs) who provide advice, support and access to follow-up services addressing the patient's medical, safeguarding, psychosocial and ongoing needs.
  - ISVAs will also support patients through the judicial process; importantly, patients supported by ISVAs are more likely to go through the full course of criminal justice proceedings, which highlights the importance of encouraging patients to access SARCs wherever possible.[11]

4.1. Access to SARCs

- **Self-referral** – patients may self-refer to SARCs by telephoning; clinicians may also call on the patient's behalf. Patients have a brief conversation with a crisis worker who helps them decide on an immediate plan and makes an appointment for them to attend. Where this appointment is immediate, subject to time constraints and local protocols, ambulance crews may transport the patient directly to the SARC or alternatively make certain the patient will be able to be taken safely by a third party.
- Local SARC contact details should be held centrally by ambulance control rooms; they are also available on NHS Choices.
- **Police referral** – the patient reports to police, who contact the SARC and arrange for the patient to be transferred.

4.2. Refusal of Care

- Patients refusing referral to support services place a duty of care on clinicians to ensure their immediate safety. Encouraging patients to call a friend or relative for support is a priority. In these cases, patients should be given details of their nearest GUM clinic and rape crisis services. These conversations require tact and sensitivity as patients may not have considered risks of STIs or pregnancy and this alone may create another crisis.
- In cases of sexual assault in vulnerable adults and children refer to **Safeguarding Adults at Risk** and **Safeguarding Children**.

5. Incidence

- Approximately 11 adults are raped every hour in England and Wales. That amounts to 85,000 women and 12,000 men becoming victims of rape every year, while nearly half a million adults are sexually assaulted.
- Of these, 90% know the perpetrator prior to the offence, and only around 15% of these will choose to report to police.[12]
- In 2012–13, 23,663 sexual offences against children were reported to police in England and Wales including 6,296 rapes, with 80% of these involving girls.[13]
- Given this incidence, as a profession, paramedics should be well versed in the care of this most vulnerable group and have a comprehensive understanding of the care pathways and services available to them.

6. Severity and Outcome

- The severity of the assault can vary from sexual touching to sustaining life-threatening injuries. The outcome of the assault can lead to long-term psychological and physical effects.

7. Pathophysiology

The Sexual Offences Act (2003) defines four offences:[14]

- Rape – penetration of the vagina, anus or mouth with a penis without consent.
- Assault by penetration – non-consensual, intentional insertion of an object (other than a penis) into the vagina or anus.
- Sexual assault – non-consensual violation of the victim's sexual anatomy, e.g. touching another person in a sexual way without consent.
- Causing a person to engage in sexual activity without consent.

8. Assessment and Management

For the assessment and management of sexual assault refer to Table 1.8.

Table 1.8 – ASSESSMENT and MANAGEMENT of:

Sexual Assault

ASSESSMENT	MANAGEMENT
● Assess **ABCD**	If any TIME CRITICAL features present major ABCD problems: ● start correcting A and B problems ● undertake a TIME CRITICAL transfer to nearest receiving hospital ● continue patient management en-route ● provide an alert/information call.
● Assess	● Limit questions to those identifying the need for medical treatment, but allow the patient to talk and document what is said. **NB** It is not appropriate to probe for details of the assault and could affect the outcome of criminal investigations. ● Manage according to condition: – Acute injury – refer to **Trauma Emergencies Overview (Adults)** and **Trauma Emergencies Overview (Children)**. – Acute illness – refer to **Medical Emergencies in Adults – Overview** and **Medical Emergencies in Children – Overview**. ● It may be appropriate to delay assessment for non-urgent injuries until transfer to a Sexual Assault Referral Centre to avoid further distress and disturbing the evidence.

Sexual Assault *continued*	
• Approach	• Rape is about power and control, not the sexual act. Listen to the patient with a sensitive and respectful manner and return control to them. • Establish the patient's safety. • Let the patient know you believe them. • If possible, ensure privacy. • Consider cultural/religious issues. • Where possible accommodate patient's requests. • Where possible avoid disturbing the scene. • Where possible avoid being alone with the patient. • Patients are not required by law to report sexual violence to police. • Healthcare professionals are not required by law to report cases of sexual violence to police unless: – the patient does not have capacity to consent – the patient is classed as 'vulnerable' – there is a clear and present danger of immediate risk to the patient or public. • No attempt should be made to persuade the patient to agree to police attendance; decision making should be facilitated by presenting available options. • Where this is requested, police should be called promptly so the scene may be secured. • Where patients decline any support or referral, they should be encouraged to obtain community support ensuring their ongoing safety is secured. These patients should be encouraged to contact their nearest GUM clinic or local rape crisis services with tact and care.
• Forensic examination	• Forensic examination will focus specifically on the areas affected, including wounds, mouth, anus and vagina and other areas where the patient has been kissed, licked or bitten, as these areas may well be contaminated with the assailant's DNA. • Clinicians should be aware of forensic windows, and where this is relevant patients should be encouraged **not** to: – wash (shower/bathe) or brush their teeth – change clothes, throw away or destroy clothes – urinate – the police will want to collect early evidence samples including a urine sample to screen for the presence of drugs, as some drugs have a very short half-life – smoke, eat or drink – a mouth swab and mouth wash may also be requested by the police – defecate. • If a blanket is required for modesty or warmth, a single-use blanket should be used and kept with the patient – the blanket needs to be retained in order to analyse cross-contamination. • If the patient is not wrapped in a single-use blanket, place a sterile sheet or single-use blanket under the patient where they sit or lie and retain for forensic examination. • Avoid cleaning any wounds unless clinically absolutely necessary – if possible keep 'washings'. • If required, lightly apply dry dressings – retain any used dressing and swabs for forensic examination; also keep the sterile packets in which they were contained in order to examine for cross-contamination. **NB** All of these recommendations are vital to conserve evidence for a successful prosecution of the offender; BUT the need for this approach must be conveyed with great sensitivity to the patient, who may well want to wash and change.

Sexual Assault *continued*	
• Care pathways	**Accident and Emergency is appropriate:** • if the patient has injuries requiring emergency care • if the level of distress makes it impossible for them to consent or coherently express their wishes. **Sexual Assault Referral Centres can provide:** • immediate care and crisis support • acute physical assessment • testing for STIs • post-infection prophylaxis • emergency contraception • access to the criminal justice system • forensic retrieval with storage where police involvement is declined • access to ISVA services • access to follow-up services addressing medical, safeguarding, psychosocial and ongoing needs. Access to SARCs, where the patient consents, is either by: • **Self referral** – the patient telephones the SARC themselves (this can easily be initiated by the ambulance crew), who give them an appointment normally within a few hours unless they are busy. There is no reason why ambulance crews – subject to local protocols and time restraints, should not transport the patient directly to the SARC or alternatively make certain the patient will be able to be taken safely by a third party. • **Police referral** – the patient reports to police, who make contact with the SARC and arrange for the patient to be transferred. **Sexual Health Clinics provide treatment for:** • sexually transmitted infections • emergency contraception • post-exposure prophylaxis. **Rape Crisis Centres provide:** • confidential telephone helpline and support • face-to-face counselling for survivors of rape or sexual assault. • ISVA services • handover to an appropriate member of staff and not in a public area. Where a patient is competent and refuses hospital treatment, advise them to seek further medical attention. They may need post-exposure prophylaxis, vaccination and/or contraception, all of which can be provided confidentially.
• Documentation	• Complete the clinical record in great detail contemporaneously and document: – only facts, not personal opinion – what the patient says – clinical findings with relevant timings – the ambulance identification number. • A police statement may be required later.

KEY POINTS

Sexual Assault

- **Sexual assault may be concurrent with other injuries that will need treating.**
- **Treatment should avoid disturbing evidence where possible.**
- **The patient's rights to autonomy should be respected unless they do not have capacity to consent or are 'vulnerable'.**
- **Leave the investigation to the police.**
- **Accommodate the patient's wishes where possible.**
- **Police may have special facilities for managing patients.**

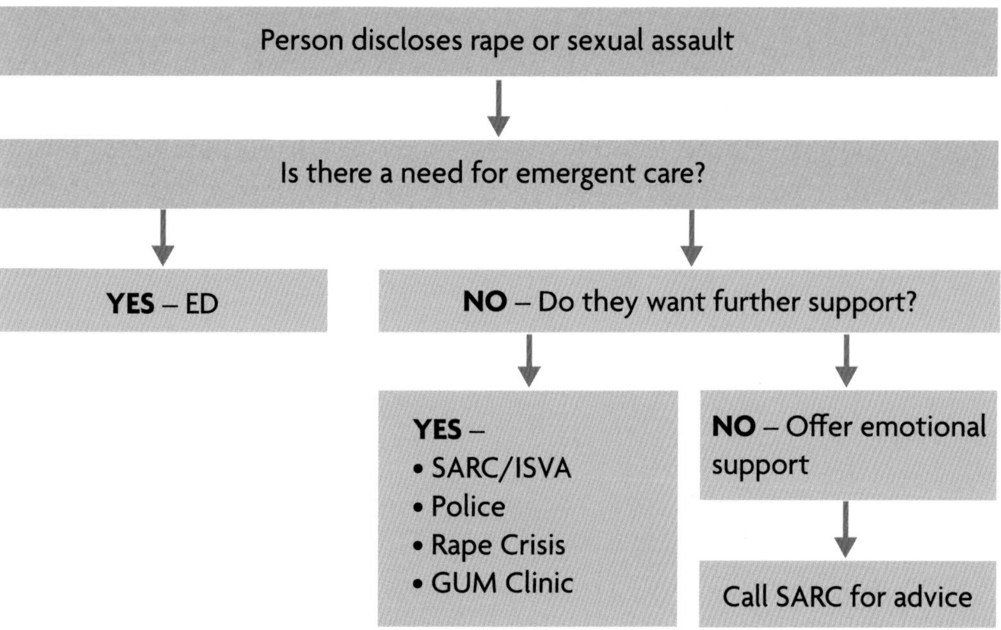

Figure 1.5 – Assessment and management of sexual assault.

Further Reading

Further important information and evidence in support of this guideline can be found in the Bibliography.[15, 16, 17, 18, 19, 20, 21, 22, 23]

Bibliography

1 World Health Organization. *Guidelines for Medico-legal Care for Victims of Sexual Violence*. Geneva: WHO, 2003. Available from: http://apps.who.int/iris/bitstream/10665/42788/1/924154628X.pdf.

2 Beckmann CR, Groetzinger LL. Treating sexual assault victims. A protocol for health professionals. *Female Patient* 1989, 14(5): 78–83.

3 Ranibar V, Speer SA. Revictimization and recovery from sexual assault: implications for health professionals. *Violence and Victims* 2013, 28(2): 274–287.

4 Dunn S, Gilchrist V. Sexual Assault. Primary Care 1993, 20: 359–373.

5 Department of Health. *Public Health Functions to be exercised by NHS England - Service Specification No 30, Sexual Assault Services*. London: HMSO, 2013. Available from: https://www.gov.uk/government/uploads/system/uploads/attachment_data/file/256501/30_sexual_assault_services.pdf.

6 British Association for Sexual Health and HIV. *UK National Guidelines on the Management of Adult and Adolescent Complainants of Sexual Assault 2011. Macclesfield: BASHH, 2011*. Available from: http://www.nordhaven.co.uk/BASHH.PDF.

7 Department of Health. *Confidentiality: NHS Code of Practice*. London: HMSO, 2003.

8 Department of Health. Confidentiality: *NHS Code of Practice Supplementary Guidance on Public Interest Disclosures*. London: HMSO, 2010.

9 Crown Prosecution Service. *Prosecution Policy and Guidance; Legal Guidance; Rape and Sexual offences: Forensic, Scientific and Medical Evidence*. Available from: http://www.cps.gov.uk/legal/p_to_r/rape_and_sexual_offences/forensic_scientific_and_medical_evidence/.

10 Department of Health, Home Office, Association of Chief Police Officers. *Revised National Service Guide – A Resource for Developing Sexual Assault Referral Centres*. London: HMSO, 2009. Available from: https://www.sericc.org.uk/pdfs/4313_sacentres.pdf.

11 Robinson AL. *Independent Sexual Violence Advisers: A process evaluation*. University of Cardiff funded by the Home Office, 2009. Available from: http://library.college.police.uk/docs/horr/horr20.pdf.

12 Ministry of Justice, Home Office and Office of National Statistics. *An Overview of Sexual Offending in England and Wales*. London: HMSO, 2013. Available from: https://www.gov.uk/government/statistics/an-overview-of-sexual-offending-in-england-and-wales.

13 Jutte S. et al. *How Safe Are Our Children?* London: NSPCC, 2014.

14 Legislation.gov.uk. Sexual Offences Act (2003). Available from: http://www.legislation.gov.uk/ukpga/2003/42/part/1.

15 Avegno J, Mills TJ, Mills LD. Sexual assault victims in the emergency department: analysis by demographic and event characteristics. *Journal of Emergency Medicine* 2009, 37(3): 328–334.

16 Dalton M. *Forensic Gynaecology: Towards better care of the female victim of sexual assault*. London: Royal College of Obstetricians and Gynaecologists Press, 2004.

17 Department of Health. *Improving Services for Women and Child Victims of Violence: The Department of Health Action Plan*. Available from: http://www.dh.gov.uk/prod_consum_dh/groups/dh_digitalassets/@dh/@en/@ps/documents/digitalasset/dh_122094.pdf, 2010.

18 Du Mont J, White D, McGregor MJ. Investigating the medical forensic examination from the perspectives of sexually

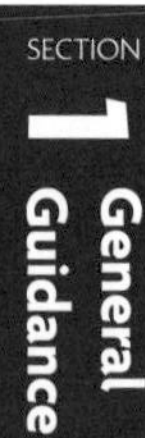

assaulted women. *Social Science and Medicine* 2009, 68(4): 774–780.

19 Martin EK, Taft CT, Resick PA. A review of marital rape. *Aggression and Violent Behavior* 2007, 12(3): 329–347.

20 Mein JK, Palmer CM, Shand MC, Templeton DJ, Parekh V, Mobbs M et al. Management of acute adult sexual assault. *Medical Journal of Australia* 2003, 178(5): 226–230.

21 Pesola GR, Westfal RE, Kuffner CA. Emergency department characteristics of male sexual assault. *Academic Emergency Medicine* 1999, 6(8): 792–798.

22 Regan L, Lovett J, Kelly L. *Forensic Nursing: An option for improving responses to reported rape and sexual assault.* London: Home Office, 2004.

23 Taskforce on the Health Aspects of Violence Against Women and Children Improving Safety. *Responding to Violence Against Women and Children – the role of the NHS.* Available from: http://www.fflm.ac.uk/wp-content/uploads/documentstore/1268669895.pdf, 2010.

1. Introduction

- Everyone has the right to live their life free from harm. Safeguarding adults at risk from significant harm is reliant on effective joint working and communication between agencies and professionals.
- This guidance is for the management of people aged 18 years and over; for those under 18 years, refer to **Safeguarding Children**.
- Ambulance clinicians are often the first professionals to make contact with an adult at risk and may identify initial concerns regarding abuse. The role of the ambulance service is not to investigate suspicions but to ensure that any suspicion is passed, with the consent of the adult (where no consent, state why), to the appropriate agency (e.g. social care or the police) in line with locally agreed procedures.
- Ambulance clinicians need to be aware of local policies and procedures relating to the abuse of vulnerable adults. The aim of this guideline is to assist ambulance clinicians to recognise and report cases (with consent) of suspected abuse of adults at risk.
- The principles of adult protection differ from those of child protection in that adults have the right to take risks and may choose to live at risk if they have the capacity to make such a decision (refer to **Mental Capacity Act 2005**).
- Anyone can be a victim of abuse.
- An abuser may be anyone, including a friend or family member, carer or professional involved in delivering care to the adult.

The introduction of the Care Act 2014[1] provides a statutory framework to safeguard adults at risk of abuse or neglect. The Care Act puts the wishes and experience of the adult at the centre of safeguarding and is a move away from the previous process-led culture.

2. Making Safeguarding Personal

2.1 'No decision about me without me'[2]

Under the Care Act 2014 there has been a move away from process-led practice to a person-centred approach that works in partnership with the adult to achieve the outcomes that they need to make them feel safe. In the words of Lord Justice Munby, 'What good is it making someone safer if it merely makes them miserable?'[3]

2.2 Six key principles

There are six key principles underpinning the Care Act guidance that put the patient at the heart of decision making:

1. **Empowerment** 'I am asked what I want as the outcome from the safeguarding process, and this directly informs what happens.'
2. **Prevention** 'I receive clear and simple information about what abuse is, how to recognise the signs and what I can do to seek help.'
3. **Proportionality** 'I am sure that the professionals will work in my interest, as I see them, and they will only get involved, as much as needed.'
4. **Protection** 'I get help and support to report abuse and neglect. I get help so that I am able to take part in the safeguarding process to the extent that I want.'
5. **Partnership** 'I know that staff treat any personal and sensitive information in confidence, only sharing what is helpful and necessary. I am confident that professionals will work together and with me to get the best result for me.'
6. **Accountability** 'I understand the role of everyone involved in my life and so do they.'

The aim of safeguarding is to:

- stop abuse or neglect wherever possible
- prevent harm and reduce the risk of abuse or neglect to adults with care and support needs
- safeguard adults in a way that supports them in making choices and having control about how they want to live
- promote an approach that concentrates on improving life for the adult concerned.

3. Definition of Adult at Risk

Not every adult will require safeguarding. To meet the criteria set out in the Care Act 2014 the adult must meet the following criteria:

- demonstrates a need for care and support (whether or not the local authority is meeting any of those needs) **and**
- is experiencing, or at risk of, abuse or neglect **and**
- as a result of those care and support needs, is unable to protect themselves from either the risk or the experience of abuse or neglect.

An adult's needs meet the eligibility criteria for care and support if:

1. the adult's needs arise from, or are related to, a physical or mental impairment or illness
2. as a result of the adult's needs, the adult is unable to achieve two or more of the outcomes
3. as a consequence there is, or is likely to be, a significant impact on the adult's well-being.

The specified outcomes are:

1. managing and maintaining nutrition
2. maintaining personal hygiene
3. managing toilet needs
4. being appropriately clothed
5. being able to make use of the adult's home safely
6. maintaining a habitable home environment
7. developing and maintaining family or other personal relationships
8. accessing and engaging in work, training, education or volunteering

9. making use of necessary facilities or services in the local community including public transport, and recreational facilities or services
10. carrying out any caring responsibilities the adult has for a child.

Table 1.9 – TYPES AND SIGNS OF ABUSE

TYPES OF ABUSE	SIGNS OF ABUSE
• **Physical**: hitting, slapping, misuse of medication, restraint.	• Multiple bruising. • Fractures. • Burns. • Bed sores. • Fear. • Depression. • Unexplained weight loss. • Assault (can be intentional or reckless).
• **Domestic violence**: incidents, or pattern of incidents, of controlling, coercive or threatening behaviour, violence or abuse by someone who is, or has been, an intimate partner or family member, regardless of gender or sexuality.	Includes: psychological, physical, sexual, financial, emotional abuse; so-called 'honour' based violence; female genital mutilation; forced marriage. Note: the age range extended down to 16 (for the purpose of the safeguarding adult arrangements, safeguarding children arrangements would be applied to a person under 18).
• **Sexual abuse**: rape, indecent exposure, subjection to pornography, not consented or pressured to consent.	• Loss of sleep. • Unexpected or unexplained change in behaviour. • Bruising. • Soreness around the genitals. • Torn, stained or bloody underwear. • Preoccupation with anything sexual. • Sexually transmitted diseases. • Pregnancy. • Rape – e.g. a male member of staff having sex with a mental health client (see Mental Health Act 1983). • Indecent assault.
• **Psychological abuse:** emotional abuse, threat of harm or abandonment, blaming, humiliation, isolation.	• Fear. • Depression. • Confusion. • Loss of sleep. • Unexpected or unexplained change in behaviour. • Deprivation of liberty could be false imprisonment. • Aggressive shouting causing fear of violence in a public place may be an offence against the Public Order Act 1986, or harassment under the Protection from Harassment Act 1997.
• **Financial or material abuse:** internet scamming, will issues, inheritance, financial transactions, theft.	• Unexplained withdrawals from the bank. • Unusual activity in bank accounts. • Unpaid bills. • Unexplained shortage of money. • Reluctance on the part of the person with responsibility for the funds to provide basic food and clothes etc. • Fraud, theft.

Table 1.9 – TYPES AND SIGNS OF ABUSE *continued*

TYPES OF ABUSE	SIGNS OF ABUSE
• **Modern slavery:** human trafficking, forced labour, domestic servitude, coerce, deceive and force individual into life of abuse.	Modern slavery is an international crime, it can include victims that have been brought from overseas, and vulnerable people in the UK. Slave masters and traffickers will deceive, coerce and force adults into a life of abuse, callous treatment and slavery.
• **Discriminatory abuse:** slurs, issues of race, gender, disability etc.	Abuse can be experienced as harassment, insults or similar actions due to race, religion, gender, gender identity, age, disability or sexual orientation.
• **Organisational abuse:** neglect or poor care within an institution or care setting. Neglect or poor professional practice as a result of policies and processes.	• Inflexible and non-negotiable systems and routines. • Lack of consideration of dietary requirements. • Name calling; inappropriate ways of addressing people. • Lack of adequate physical care – an unkempt appearance.
• **Neglect and acts of omission:** ignoring medical, emotional or physical care needs. Failure to provide access to appropriate health care.	• Malnutrition. • Untreated medical problems. • Bed sores. • Confusion. • Over-sedation. • Deprivation of meals may constitute 'wilful neglect'.
• **Self-neglect:** wide-ranging neglect for one's personal hygiene, health or surroundings and includes behaviour such as hoarding.	This includes various behaviours: disregarding one's personal hygiene, health or surroundings, resulting in a risk that impacts on the adult's wellbeing – this could consist of behaviours such as hoarding.
Incidents can be a one-off or multiple and may affect one person or more.	

4. Wellbeing

Ambulance clinicians often come across adults who have an unmet or increasing care need. Whilst these are unlikely to meet the threshold for safeguarding, raising an alert is still possible with the patient's consent. Please follow your local reporting procedures.

5. Consent

Adults at risk should, where possible, be given full information about any concerns for their safety to enable them to give informed consent to the ambulance service raising a safeguarding alert with the local authority or other appropriate agency. Where the adult does not have capacity (refer to **Mental Capacity Act 2005**), or having a discussion may increase the risk to the adult, ambulance clinicians can raise an alert in the patient's best interest.

If there is a risk to others (i.e. other residents in a care setting or an identified fire or public health risk), ambulance clinicians can share information without consent (refer to **Mental Capacity Act 2005**).

6. Mandatory reporting of Female Genital Mutilation (FGM)

From 31st October 2015 the FGM Act introduces a mandatory reporting duty which requires health and social care professionals as well as teachers to report known cases of FGM in those under 18 years of age to the police.

FGM is child abuse and the current procedure is set out below:

- **Children and vulnerable adults**: if any child (under 18) or vulnerable adult in your care has symptoms or signs of FGM, or if you have good reason to suspect they are at risk of FGM having considered their family history or other relevant factors, they **must** be referred using existing safeguarding procedures as with all instances of child abuse. This will involve referral to police and social care in the usual way.
- **Adults**: there is no requirement for automatic referral of adult women with FGM to adult services or the police. Ambulance clinicians should be aware that a disclosure may be the first time that a woman has discussed her FGM with anyone. Referral to police must not be introduced as an automatic response when identifying adult women with FGM, and each case must be individually assessed. Ambulance clinicians should seek to assist women by offering referral to community groups for support, clinical intervention or other services as appropriate, for example through an NHS FGM clinic. The wishes of the woman must be respected at all times. If she is pregnant, the welfare of the unborn child or others in her extended family must be considered at this point as they are potentially at risk, and action taken accordingly.
- In all cases where staff are unsure of their actions, they should seek the advice of the Trust Safeguarding Service.

7. Prevent

7.1 Introduction

- The NHS, including the ambulance service, has a statutory responsibility to comply and engage with *Prevent*.[a]
- This involves the formulation of policy and procedures, the training of staff and, importantly, having appropriate mechanisms in place to ensure that concerns are noted and shared.

The three key objectives of the national *Prevent* strategy are to:

1. Challenge the **ideology** that supports terrorism and those who promote it.
2. Prevent vulnerable **individuals** from being drawn into terrorism, and ensure that they are given appropriate advice and support.
3. Work with sectors and **institutions** where there are risks of radicalisation.

It remains clear that while the focus is an imminent threat from Al-Qaida or Islamic State (IS), it should be noted that radicalisation of vulnerable individuals can be undertaken by any extremist group. These forms of terrorism include (but are not limited to):

- far-right extremists, e.g. English Defence League
- Al-Qaida-influenced groups
- environmental extremists
- animal rights extremists.

7.2 Definitions

The following examples of vulnerability are included within 'Building Partnerships, Staying Safe' (DoH 2011).

Identity crisis Adolescents/vulnerable adults who are exploring issues of identity can feel both distant from their parents/family and cultural and religious heritage, and uncomfortable with their place in the society around them. Radicalisers can exploit this by providing a sense of purpose or feelings of belonging. Where this occurs, it can often manifest itself in a change in a person's behaviour, their circle of friends, and the ways in which they interact with others and spend their time.

Personal crisis This may, for example, include significant tensions within the family, which produce a sense of isolation in the vulnerable individual from the traditional certainties of family life.

Personal circumstances The experiences of migration, local tensions or events affecting families in countries of origin may contribute to alienation from UK values and a decision to cause harm to symbols of the community or state.

Unemployment or under-employment Individuals may perceive their aspirations for career and lifestyle to be undermined by limited achievements or employment prospects. This can translate into a generalised rejection of civic life and the adoption of violence as a symbolic act.

Criminality In some cases, a vulnerable individual may have been involved in a group that engages in criminal activity or, on occasion, a group that has links to organised crime, and be further drawn to engagement in terrorist-related activity.

An additional vulnerability is around young people moving from childhood into adulthood, and, in particular, those children known to children's services as they transition into adult services.

7.3 Duties/Responsibility

- Any member of staff identifying concerns that vulnerable people may be radicalised, should report to the safeguarding service, their *Prevent* lead or their line manager in the Trust.
- If the incident occurs outside of office hours, staff should contact police for advice.

8. Assessment and Management

- Identify an adult(s) at risk.
- Report concerns following local guidelines:
  - Ascertain the patient's wishes wherever possible.
  - Gain consent if it is safe and appropriate to do so.
  - Consider the use of the Mental Capacity Act (MCA) if needed.
- Ensure concerns are clearly and concisely documented and jargon free.

KEY POINTS

Safeguarding Adults at Risk

- **Stop abuse and neglect wherever possible.**
- **Respect the adults wishes wherever possible.**
- **Concerns of suspected abuse must be reported as soon as possible following trust policy and procedures.**
- **Ambulance clinicians must document fully the reasons for concern and any action taken.**
- **Documentation of consent or the reason it has not been obtained must be clearly recorded.**
- **Ambulance clinicians should not investigate concerns, but should identify and report appropriately.**

a Section 26 of the Counter-Terrorism and Security Act 2015 places a duty on certain bodies (including the NHS) in the exercise of their functions to have 'due regard to the need to prevent people from being drawn into terrorism'.

Further Reading

Further important information and evidence in support of this guideline can be found in the Bibliography.[4, 5, 6, 7, 8, 9, 10, 11]

Bibliography

1 Department of Health. *Care Act 2014*. London: HMSO, 2014. Available from: http://www.legislation.gov.uk/ukpga/2014/23/pdfs/ukpga_20140023_en.pdf.

2 Department of Health. *Liberating the NHS: No decision about me without me*. London: HMSO, 2012.

3 Munby J. *Safeguarding Adults: Advice and guidance to directors of adult social services*, March 2013. Available from: https://www.adass.org.uk/safeguarding-adults/public-content/advice-and-guidance-to-directors-of-adults-social-services-march-2013.

4 Office of the Public Guardian. *Office of the Public Guardian and Local Authorities: A protocol for working together to safeguard vulnerable adults*. London: HMSO, 2008.

5 Office of the Public Guardian. *Safeguarding Policy: Protecting vulnerable adults*. Available from: https://www.gov.uk/government/publications/safeguarding-policy-protecting-vulnerable-adults, 2015.

6 Lord Chancellor's Department. *Who Decides? Making decisions on behalf of mentally incapacitated adults*. London: HMSO, 1997.

7 Department of Health. *Clinical Governance and Adult Safeguarding: An integrated process*. London: HMSO, 2010. Available from: http://webarchive.nationalarchives.gov.uk/20130107105354/http:/www.dh.gov.uk/en/Publicationsandstatistics/Publications/PublicationsPolicyAndGuidance/DH_112361.

8 Department of Health. *Safeguarding Adults: Report on the consultation on the review of No Secrets*. London: HMSO, 2009. Available from: http://webarchive.nationalarchives.gov.uk/20130107105354/http:/www.dh.gov.uk/prod_consum_dh/groups/dh_digitalassets/documents/digitalasset/dh_102981.pdf.

9 Department of Health. *No Secrets: Guidance on developing and implementing multi-agency policies and procedures to protect vulnerable adults from abuse*. London: HMSO, 2000. Available from: https://www.gov.uk/government/uploads/system/uploads/attachment_data/file/194272/No_secrets__guidance_on_developing_and_implementing_multi-agency_policies_and_procedures_to_protect_vulnerable_adults_from_abuse.pdf.

10 Department of Health. *Safeguarding Adults: The role of health services*. London: HMSO, 2011. Available from: http://www.dh.gov.uk/en/Publicationsandstatistics/Publications/PublicationsPolicyAndGuidance/DH_124882.

11 Biarent D, Bingham R, Eich C, López-Herce J, Maconochie I, Rodriguez-Nunez A, et al. European Resuscitation Council Guidelines for Resuscitation 2010 Section 6: Paediatric life support. *Resuscitation* 2010, 81(10): 1364–88.

Domestic Abuse

1. Introduction

- Domestic abuse includes any threatening behaviour, violence or abuse between adults, young people, intimate partners, family members or extended family members, regardless of gender or sexuality.
- Domestic abuse is extremely distressing; managing such cases demands sensitive, non-judgemental medical and emotional care and an awareness of the forensic requirements.
- In December 2015 a new criminal offence of domestic abuse, 'coercive and controlling behaviour', came into force, making all domestic abuse a reportable crime.
- Patients are likely to be very distressed about the events surrounding domestic abuse. They may not want to involve anybody else, and may not consent to disclosure of information to other parties such as the police. Do not judge, or give the appearance of judging the patient. Be kind and considerate, and allow the patient space, and as much choice about options for their treatment as possible.
- Alcohol and drugs may also be involved.
- **Further care** – it is important to encourage all victims of domestic abuse to seek medical help, and inform the police. Both will be able to provide physical, medical and emotional support.
- In cases of domestic abuse in vulnerable adults and children refer to **Safeguarding Adults at Risk** and **Safeguarding Children**.

2. Incidence

- Domestic abuse affects approximately 28% of women and 13% of men. 52% of child protection cases involve domestic abuse. Each week, 2–3 women or men are killed by their current or former partner. Disabled women are raped twice as often as non-disabled women, and 50% have experienced domestic abuse. Of teenagers, 1 in 5 have been physically abused by their boyfriend or girlfriend.
- The average length of time someone is in an abusive relationship before leaving is 8 years.
- The number of women convicted of perpetrating domestic abuse has more than quadrupled in the past ten years.
- A third of all domestic abuse starts or escalates during pregnancy.
- In 90% of domestic abuse cases, children are in the same or the next room.

3. Severity and Outcome

- The severity of the abuse can vary from verbal abuse to sustaining life-threatening injuries or death. The outcome of the abuse can lead to long-term psychological and physical effects.

4. Pathophysiology

- Domestic abuse is an incident or pattern of incidents of controlling, coercive or threatening behaviour, violence or abuse to those aged 16 or over. These types of abuse include: psychological, physical, sexual, financial and emotional.
- Domestic abuse also includes 'honour' based violence, forced marriage and female genital mutilation (for FGM also refer to **Safeguarding Adults at Risk** and **Safeguarding Children**).

5. Assessment and Management

For the assessment and management of domestic abuse refer to Table 1.10.

Further Reading

Other useful resources include:

https://www.gov.uk/government/uploads/system/uploads/attachment_data/file/211018/9576-TSO-Health_Visiting_Domestic_Violence_A3_Posters_WEB.pdf.

Mankind Initiative: information and support for male victims of domestic abuse or violence – http://.mankind.org.uk/.

Broken Rainbow: Support for lesbians, gay men, bisexuals and transgender people suffering domestic violence throughout UK – 0300 999 5428, www.broken-rainbow.org.uk.

Refuge – National helpline: 0808 2000 247, email: helpline@refuge.org.uk.

Every Child Matters – www.everychildmatters.gov.uk/resourses-and-practice/IG00042/.

FCO – www.fco.gov.uk/en/travel-and-living-abroad/when-things-go-wrong/forced-marriage.

KEY POINTS

Domestic Abuse

- **If staff suspect a crime has been committed resulting in harm to the patient, the police must be called.**
- **Listen closely to the patient for disclosure, and document this on the patient record.**
- **If possible, take the patient away from the scene.**
- **Treatment should avoid disturbing evidence where possible.**
- **Take into account any information that is disclosed by children.**
- **Never leave a child with an alleged perpetrator if transporting the patient to hospital.**
- **Accommodate patient wishes where possible.**

Table 1.10 – ASSESSMENT and MANAGEMENT of:

Domestic Abuse

ASSESSMENT	MANAGEMENT
• Assess **ABCD**	If any **TIME CRITICAL** features present major **ABCD** problems: • start correcting **A** and **B** problems • undertake a **TIME CRITICAL** transfer to nearest receiving hospital • continue patient management en-route • provide an alert/information call.
• Assess	• Limit questions to those identifying the need for medical treatment, but allow the patient to talk and document what is said. **NB** It is not appropriate to probe for details of the abuse and could affect the outcome of criminal investigations. • Manage according to condition: – Acute injury – refer to **Trauma Emergencies Overview (Adults)** and **Trauma Emergencies Overview (Children)**. – Acute illness – refer to **Medical Emergencies in Adults – Overview** and **Medical Emergencies in Children – Overview**. **Indicators in the patient:** • Seem afraid or anxious to please their partner. • Agreeing with everything their partner says. • Checking everything first with their partner. • Talk about their partner's temper or jealousy. • Have frequent injuries, often described as 'accidents'. • Dress in clothing designed to hide bruises or scars. • Restricted from seeing family and friends. • Have limited access to money, credit cards etc. • Have low self-esteem. • Depressed, anxious or have suicidal thoughts/action.
• Approach	• Use a sensitive and respectful manner. • Focus on your care but be mindful of your surroundings and the information that is being passed to you, both verbal and non-verbal. • If possible, ensure privacy. • Consider cultural/religious issues. • Where possible accommodate the patient's requests. • Where possible avoid disturbing the scene. • Where possible try to get the patient on their own so that they can be open and honest with you.
• Criminal offence/ forensic examination	• Many forms of domestic violence are criminal offences and staff must report all serious crimes to the police, particularly if: – the patient has suffered from abuse involving a weapon/strangulation/ smothering or has sustained a significant injury – the patient is in fear of the perpetrator – the abuse is escalating – the alleged perpetrator is stalking the patient – there is an immediate risk to the patient or any children in the household. • Forensic examination may be required if a physical assault has taken place. Domestic abuse is a criminal offence and the police must be informed immediately (refer to **Sexual Assault**).

Domestic Abuse *continued*	
• Transfer[a]	• Encourage all patients to attend further care and to inform the police. • Transfer patients to further care according to local guidelines. • Where a patient is competent and refuses hospital treatment, advise them to seek further medical attention. • If safe to do so, provide information on where the patient may seek further support in relation to domestic abuse. • If children are involved, a safeguarding notification of concern must be made using local ambulance procedures. • If the patient is transported to hospital, do not leave children in the care of the alleged perpetrator. • Always try to speak to the patient alone. • Remember consent is not always required from the patient to report the crime, particularly if the patient remains at risk. • Share concerns at the receiving hospital.
• Documentation	• Complete the clinical record in great detail contemporaneously and document: – only facts, not personal opinion – what the patient says – clinical findings with relevant timings – the ambulance identification number. • A police statement may be required later. • Consideration must be given with regard to leaving any documentation (such as a clinical record) with a victim, which could potentially increase the risk of harm.

Bibliography

1 Department of Health. *Improving Services for Women and Child Victims of Violence: The Department of Health Action Plan*. Available from: http://www.dh.gov.uk/prod_consum_dh/groups/dh_digitalassets/@dh/@en/@ps/documents/digitalasset/dh_122094.pdf, 2010.

2 Taskforce on the Health Aspects of Violence Against Women and Children Improving Safety. *Responding to Violence Against Women and Children – the role of the NHS*. Available from: http://www.fflm.ac.uk/wp-content/uploads/documentstore/1268669895.pdf, 2010.

3 Department of Health. *Guidance for Health Professionals on Domestic Violence*. Available from: https://www.gov.uk/government/publications/guidance-for-health-professionals-on-domestic-violence, 2013.

4 National Institute for Health and Clinical Excellence. *Domestic Violence and Abuse: Multi-agency working* (PH50). London: NICE, 2014. Available from: https://www.nice.org.uk/guidance/ph50/chapter/introduction.

5 National Institute for Health and Clinical Excellence. *Domestic Violence and Abuse Overview Pathways*. Available from: http://pathways.nice.org.uk/pathways/domestic-violence-and-abuse, 2014.

6 British Crime Survey (2008–2009). Available from: www.crimereduction.homeoffice.gov.uk/dv/dv01.htm.

7 Department of Health. *Responding to Domestic Abuse: A handbook for professionals*. London: HMSO, 2005.

8 Department of Health. *Improving Safety, Reducing Harm – A practical toolkit for front-line practitioners*. London: HMSO, 2009.

9 Department of Health. *Multi–Agency Practice Guidelines – Handling cases of forced marriage*. London: HMSO, 2009.

10 Edelson JL. The overlap between child maltreatment and women battering. *Violence Against Women* 1999, 5(2): 134–154.

11 Home Office. *Female Genital Mutilation Act 2003*. London: HMSO, 2003. Available from: http://www.legislation.gov.uk/ukpga/2003/31/pdfs/ukpga_20030031_en.pdf.

12 Home Office, *Domestic Violence: A National Report*. Available from: http://webarchive.nationalarchives.gov.uk/+/http:/www.crimereduction.homeoffice.gov.uk/domesticviolence/domesticviolence51.pdf, 2004.

13 McAfee RE. *Domestic Abuse as a Woman's Health Issue*. Chicago: Elservier Science Inc, 2001.

14 McWilliams M, McKiernan S. *Bringing It Out in the Open*. Belfast: HMSO, 1999.

15 Department of Health. *National Service Framework for Children, Young People and Maternity Services*. London: HMSO, 2004.

a In some areas arrangements exist for patients to be examined and interviewed in police or other facilities.

3

Medical

Altered Level of Consciousness

1. Introduction

- Patients presenting in pre-hospital care with an altered level of consciousness (ALoC) provide a major challenge.
- In patients with ALoC it is important to undertake a rapid assessment for **TIME CRITICAL** conditions.
- It is important to understand, where possible, the cause of altered consciousness which can range from diabetic collapse, to factitious illness (refer to Table 3.1 and Table 3.2).
- The patient history may provide valuable insight into the cause of the current condition. Consider the following in formulating your diagnosis; ask relatives or bystanders:
  - is there any history of recent illness or pre-existing chronic illness (e.g. diabetes, steroid-dependent adrenal insufficiency or epilepsy)?
  - any past history of mental health problems?
  - any preceding symptoms such as headache, fits, confusion?
  - any history of trauma?

NOTE: Remember, an acute condition may be an exacerbation of a chronic condition or a 'new' illness superimposed on top of a pre-existing problem, such as adrenal crisis triggered by infective gastroenteritis.

However, often there is little available information – in these circumstances the scene may provide clues to assist in formulating a diagnosis:

- Environmental factors (e.g. extreme cold, possible carbon monoxide sources)?
- Evidence of tablets, ampoules, pill boxes, syringes, including domiciliary oxygen (O_2), or administration devices (e.g. nebuliser machines)?
- Evidence of alcohol, or medication abuse?

Table 3.1 – RED FLAG CONDITIONS

Condition
Adrenal insufficiency (risk of adrenal crisis with hypoglycaemia) (refer to **Hydrocortisone**).
Epilepsy (refer to **Convulsions (Adult)** and **Convulsions (Child)**).
Head injury (refer to **Head Injury**).
Hyperglycaemia (refer to **Glycaemic Emergencies (Adults)** and **Glycaemic Emergencies (Children)**).
Hypoglycaemia (refer to **Glycaemic Emergencies (Adults)** and **Glycaemic Emergencies (Children)**).
Overdose (refer to **Overdose and Poisoning (Adults)** and **Overdose and Poisoning (Child)**).
Stroke/TIA (refer to **Stroke/TIA**).
Subarachnoid haemorrhage (refer to **Headache**).

Table 3.2 – SOME CONDITIONS THAT MAY RESULT IN DLoC (Decreased level of consciousness)

Alterations in pO_2 (hypoxia) and/or pCO_2 (hyper/hypocapnia)
Inadequate airway.
Inadequate ventilation or depressed respiratory drive.
Persistent hyperventilation.
Inadequate perfusion
Cardiac arrhythmias.
Distributive shock.
Hypovolaemia.
Neurogenic shock.
Raised intracranial pressure.
Altered metabolic states
Hypoglycaemia and hyperglycaemia.
Intoxication or poisoning
Alcohol intoxication.
Carbon monoxide poisoning.
Drug overdose.
Medical conditions
Adrenal crisis.
Epilepsy.
Hypo/hyperthermia.
Meningitis.
Stroke.
Subarachnoid haemorrhage.
Head injury

This guideline contains guidance for managing patients with transient loss of consciousness (section 1) and coma (section 2).

2. SECTION 1 – Transient Loss of Consciousness (TLoC)

- Transient loss of consciousness (TLoC) may be defined as spontaneous loss of consciousness with complete recovery i.e. full recovery of consciousness without any residual neurological deficit.
- An episode of TLoC is often described as a 'blackout' or a 'collapse'. There are various causes of TLoC, including:
  - cardiovascular disorders (which are the most common)
  - neurological conditions such as epilepsy, and psychogenic attacks.
- The diagnosis of the underlying cause of TLoC is often inaccurate and delayed.

2.1 Assessment and Management

For the assessment and management of transient loss of consciousness refer to Table 3.3.

Table 3.3 – ASSESSMENT and MANAGEMENT of:

Transient Loss of Consciousness	
ASSESSMENT (ADULTS)	**MANAGEMENT (ADULTS)**
• Assess ABCD	• If any of the following **TIME CRITICAL** features are present: – major **ABCD** problems – unexpected OR persistent loss of consciousness, then: • Start correcting any **ABCD** problems. • Undertake a **TIME CRITICAL** transfer to nearest appropriate receiving hospital. • Continue patient management en-route. • Provide an alert/information call.
• Assess for **TIME CRITICAL** features	
• Ascertain from the patient or witnesses what happened before, during and after the event	**Record details about:** • Circumstances of the event. • The patient's posture immediately before loss of consciousness. • Prodromal symptoms (such as sweating or feeling warm/hot). • Appearance (whether eyes were open or shut) and colour of the patient during the event. • Presence or absence of movement during the event (limb-jerking and its duration). • Any tongue-biting (record whether the side or the tip of the tongue was bitten). • Injury occurring during the event (record site and severity). • Duration of the event (onset to regaining consciousness). • Presence or absence of confusion during the recovery period. • Weakness down one side during the recovery period.
• If TLoC is confirmed:	Assess and record: • Details of any previous TLoC, including number and frequency. • The patient medical history and any family history of cardiac disease (personal history of heart disease or family history of sudden cardiac death). • Current medication that may have contributed to TLoC (diuretics). • Routine observations (pulse rate, respiratory rate and temperature) – repeat if clinically indicated. • Lying and standing blood pressure if clinically appropriate. • Other cardiovascular and neurological signs.
• Assess for concomitant injuries	• Refer to relevant guideline.
• Assess heart rhythm	• Undertake a 12-lead ECG using automated interpretation (refer to local guidelines).
• If an underlying cause is suspected	• Undertake relevant examinations and investigations, for example, check blood glucose levels if hypoglycaemia is suspected – refer to relevant guideline.

Transient Loss of Consciousness *continued*	
• Assess for uncomplicated faint and situational syncope	Diagnose uncomplicated faint (uncomplicated vasovagal syncope) on the basis of the initial assessment when: • There are no features that suggest an alternative diagnosis (NOTE: that brief seizure activity can occur during uncomplicated faints and is not necessarily diagnostic of epilepsy). **AND** • There are features suggestive of uncomplicated faint (the 3 'P's) such as: – **posture** – prolonged standing, or similar episodes that have been prevented by lying down – **provoking** factors (such as pain or a medical procedure) – **prodromal** symptoms (such as sweating or feeling warm/hot before TLoC). Diagnose situational syncope on the basis of the initial assessment when: • There are no features from the initial assessment that suggest an alternative diagnosis. **AND** • Syncope is clearly and consistently provoked by straining during micturition (usually while standing) or by coughing or swallowing.
• Care pathway	• Only patients with a GCS 15, with normal blood sugar and responsible adult supervision present may be left at scene, for example if a diagnosis of uncomplicated faint or situational syncope is made, and there is nothing in the initial assessment to raise clinical or social concern. • **Advise the patient to take a copy of the clinical record and the ECG record to their GP and follow local protocols to safely hand over clinical responsibility.**

3. SECTION 2 – Coma

3.1 Introduction

- Coma is defined as U on the AVPU scale or a Glasgow Coma Score (GCS) (refer to Appendix) of 8 or less; however, any patient presenting with a decreased level of consciousness (GCS<15) mandates further assessment and, possibly, treatment.
- There are a number of causes of coma; refer to Tables 3.1 and 3.2.

3.2 Assessment and Management

For the assessment and management of coma refer to Table 3.4.

Table 3.4 – ASSESSMENT and MANAGEMENT of:

Coma (GCS <8)	
ASSESSMENT (ADULTS)	**MANAGEMENT (ADULTS)** NOTE: TAKE A DEFRIBILLATOR TO THE INCIDENT – many calls to unconscious patients are cardiac arrests.
• Assess **ABCD**	• Start correcting any **ABCD** problems. • Undertake a **TIME CRITICAL** transfer to the nearest appropriate receiving hospital. • Continue patient management en-route. • Provide an alert/information call.
• Oxygen	• Administer high levels of supplementary oxygen and aim for a target saturation within the range of 94–98% (refer to **Oxygen**).
• Assess for hypoxia	• Apply pulse oximetry. • Obtain IV access if appropriate.
• Assess heart rhythm for arrhythmias	• Undertake a 12-lead ECG.

Coma (GCS <8) *continued*	
• Assess level of consciousness	• Assess using the AVPU scale or Glasgow Coma Scale (GCS) (refer to Appendix): A – Alert V – Response to voice P – Responds to painful stimulus U – Unresponsive. • Assess and note pupil size, equality and response to light. • Check for purposeful movement in all four limbs and note sensory function.
• Assess blood glucose level	• If hypoglycaemic (<4.0 mmol/l) or suspected, refer to **Glycaemic Emergencies (Adult)** and **Glycaemic Emergencies (Children)**.
• Blood pressure	• Measure blood pressure.
• Assess for significant injury especially to the head	• If trauma detected or suspected, immobilise spine and refer to **Spinal Injury and Spinal Cord Injury**.
• Assess for other causes	• Breath for ketones, alcohol and solvents. • Evidence of needle tracks/marks. • MedicAlert® type jewellery (bracelets or necklets) which detail the patient's primary health risk (e.g. diabetes, anaphylaxis, Addison's disease etc) – also list a 24-hour telephone number to obtain a more detailed patient history. • Warning stickers, often placed by the front door or the telephone, directing the health professional to a source of detailed information (one current scheme involves storing the patient details in a container in the fridge, as this is relatively easy to find in the house). • Patient-held warning cards, for example, those taking monoamine oxidase inhibitor (MAOI) medication. **For management refer to relevant guideline(s).**
• Assess for respiratory depression	• In cases of severe respiratory depressions, refer to **Airway and Breathing Management**. • If the level of consciousness deteriorates or respiratory depression develops in cases where an overdose with opiate-type drugs may be a possibility, consider naloxone (refer to **Naloxone**). • In a patient with fixed pinpoint pupils suspect opiate use/overdose. NOTE: any patient with a decreased level of consciousness may have a compromised airway.
• Re-assess ABCD	• Document any changes/note trends in: – GCS – altered neurological function – base line observations.

KEY POINTS

Decreased Level of Consciousness

- **Maintain patent airway.**
- **Support ventilation if required.**
- **Address treatable causes.**
- **History – obtain as much information as possible.**
- **Consider an alert/information call.**

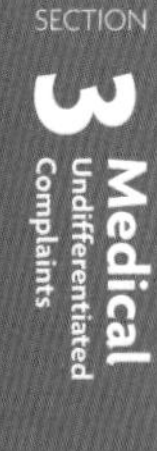

Appendix

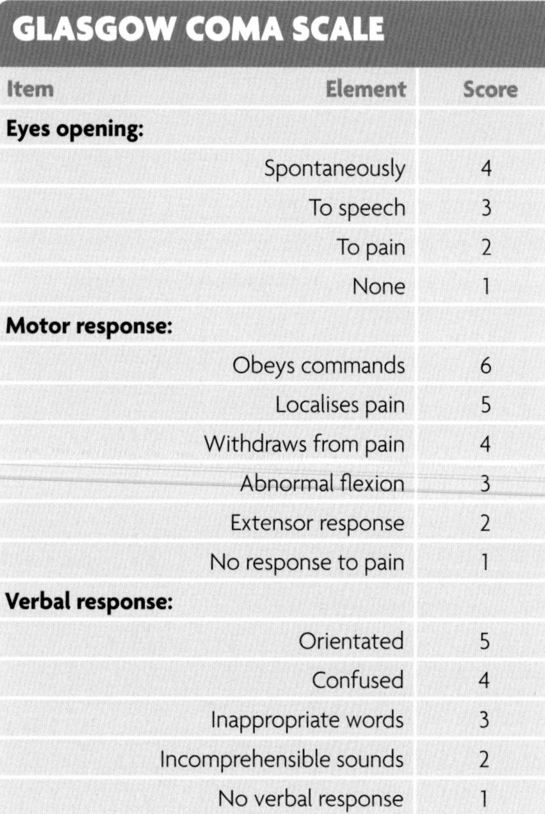

GLASGOW COMA SCALE

Item	Element	Score
Eyes opening:		
	Spontaneously	4
	To speech	3
	To pain	2
	None	1
Motor response:		
	Obeys commands	6
	Localises pain	5
	Withdraws from pain	4
	Abnormal flexion	3
	Extensor response	2
	No response to pain	1
Verbal response:		
	Orientated	5
	Confused	4
	Inappropriate words	3
	Incomprehensible sounds	2
	No verbal response	1

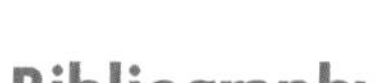

Bibliography

1 National Collaborating Centre for Acute Care. *Head Injury: Triage, assessment, investigation and early management of head injury in infants, children and adults* (CG56). London: National Collaborating Centre for Acute Care at The Royal College of Surgeons of England, 2007. Available from: https://www.nice.org.uk/guidance/cg176.

2 National Institute for Health and Clinical Excellence. *Stroke: The diagnosis and initial management of acute stroke and transient ischaemic attack* (CG68). London: NICE, 2008.

3 National Institute for Health and Clinical Excellence. *The Epilepsies: The diagnosis and management of the epilepsies in adults and children in primary and secondary care* (CG137). London: NICE, 2012. Available from: https://nice.org.uk/guidance/CG137.

4 National Institute for Health and Clinical Excellence. *Transient Loss of Consciousness in Adults and Young People* (CG109). London: NICE, 2012. Available from: https://www.nice.org.uk/guidance/qs71.

5 Task Force for the Diagnosis and Management of Syncope, European Society of Cardiology, European Heart Rhythm Association, Heart Failure Association, Heart Rhythm Society, Moya A, Sutton R, Ammirati F, Blanc JJ, Brignole M, Dahm JB, et al. Guidelines for the diagnosis and management of syncope (version 2009). *European Heart Journal* 2009, 30(21): 2631–71.

1. Introduction

Although the care of a wide range of medical conditions will be quite specific to the presenting condition, there are general principles of care that apply to most medical cases, regardless of underlying condition(s).

2. Patient Assessment

In order to gather as much relevant information as possible, without delaying care, the accepted format of history taking is as follows:

- Presenting complaint – why the patient or carer called for help at this time.
- The history of presenting complaint – details of when the problem started, exacerbating factors and previous similar episodes.
- Direct questioning about associated symptoms, by system. Ask about all appropriate systems.
- Past medical history, including current medication.
- Family history.
- Social history.

Combined with a good physical examination (primary and secondary survey), this format of history taking should ensure that you correctly identify those patients who are time critical, urgent or routine. The history taken must be fully documented. In many cases, a well-taken history will point to the diagnosis.

The presence of 'MedicAlert®' type jewellery (bracelets or necklets) can provide information on the patient's pre-existing health risk that may be relevant to the current medical emergency.

1. A primary survey should be undertaken for **ALL** patients as this will rapidly identify patients with actual or potential **TIME CRITICAL** conditions.
2. A secondary survey is a more thorough 'head-to-toe' assessment of the patient. It should be undertaken following completion of the primary survey, where time permits. The secondary survey will usually be undertaken during transfer to further care; however, in some patients with time critical conditions, it may not be possible to undertake the secondary survey before arrival at further care.

2.1 Primary Survey

- The primary survey should take 60–90 seconds for assessment and follow **ABCD** approach (Table 3.6). Document the vital signs and the time the observations were taken.
- Assessment and management should proceed in a 'stepwise' manner and abnormalities should be managed as they are encountered, that is do not move onto breathing and circulation until the airway is managed (refer to **Airway and Breathing Management**). Every time an intervention has been carried out, re-assess the patient.
- If any of the features/conditions listed in Table 3.5 are identified during the primary survey or immediately uncorrectable ABCD problems, then the patient should be considered **TIME CRITICAL. CORRECT A AND B PROBLEMS ON SCENE, THEN UNDERTAKE A TIME CRITICAL** transfer **TO NEAREST SUITABLE RECEIVING HOSPITAL.**
- If airway and breathing cannot be corrected, or haemorrhage cannot be controlled, evacuate immediately, continuing resuscitation as appropriate en-route.
- Provide an alert/information call.
- Continue patient assessment and management en-route.

Table 3.5 – TIME CRITICAL FEATURES/ CONDITIONS

- **Adrenal crisis (including Addisonian crisis)** – is a life-threatening condition resulting from adrenal insufficiency – refer to **Hydrocortisone**.
- **Airway impairment.**
- **Anaphylaxis** – is a life-threatening condition resulting from an immune response to an allergen – refer to **Allergic Reactions including Anaphylaxis**.
- Any patient with **GCS <15** – check the airway and blood glucose levels in all patients with a decreased GCS.
- **Cardiac chest pain.**
- **Cardiogenic shock.**
- **Sepsis** – is a life-threatening condition resulting from infection. Suspect sepsis in anyone that presents with fever/feeling unwell, and NEWS greater than or equal to 5, and/or looks unwell with a history of infection – refer to **Intravascular Fluid Therapy**.
- **Failing ventilation.**
- **Severe breathlessness** – unable to complete a sentence.
- **Severe haemorrhage** – refer to **Trauma Emergencies Overview** and gastrointestinal bleeding.
- **Severe hypotension** – due to bradycardia or extreme tachycardia. For hypovolaemic hypotension with adrenal crisis, give parenteral hydrocortisone prior to transportation.
- **Status epilepticus** – is a life-threatening condition defined as a convulsion lasting >30 minutes – refer to **Convulsion**.

NB This list is not inclusive; patients with other signs may also be time critical; this is where the clinical judgement of the paramedic is important.

Table 3.6 – ASSESSMENT and MANAGEMENT of:

Medical Emergencies

STAGE	ASSESSMENT	MANAGEMENT
	● All stages should be considered but some may be omitted if not considered appropriate and only if waveform capnography is available.	At each stage consider the need for: ● **TIME CRITICAL** transfer to further care. ● Early senior clinical support.
A	**AIRWAY** – assess the airway (refer to Airway and Breathing Management). **Look for** obvious obstructions, e.g. teeth/dentures, foreign bodies, vomit, blood. **Listen for** noisy airflow, e.g. snoring, gurgling or no airflow. **Feel for** air movement.	Correct any airway problems immediately by: ● Positioning – head tilt, chin lift, jaw thrust. ● Suction (if available and appropriate). ● Oropharyngeal airway. ● Nasopharyngeal airway. ● Laryngeal mask airway (if appropriate). ● Endotracheal intubation (if appropriate and only if waveform capnography is available). ● Needle cricothyroidotomy.
B	**BREATHING** – expose the chest and assess (refer to Airway and Breathing Management). **Look for:** ● Respiratory rate (<10 or >30). ● Respiratory depth. ● Breaths per minute. ● Adequacy and depth of chest movements. ● Symmetry of chest movement. ● Equality of air entry. ● Effectiveness of ventilation. ● Cyanosis or pallor peripherally and centrally. ● Position of trachea in suprasternal notch. **Feel for:** ● Any instability of chest wall and note any areas of tenderness and note depth and equality of chest movement. **Note any:** ● Wheezing, noisy respiration on inspiration or expiration. ● Stridor (higher pitched noise on inspiration), suggestive of upper respiratory obstruction. **Listen for:** ● Altered breathing patterns with a stethoscope – ask the patient to take deep breaths in and out briskly through their mouth if possible – listen on both sides of the chest: – above the nipples in the mid-clavicular line – laterally in the mid-axillary line – below the shoulder blade (front and back). ● Auscultate to assess air entry and compare sides. ● Wheezing on expiration. ● Crepitations at the rear of the chest (crackles, heard low down in the lung fields at the rear – may indicate fluid in the lung in heart failure). ● Additional crackles and wheeze on inspiration may be associated with inhalation of blood or vomit. **Percuss for:** ● Dullness or hyperresonance.	● Correct any breathing problems immediately. ● If breathing is absent refer to appropriate resuscitation guidelines. If the breathing is inadequate refer to Airway and Breathing Management. ● Treat underlying cause of unilateral chest movement if tension pneumothorax. ● Administer supplemental oxygen if the patient is hypoxaemic – aim for target saturation (SpO_2) within the range of 94–98% except for patients with COPD or other risk factors for hypercapnia (refer to Oxygen). ● In patients with a decreased level of consciousness (Glasgow Coma Scale (GCS) <15) administer the initial supplemental oxygen dose until the vital signs are normal, then reduce the oxygen dose and aim for a target saturation (SpO_2) within the range of 94–98%. ● In patients with sickle cell crisis administer supplemental oxygen via an appropriate mask/nasal cannula until a reliable SpO_2 measurement is available; then adjust the oxygen flow to aim for target saturation within the range of 94–98%. Consider assisted ventilation at a rate of 12–20 respirations per minute if any of the following are present: ● Oxygen saturation (SpO_2) <90% on levels of supplemental oxygen. ● Respiratory rate <10 or >30 bpm. ● Inadequate chest expansion. **NB Restraint (positional) asphyxia** – If the patient is required to be physically restrained (e.g. by police officers) in order to prevent them injuring themselves or others, or for the purpose of being detained under the Mental Health Act, then it is paramount that the method of restraint allows both for a patent airway and adequate respiratory volume. **Under these circumstances it is essential to ensure that the patient's airway and breathing are adequate at all times.**

Medical Emergencies *continued*

<table>
<tr><th>STAGE</th><th>ASSESSMENT</th><th>MANAGEMENT</th></tr>
<tr><td>C</td><td>
<ul><li>Assess for evidence of external haemorrhage (e.g. epistaxis, haemoptysis, haematemesis, melaena).</li></ul>
<ul><li>Assess skin colour and temperature.</li>
<li>Palpate for a radial pulse – if present this implies adequate perfusion of vital organs, but this is highly variable. If absent feel for a carotid pulse. NB The estimation of blood pressure by pulse is inaccurate and unreliable; however, the presence of a radial suggests adequate perfusion of major organs. The presence of a femoral pulse suggests perfusion of the kidneys, while a carotid pulse and coherent mentation suggests adequate perfusion of the brain.</li>
<li>Assess pulse rate, volume and rhythm.</li>
<li>Check capillary refill time centrally (forehead or sternum – normal <2 seconds).</li></ul>
Consider hypovolaemic shock and be aware of its early signs:
<ul><li>Pallor.</li>
<li>Cool peripheries.</li>
<li>Anxiety, abnormal behaviour.</li>
<li>Increased respiratory rate.</li>
<li>Tachycardia.</li></ul>
Recognition of shock
Shock is difficult to diagnose. In certain groups of patients the signs of shock may appear late (e.g. patients with acute adrenal insufficiency (adrenal crisis), pregnant women, patients on medication such as beta-blockers, and the physically fit).
Blood loss of 750–1000 ml will produce little evidence of shock; blood loss of 1000–1500 ml is required before more classical signs of shock appear. NB This loss is from the circulation NOT necessarily visible externally.
</td><td>
<ul><li>Arrest external haemorrhage.</li>
<li>In cases of internal or uncontrolled haemorrhage undertake a TIME CRITICAL transfer to further care; provide an alert/information call.</li>
<li>Patients with acute adrenal insufficiency (adrenal crisis) and/or sepsis will usually benefit from early fluid therapy and an appropriate hospital alert/information call. Adrenal insufficiency patients with hypotension and hypovolaemia must be given IV fluids and injected hydrocortisone prior to transportation, to minimise the risk of circulatory collapse.</li>
<li>Adrenal crisis may also occur in undiagnosed adrenal patients and patients with pituitary deficiency (secondary adrenal insufficiency). Adrenal suppression may occur in patients who have been receiving either long-term inhaled steroids or opiates.</li>
<li>Hypoadrenal patients can look well for a while after steroid withdrawal and often score low on NEWS until hypocortisolaemia is advanced, at which point they may rapidly deteriorate into circulatory collapse or organ failure, with or without hypoglycaemia. This is particularly so in very young patients who are more likely to develop severe hypoglycaemia.</li></ul>
<ol><li>It is advisable to stabilise the patient with IV fluids AND injected hydrocortisone prior to transportation.</li>
<li>Patients may become profoundly hypotensive when sitting upright.</li>
<li>Where the patient cannot be transported flat on a stretcher (e.g. domestic stairs) they must not be moved until circulatory volume has been restored with IV fluids and they have received injected hydrocortisone.</li></ol>
Fluid therapy
<ul><li>If fluid replacement is indicated refer to Intravascular Fluid Therapy.</li>
<li>Rapid fluid replacement into the vascular compartment can overload the cardiovascular system particularly where there is pre-existing cardiovascular disease and in older people. Gradual rehydration over many hours rather than minutes is indicated. NB Monitor fluid replacement closely in these cases.</li></ul>
</td></tr>
</table>

Medical Emergencies *continued*

D	**DISABILITY (mini neurological examination)** Note the initial level of responsiveness on AVPU scale, and time of assessment. • **A** – Alert • **V** – Responds to voice • **P** – Responds to painful stimulus • **U** – Unresponsive	• Check blood glucose level to rule out hypo or hyperglycaemia as the cause – refer to **Glycaemic Emergencies**.
	• Assess and note pupil size, equality and response to light.	
	• Check for purposeful movement in all four limbs. • Check sensory function.	
	• Assess blood glucose levels in all patients with diabetes, impaired consciousness, convulsions, collapse or alcohol consumption, a history of Addison's disease or other forms of adrenal insufficiency.	

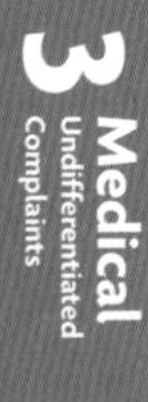

2.2 Secondary survey

- A secondary survey should only commence after the primary survey has been completed and an assessment of the patient's critical status has been made.
- The secondary survey is a more thorough 'head-to-toe' assessment of the patient including their past medical history (refer to Table 3.7). It is important to monitor the patient's vital signs during the survey.
- The secondary survey will usually be undertaken during transfer to hospital; however, in some patients with critical conditions, it may not be possible to undertake the secondary survey before arrival at further care.

Table 3.7 – SECONDARY SURVEY

Assessment

HEAD

- Re-assess airway, breathing, and circulation.
- Re-assess levels of consciousness (AVPU), pupil size and activity.
- Establish Glasgow Coma Scale (refer to Table 3.8).

CHEST

- Re-assess rate and depth of breathing.
- Re-listen for breath sounds in all lung fields, and record.
- Assess for pneumothorax – in small pneumothorax no clinical signs may be detected. A pneumothorax causes breathlessness, reduced air entry and chest movement on the affected side. If this is a tension pneumothorax, then the patient will have increasing respiratory distress, distended neck veins, and tracheal deviation (late sign) away from affected side may also be present.
- Assess skin colour, temperature, and record.
- Assess heart sounds and heart rate.
- Obtain a blood pressure reading using a sphygmomanometer.
- Document and record all results.
- Record pulse oximeter reading.
- Re-assess and continue management as appropriate en-route to further care.

ABDOMEN

- Feel for tenderness and guarding in all four quadrants.
- Check for bowel sounds.
- Listen and auscultate.

LOWER/UPPER LIMBS

Check for MSC in **ALL** four limbs:

- **MOTOR** – Test for movement and power.
- **SENSATION** – Apply light touch to evaluate sensation.
- **CIRCULATION** – Assess pulse and skin temperature.

MANAGEMENT

Correct:

- Airway.
- Breathing.
- Circulation.
- Disability (mini neurological examination).
- Ensure adequate oxygen therapy and support ventilation if required.
- Apply ECG and pulse oximetry monitoring, as required.

Consider ECG monitoring for patients on dialysis to check for the presence of hyperkalaemia.

- Consider patient positioning (e.g. sitting upright for respiratory problems).
- Check blood glucose levels in all patients with diabetes, impaired consciousness, seizures, collapse or alcohol/drug consumption, history of Addison's disease or other forms of adrenal insufficiency. Provide drug therapy as required; refer to appropriate drug guidelines. In adrenal crisis refer to **Hydrocortisone**.
- If the level of consciousness deteriorates or respiratory depression develops in cases where an overdose with opiate type drugs may be a possibility, consider administering naloxone (refer to **Naloxone**).
- In patients with fixed pinpoint pupils suspect opiate use. Follow ADDITIONAL MEDICAL guidelines as indicated by the patient's condition (e.g. cardiac rhythm disturbance):
  - correct A and B problems on scene
  - undertake a **TIME CRITICAL** transfer to nearest suitable further care
  - provide an alert/information call
  - provide a comprehensive verbal hand-over and a completed clinical record to the receiving staff.

ADDITIONAL INFORMATION

- The patient history can provide valuable insight into the cause of the current condition.

The following may assist in determining the diagnosis:

- Relatives, carers or friends with knowledge of the patient's history.
- Packets or containers of medication (including domiciliary oxygen) or evidence of administration devices (e.g. nebuliser machines).
- Medical alert type jewellery (bracelets or necklets) which detail the patient's primary health risk (e.g. diabetes, anaphylaxis, Addison's disease and other forms of adrenal insufficiency etc). May also list:
  - the patient's date of birth and NHS (England and Wales) or CHI (Scotland and Northern Ireland) number. Medical summary available by phone from NHS 111 and other providers.
  - a 24-hour telephone number for the medical jewellery provider to obtain next of kin and/or a more detailed patient history
- Warning stickers, often placed by the front door or the telephone, directing the health professional to a source of detailed information (one current scheme involves storing the patient details in a container in the fridge, as this is relatively easy to find in the house).
- Patient-held condition-specific warning cards (e.g. previous thrombolysis, at-risk COPD patients, those taking monoamine oxidase inhibitor (MAOI) medication, Addison's disease or other forms of adrenal insufficiency).
- Patients' individualised treatment plans.
- Patients on long-term steroids or who have adrenal insufficiency may deteriorate rapidly because of steroid insufficiency. If significantly unwell, the patient should be given hydrocortisone and fluids as soon as practical.

Appendix

Table 3.8 – GLASGOW COMA SCALE

Item	Element	Score
Eyes Opening:		
	Spontaneously	4
	To speech	3
	To pain	2
	None	1
Motor Response:		
	Obeys commands	6
	Localises pain	5
	Withdraws from pain	4
	Abnormal flexion	3
	Extensor response	2
	No response to pain	1
Verbal Response:		
	Orientated	5
	Confused	4
	Inappropriate words	3
	Incomprehensible sounds	2
	No verbal response	1

KEY POINTS

Medical Emergencies in Adults (Overview)

- **Detect TIME CRITICAL problems early.**
- **Minimise time on scene.**
- **Continuously re-assess ABCD, AVPU.**
- **Initiate treatments en-route if there is deterioration.**
- **Provide an alert/information call for TIME CRITICAL patients.**

Sepsis

1. Introduction

1.1 Terminology

- Suspected sepsis is not a specific illness but rather a syndrome encompassing a pathophysiology of which understanding is changing on a yearly basis. It is identified by a constellation of clinical signs and symptoms in a sick patient with an infection.
- The final diagnosis of sepsis is usually only confirmed at the end of an admission, when all the evidence becomes available.
- National Early Warning Scores (NEWS) are the best physiological scoring system for assessing sepsis and all causes of deterioration.
- A NEWS score greater than or equal to 5 highlights a sick patient who needs urgent clinical review; it does not represent a diagnosis, only a patient at significant risk.

1.2 Clinical Judgement

- Clinical judgement in determining what is or is not suspected sepsis is critical.
- Clinicians can rule out suspected sepsis in mimic conditions (e.g. asthma, diabetic ketoacidosis, mental health crisis), and rule in suspected sepsis when they are concerned.
- Over 70% of cases arise in the community, and ambulance clinicians are often the first point of contact for these patients.
- If left untreated, sepsis can lead to shock, multi-organ failure and death.
- Ambulance clinicians can help improve the outcomes by recognising sepsis early and providing a pre-alert and time critical transfer to the ED. Management should include (if indicated) high-flow oxygen, fluid resuscitation and benzylpenicillin if meningitis or meningococcal septicaemia is suspected.
- **Suspect sepsis in:**
  - anyone that presents with fever/feeling unwell
  - **and** NEWS greater than or equal to 5
  - **and/or** looks unwell with a history of infection.

2. Sepsis Definitions

2.1 Surviving Sepsis Campaign (2016)

- Sepsis is defined as life-threatening organ dysfunction caused by a dysregulated host response to infection.[1]

2.2 NICE (2016)

- Sepsis is a clinical syndrome caused by the body's immune and coagulation systems being switched on by an infection. Sepsis with shock is a life-threatening condition that is characterised by low blood pressure despite adequate fluid replacement, and organ dysfunction or failure.

3. Incidence

- There are an estimated 150,000 cases of sepsis each year in the UK with approximately 44,000 deaths attributed to sepsis. Half of ED sepsis patients arrive by ambulance.[2, 3] Sepsis patients arriving at the ED by ambulance are 'sicker' than patients arriving by other means.[4, 5, 6] Of patients admitted to ITU from the ED, 80–90% will have arrived by ambulance.[7, 8]

4. Severity and Outcome

- Sepsis has a high mortality rate and this can be as high as 50% in some patients.[9]
- Sepsis cases are responsible for 27% of all intensive care unit beds in England and Wales, and costs the NHS an estimated £2.5 billion per year.[10]
- Having a high index of suspicion, early recognition and rapid transport to hospital ensures early treatment with antibiotics and access to expert-led care.
- Survivors can suffer from long-term physical and psychological problems, resulting in significantly reduced quality of life.[1]
- Each hour of delay in giving antibiotics to a patient with septic shock has an increased mortality rate of 7.6%.[11] Treatment within one hour is considered best practice.

5. Pathophysiology

Sepsis is a multifaceted host response to the invasion of normally sterile tissue by pathogenic, or potentially pathogenic, micro-organisms.[1, 12, 13] The clinical manifestations of sepsis are highly variable between individuals due to age, underlying comorbidities, the causative pathogen and medications.[1, 14] Small amounts of cytokines are released into the circulation, leading to recruitment of inflammatory cells and an acute-phase response normally limited by anti-inflammatory mediators. In sepsis, there is a failure to control the inflammatory cascade, leading to a loss of capillary integrity, maldistribution of microvascular blood flow and stimulation of nitric oxide production, all leading towards organ injury and dysfunction.[12, 13]

6. Risk Factors for Sepsis[10]

The following groups of patients are at higher risk of developing sepsis:

- The very young (under 1 year) and older people (over 75 years) or people who are very frail.
- People who have impaired immune systems because of illness or drugs, including those:
  - being treated for cancer with chemotherapy (refer to Section 7 below on neutropaenic sepsis)
  - who have impaired immune function (for example, people with diabetes, people who have had a splenectomy, or people with sickle cell disease)
  - taking long-term steroids
  - taking immunosuppressant drugs to treat non-malignant disorders, such as rheumatoid arthritis.

- People who have had surgery, or other invasive procedures, in the past 6 weeks.
- People with any breach of skin integrity (for example, cuts, burns, blisters or skin infections).
- People who misuse drugs intravenously.
- People with indwelling lines or catheters.
- Pregnant women (refer to Section 8 below).

Take into account the following risk factors for sepsis in a newborn baby:

- History of maternal fever during labour or in the 24 hours before and after birth or maternal treatment with intravenous antibiotics for suspected infection.
- History of previous baby with sepsis during the newborn period.
- History of ruptured membranes before labour.
- Preterm birth following spontaneous labour (before 37 weeks gestation).
- Suspected or confirmed sepsis in another baby in the case of a multiple pregnancy.

7. Neutropaenic Sepsis

- Neutropaenic sepsis is a potentially fatal complication of cancer treatments, such as chemotherapy. Mortality rates as high as 21% have been reported in adults.[15] Patients can have neutropaenia as a result of the cancer therapy, which increases their risk of developing severe infections. Cancer patients can become neutropaenic, and not develop severe infections or sepsis. If a patient is neutropaenic and not showing signs of infection but is unwell, this should be taken seriously. Many patients develop this serious complication; therefore, always suspect neutropaenic sepsis in patients having cancer treatment who become unwell.
- Patients may have been given an advice line number to ring by their oncology service. Consider ringing advice lines such as this in line with your local procedures, as it may inform the appropriate destination or care pathway for the patient.
- Any of the following features could indicate that a neutropaenic patient has an infection and is at risk of sepsis:
  - tachypnoea
  - tachycardia
  - hypotension
  - temperature greater than 37.5°C
  - pleuritic chest pain
  - shivering episodes
  - flu-like symptoms
  - catheter site infections.
- Note that neutropaenic patients are unable to produce the pus normally associated with skin infections.
- A neutropaenic patient at risk of sepsis can look deceptively well and can deteriorate rapidly. A high index of suspicion is necessary, particularly if a patient who has recently undergone chemotherapy has an increased temperature. Patients who have received treatment within 6–8 weeks are at risk and at higher risk within the first 10 days after treatment.
- Neutropaenic sepsis is a medical emergency and all patients should be transported to the nearest emergency department or locally agreed pathway (oncology) with a hospital pre-alert.

8. Women and Pregnancy

- Have a very high index of suspicion for pregnant women who are unwell and have signs of infection.
- Take into account that women who are pregnant, have given birth or had a termination of pregnancy or miscarriage in the past 6 weeks are in a high-risk group for sepsis.[10] In particular, women who:
  - have impaired immune systems because of illness or drugs
  - have gestational diabetes, diabetes or other comorbidities
  - needed invasive procedures (for example, caesarean section, forceps delivery, removal of retained products of conception)
  - had prolonged rupture of membranes
  - have or have been in close contact with people with group A streptococcal infection, for example, scarlet fever
  - have continued vaginal bleeding or an offensive vaginal discharge.
- Note that the baseline heart rate in pregnancy is 10–15 beats per minute more than normal and there may be a decrease in systolic and diastolic blood pressure by an average of 10–15 mmHg. Therefore, this should be taken into account when considering sepsis, and rapid transport to definitive care is the priority and not extended on-scene times.
- These physiological changes in pregnancy can mask signs of significant sepsis and shock. Therefore, a strong index of suspicion must be maintained and transfer to hospital considered when underlying sepsis is suspected during or after pregnancy.
- Refer to **Maternity Care** for other changes in pregnancy.

9. Assessment

- Assess **ABCD** (refer to **Medical Emergencies in Adults Overview** and **Medical Emergencies in Children Overview**).
- Take extra care if the patient cannot provide a reliable history.
- Consider sepsis in all patients with non-specific, non-localised presentations, for example feeling very unwell, with a low or high temperature.
- Think about potential infection causing general deterioration, particularly in older patients presenting with new confusion (delirium), falls or new immobility.
- Pay particular attention if concerns are expressed by the patient, or their family/carers, regarding changes in behaviour.

- Examine people with suspected sepsis for mottled or ashen appearance, cyanosis of the skin, lips or tongue, non-blanching rash of the skin, any breach of skin integrity (for example, cuts, burns or skin infections) or other rash indicating potential infection.
- If possible, try to identify a source of infection.
- Be highly suspicious of neutropaenic sepsis in patients having cancer treatment who become unwell.
- Use a structured screening tool and NEWS score to stratify risk if sepsis is suspected.

10. Signs of Infection

Look for signs of infection by conducting a systems assessment, with particular regard for the areas covered in Table 3.9.

Table 3.9 – SIGNS OF INFECTION

The review of systems should cover the following areas:	
General	Lethargy, fever/rigors.
Neurological system	Severe headaches, new confusion. Signs of meningitis or encephalitis (neck stiffness/photophobia).
Cardiovascular	Shortness of breath, shortness of breath on exertion.
Respiratory	Pleurisy, shortness of breath, shortness of breath on exertion, cough, sputum, haemoptysis, increased respiratory rate or effort.
Gastrointestinal	Abdominal pain/distension, diarrhoea/vomiting
Genito-urinary	UTI symptoms (offensive urine, frequency, dysuria), reduced urine output, abdominal, flank and back pain.
Musculoskeletal	Hot painful joint, non-weight bearing.
Skin	Rapidly progressive cellulitis, diabetic foot and ulcers, burns, purpuric rash/ mottling.
Other	Dental problems, foreign travel, exposure to other unwell contacts.
NB This is not an exhaustive list and clinical judgement should be used when considering whether a sign or symptom of a serious bacterial infection is present.	

11. Respiratory Rate

- An increased respiratory rate is an early indicator of illness, and can be one of the first clinical observations to become abnormal. Therefore, accurately measuring respiratory rate (e.g. over 30 seconds) is essential. The respiratory rate will increase due to a compensatory mechanism to reduce metabolic acidosis, a consequence of sepsis. Development of sepsis screening tools has demonstrated that respiration rate will be higher in septic patients compared to non-septic patients.[16, 17]
- Respiratory rate is particularly important in children, and is a very early sign of illness. It is recommended that children presenting with signs and symptoms of an infection have an accurate respiration rate measured as it can be an important marker for serious illness.[18]
- Always refer to the relevant 'Page for Age' for vital signs of normal parameters.

12. Oxygen Saturation in Suspected Sepsis

- Take into account that if peripheral oxygen saturation is difficult to measure in a person with suspected sepsis, this may indicate poor peripheral circulation because of shock.
- In some groups of patients, pulse oximetry may be difficult, for example in children, or those with existing chronic respiratory disease, due to lack of appropriate or suitable equipment, chronic low saturations or patient compliance.

13. Heart Rate in Suspected Sepsis[10]

Interpret the heart rate of a person with suspected sepsis in context, taking into account that:

- baseline heart rate may be lower in young people and adults who are fit
- older people with an infection may not develop an increased heart rate
- older people may develop a new arrhythmia in response to infection rather than an increased heart rate
- heart rate response may be affected by medicines, such as beta-blockers.

Always refer to the children's 'Page for Age' for vital signs of normal parameters.

14. Blood Pressure in Suspected Sepsis[10]

- Interpret blood pressure in the context of a person's usual blood pressure, if known.
- Patients may present with a normal BP but still have sepsis, particularly children and young people.

15. Confusion, Mental State and Cognitive State in Suspected Sepsis[10]

- Interpret a person's mental state in the context of their normal function and treat changes as being significant.
- Be aware that changes in cognitive function may be subtle and assessment should include history from the patient and family or carers.
- Changes in cognitive function may present as changes in behaviour or irritability in both children and in adults with dementia.
- Changes in cognitive function in older people may present as acute changes in functional abilities.

16. Temperature in Suspected Sepsis[10]

- Do not use a person's temperature as the sole predictor of sepsis.
- Do not rely on fever or hypothermia to rule sepsis either in or out.
- Ask the person with suspected sepsis and their family or carers about any recent fever or rigors.
- Take into account that some groups of people with sepsis may not develop a raised temperature. These include:
  - people who are older or very frail
  - people having treatment for cancer
  - people deteriorating with sepsis
  - infants or young children.

Do not ignore a high temperature or symptoms of fever/ rigors as they are useful in highlighting patients with infection.

17. Pre-hospital Sepsis Screening Tools

- Exclusion or diagnosis of sepsis is only possible by obtaining complete blood test results from a laboratory or after urine output monitoring.
- Several pre-hospital sepsis screening tools have been proposed/developed; however, none have been validated in pre-hospital clinical practice.
- JRCALC recommends using tools that have been agreed locally in your own organisation, or across a network or region, and use of a NEWS score.
- Several additional screening tools have been proposed internationally, the PreSep score, PRESS score, and BAS 90-30-90 score have been proposed specifically to identify sepsis in the pre-hospital environment, but none have been validated clinically.[16, 19, 20] The Critical Illness Score was developed to identify all critically ill patients attended by EMS (not just sepsis patients). Again, this score has not been validated clinically.[21]

18. National Early Warning Score (NEWS)

- NEWS should be undertaken for all patients who are ill, including suspected sepsis.
- NEWS is designed as a system to help to identify a seriously ill or deteriorating patient in a standardised way across the NHS. It is not designed to identify the cause of the clinical deterioration. Its strength is its simplicity and pragmatism – using routine physiological measurements.
- NEWS allows healthcare workers to communicate in a common language.
- With regard to sepsis, a NEWS score of 5 or more predicts at least a twofold increase in the risk of adverse outcomes, **BUT** NEWS does not diagnose sepsis – it simply identifies sick patients who need urgent senior medical review and intervention. The nature of the intervention requires confirmation of the diagnosis.
- NEWS is the first step in a two-step process: (1) identification of the sick and/or deteriorating patient, and (2) a timely and competent clinical response.
- NEWS scores may be masked in patients who are taking beta-blockers and/or steroids.
- NEWS 2 is in development and this guideline will be updated to incorporate it.

National Early Warning Score (NEWS)*

PHYSIOLOGICAL PARAMETERS	3	2	1	0	1	2	3
Respiration Rate	≤8		9 - 11	12 - 20		21 - 24	≥25
Oxygen Saturations	≤91	92 - 93	94 - 95	≥96			
Any Supplemental Oxygen		Yes		No			
Temperature	≤35.0		35.1 - 36.0	36.1 - 38.0	38.1 - 39.0	≥39.1	
Systolic BP	≤90	91 - 100	101 - 110	111 - 219			≥220
Heart Rate	≤40		41 - 50	51 - 90	91 - 110	111 - 130	≥131
Level of Consciousness				A			V, P, or U

*The NEWS initiative flowed from the Royal College of Physicians' NEWS Development and Implementation Group (NEWSDIG) report, and was jointly developed and funded in collaboration with the Royal College of Physicians, Royal College of Nursing, National Outreach Forum and NHS Training for Innovation

Figure 3.1 – NEWS chart. © Royal College of Physicians 2012. Available at: https://www.rcplondon.ac.uk/projects/outputs/national-early-warning-score-news

Suspect sepsis in:

- anyone that presents with fever/feeling unwell

  and

- NEWS greater than or equal to 5
- **and/or** looks unwell with history of infection.

Table 3.10 – ADULT 'RED FLAG' SEPSIS – TIME CRITICAL EMERGENCY

The following markers are suggestive of 'red flag' sepsis:

- Responds only to voice or pain/is unresponsive.
- Systolic BP ≤90 mmHg (or drop ≥40 from normal) or mean arterial pressure less than 65 mmHg.
- Heart rate ≥130 per minute.
- Respiratory rate ≥25 per minute.
- Needs oxygen to keep SpO_2 ≥92%.
- Non-blanching rash, mottled/ashen/cyanotic.
- Not passed urine in last 18 hours.
- Recent chemotherapy (in past 6 weeks).

Table 3.11 – ADULT 'AMBER SUSPECT' SEPSIS –

The following are markers to indicate sepsis is likely:

- History from friend/family of new altered mental behaviour/state.
- Impaired immune system.
- Trauma/surgery in past 6 weeks.
- Respiration rate 21–24 per minute or increased work of breathing.
- Heart rate 91–130 per minute.
- Systolic BP 91–100 mmHg.
- Not passed urine in the last 12–18 hours.
- Tympanic temperature <36°C/axillary temperature <35°C.
- Signs of potential infection at wound (increased redness/discharge).

19. Children and Sepsis

Suspect sepsis in:

- children <12 years that present with fever/feeling unwell

  OR

- children with abnormal observations

  OR

- children with very worried parents/carers.

Table 3.12 – CHILD 'RED FLAG' SEPSIS – TIME CRITICAL EMERGENCY

High risk criteria suspect 'Red flag' sepsis:	
Colour	● Pale/mottled/ashen/blue.
Activity	● No response to social cues. ● Appears very ill to a healthcare professional. ● Does not wake or, if roused, does not stay awake. ● Weak, high-pitched or continuous cry.
Respiratory	● Grunting. ● Severe tachypnoea. ● Moderate or severe chest indrawing. ● Oxygen saturations ≤90% on air.
Hydration	● Reduced skin turgor. ● Severe tachycardia (see below). ● Bradycardia <60. ● Not passed urine/no wet nappies in last 18 hours.
Other	● Temperature <36°C. ● Non-blanching rash. ● Bulging fontanelle. ● Neck stiffness. ● Status epilepticus. ● Focal neurological signs. ● Focal seizures.

Table 3.13 – CHILD 'AMBER SUSPECT' SEPSIS –

Sepsis likely/intermediate risk for sepsis (if history suggestive of infection):	
Colour	● Pallor reported by parent/carer.
Activity	● Not responding normally to social cues/not wanting to play. ● Wakes only with prolonged stimulation. ● Significantly decreased activity. ● No smile.
Respiratory	● Nasal flaring. ● Moderate tachypnoea (see below). ● Oxygen saturations ≤92% on air. ● Crackles.
Hydration	● Dry mucous membranes. ● Moderate tachycardia (see below). ● Poor feeding in infants. ● CRT ≥3 seconds. ● Reduced urine output. ● Cold feet or hands.
Other	● Age 0–3 months ≥38°C. ● Age 3–6 months ≥39°C. ● Fever for ≥5 days. ● Rigors. ● Swelling of a limb or joint. ● Leg pain. ● Non-weight bearing/not using an extremity.

Table 3.14 – CHILD LOW RISK FOR SEPSIS	
Colour	Normal colour of skin, lips and tongue.
Activity	Responds normally to social cues. Content/smiles. Stays awake or awakens quickly. Strong normal cry/not crying.
Hydration	Normal skin and eyes. Moist mucous membranes.
Other	Child >2 years.

Clinical observations in children <12 years with suspected sepsis:

- Assess temperature, heart rate, respiratory rate, level of consciousness, oxygen saturation and capillary refill time.
- Only measure blood pressure in children <12 years in community settings if facilities to measure blood pressure, including a correctly-sized cuff, are available and taking a measurement does not cause a delay in assessment or treatment.

Table 3.15– SEPSIS RISK IN CHILDREN IN RELATION TO RESPIRATORY AND HEART RATES

AGE	TACHYPNOEA		TACHYCARDIA	
	Moderate	**Severe**	**Moderate**	**Severe**
1 year	50–59	≥60	150–159	≥160
1–2 years	40–49	≥50	140–149	≥150
3–4 years	35–39	≥40	130–139	≥140
5 years	27–28	≥29	120–129	≥130
6–7 years	24–26	≥27	110–119	≥120
8–11 years	22–24	≥25	105–114	≥115

20. Management

Table 3.16– MANAGEMENT of:

Sepsis	
Oxygen therapy	Sepsis is categorised as critical illness and requires supplemental oxygen regardless of initial oxygen saturation reading (SpO_2). Give oxygen to achieve a target saturation of 94–98% for adult patients or 88–92% for those at risk of hypercapnic respiratory failure (COPD). Oxygen should be given to children with suspected sepsis who have signs of shock or oxygen saturation (SpO_2) of less than 91% when breathing air. Treatment with oxygen should also be considered for children with an SpO_2 of greater than 92%, as clinically indicated.[14]
Fluid therapy	The choice of fluid is crystalloid. For adults, children and young people aged ≥12 years with suspected sepsis and systolic blood pressure less than 90 mmHg or mean arterial pressure (MAP) less than 65 mmHg, give an intravenous fluid bolus of 500 ml over 15 minutes and monitor response. Regularly reassess the patient after completion of the intravenous fluid bolus, and titrate response up to a maximum of 2000 ml if the systolic blood pressure remains below 90 mmHg and MAP below 65. IV fluids should be given to children if haemodynamically shocked or unresponsive. Give a bolus of 20 ml/kg over less than 10 minutes up to a maximum of 40 ml/kg. Assess response to fluids. Take into account pre-existing conditions (for example, cardiac disease or kidney disease), because smaller fluid volumes may be needed.

Sepsis *continued*	
• **Rapid transport to hospital with pre-alert**	• Keep on-scene times to a minimum. • Make a **TIME CRITICAL** transfer. • Provide a pre-alert and NEWS score to the receiving hospital – 'patient has suspected sepsis' – in line with local arrangements. • Handover to hospital using local handover tools, such as SBAR, and give a NEWS score: **S** – Situation **B** – Background **A** – Assessment **R** – Recommendation.

20.1 Further Management Considerations

Antibiotic Therapy

- If meningococcal disease is specifically suspected (fever and purpuric rash) give appropriate doses of parenteral benzylpenicillin and refer to **Meningococcal Meningitis and Septicaemia**.
- Any organisation considering pre-hospital antibiotic therapy for sepsis, particularly where journey times to hospital are more than one hour, should seek agreement from their relevant clinical networks.
- Early studies suggested significant survival benefit from early antibiotic administration in sepsis.[11] However, more recent studies fail to demonstrate such significant benefit. A recent meta-analysis indicated no survival benefit for antibiotics within the first hour of severe sepsis and septic shock.[22]
- Very few studies addressing pre-hospital antibiotic therapy have been undertaken. Some studies have also failed to demonstrate any survival benefit.[23] A recent study suggests that each hour of delay in giving antibiotics to a patient with septic shock increases mortality[24, 25, 26]At present there is insufficient evidence to make a robust recommendation in favour of, or against, pre-hospital antibiotic therapy.

Paracetamol

- Paracetamol should not to be given solely for reducing a high temperature but may be considered if the patient is in pain or to relieve distressing symptoms such as rigors.
- Paracetamol should be given intravenously only if the patient is unable to take anything orally or is in severe pain, otherwise oral paracetamol remains the first-line choice.
- Anti-pyretics such as paracetamol are often used in ICUs to manage fever in critically unwell patients by reducing the physiological stress fever causes; however, there is limited evidence to show any improvement in mortality.[27, 28, 29] Paracetamol is not part of any agreed sepsis pathway,[30] therefore may not be beneficial and does not improve outcomes in septic patients.[28, 31]
- It should be noted that paracetamol may mask the abnormal physiology and therefore treatment opportunities for sepsis may be missed in hospital due to dampening of the sepsis signs.
- If paracetamol is used it should be highlighted in the SBAR handover at hospital.

Measurement of Lactate

- Currently there is insufficient evidence to make a robust recommendation in favour of changing current practice to include pre-hospital lactate measurement.
- NICE have not recommended measuring pre-hospital lactate for suspected sepsis so at this time we do not recommend it for pre-hospital use.
- Lactate itself is not a predictor of sepsis. Lactate may be elevated in a number of clinical conditions, and indeed may be normal in cases of septic shock.

KEY POINTS

Sepsis

- **Suspect sepsis in:**
  - **anyone that presents with fever/feeling unwell**
  - **and NEWS greater than or equal to 5**
  - **and/or looks unwell with a history of infection.**
- **NEWS does not diagnose sepsis – it simply identifies sick patients who need urgent senior medical review and intervention.**
- **Keep on-scene times to a minimum.**
- **Provide a pre-alert and NEWS score to the receiving hospital – 'patient has suspected sepsis' – in line with local arrangements.**

Further Reading

Further important information and evidence in support of this guideline can be found in the Bibliography.[32, 33, 34, 35] Other useful resources include:

http://sepsistrust.org/

https://www.nice.org.uk/guidance/ng51

Bibliography

1 Singer M, Deutschman CS, Seymour CW, Shankar-Hari M, Annane D, Bauer M, Bellomo R et al. The Third International Consensus definitions for sepsis and septic shock (Sepsis-3). *JAMA* 2016, 315**:** 801–810.

2 Wang HE, Weaver MD, Shapiro NI, Yealy DM. Opportunities for emergency medical services care of sepsis. *Resuscitation* 2010, 81**:** 193–197.

3 Guerra WF, Mayfield TR, Meyers MS, Clouatre AE, Riccio JC. Early detection and treatment of patients with severe sepsis by prehospital personnel. *Journal of Emergency Medicine* 2013, 44**:** 1116–1125.

4 Van der Wekken LC, Alam N, Holleman F, Van Exter P, Kramer MH, Nanayakkara PW. Epidemiology of sepsis and its recognition by emergency medical services personnel in the Netherlands. *Prehosp Emerg Care* 2016, 20(1): 90–96.

5 Groenewoudt M, Roest AA, Leijten FMM, Stassen PM. Septic patients arriving with emergency medical services: A seriously ill population. *European Journal of Emergency* Medicine 2014, 21**:** 330–335.

6 Roest AA, Stoffers J, Pijpers E, Jansen J, Stassen PM. Ambulance patients with nondocumented sepsis have a high mortality risk: a retrospective study. *Eur J Emerg Med* 2017, 24(1): 36–43.

7 Gray A, Ward K, Lees F, Dewar C, Dickie S, McGuffie C, Committee SS. The epidemiology of adults with severe sepsis and septic shock in Scottish emergency departments. *Emergency Medicine Journal* 2013, 30: 397–401.

8 Ibrahim I, Jacobs IG. Can the characteristics of emergency department attendances predict poor hospital outcomes in patients with sepsis? *Singapore Med J* 2013, 54**:** 634–638.

9 Martin GS, Mannino DM, Eaton S, Moss M. The epidemiology of sepsis in the United States from 1979 through 2000. *N Engl J Med* 2003, 348(16): 1546–1554.

10 National Institute for Health and Clinical Excellence. *Sepsis: Recognition, Diagnosis and Early Management* (NG51). London: NICE, 2017.

11 Liu VX, Fielding-Singh V, Greene JD, Baker JM, Iwashyna TJ, Bhattacharya J, Escobar GJ. The timing of early antibiotics and hospital mortality in sepsis. *American Journal of Respiratory and Critical Care Medicine*, 2017. Available from: http://atsjournals.org/doi/abs/10.1164/rccm.201609-1848OC.

12 Bone RC, Balk RA, Cerra FB, Dellinger RP, Fein AM, Knaus WA, Schein RM, Sibbald WJ. Definitions for sepsis and organ failure and guidelines for the use of innovative therapies in sepsis. The ACCP/SCCM Consensus Conference Committee. American College of Chest Physicians/Society of Critical Care Medicine. *Chest* 1992, 101**:** 1644–1655.

13 Bone RC, Sibbald WJ, Sprung CL. The ACCP-SCCM consensus conference on sepsis and organ failure. *Chest* 1992, 101**:** 1481–1483.

14 Angus DC, Van der Poll T. Severe sepsis and septic shock. *N Engl J Med* 2013, 369**:** 2063.

15 Herbst C, Naumann F, Kruse EB, Monsef I, Bohlius J, Schulz H, Engert A. Prophylactic antibiotics or G-CSF for the prevention of infections and improvement of survival in cancer patients undergoing chemotherapy, *Cochrane Database Syst Rev* 2009, 21(1): CD007107.

16 Polito CC, Isakov A, Yancey AH, Wilson DK, Anderson BA, Bloom I, Martin GS, Sevransky JE. Prehospital recognition of severe sepsis: development and validation of a novel emergency medical services screening tool. *Am J Emerg Med* 2015, 33(9):1119–1125.

17 Goerlich CE, Wade CE, McCarthy JJ, Holcomb JB, Moore LJ. Validation of sepsis screening tool using StO_2 in emergency department patients. *J Surg Res* 2014, 190**:** 270–275.

18 Davis T. NICE guideline: feverish illness in children--assessment and initial management in children younger than 5 years. *Arch Dis Child Educ Pract Ed* 2013, 98**:** 232–235.

19 Bayer O, Schwarzkopf D, Stumme C, Stacke A, Hartog CS, Hohenstein C, Kabisch B, Reichel J, Reinhart K, Winning J. An early warning scoring system to identify septic patients in the prehospital setting: The PRESEP Score. *Acad Emerg Med* 2015, 22**:** 868–871.

20 Wallgren UM, Castren M, Svensson AE, Kurland L. Identification of adult septic patients in the prehospital setting: a comparison of two screening tools and clinical judgment. *Eur J Emerg Med* 2014, 21**:** 260–265.

21 Seymour CW, Kahn JM, Cooke CR, Watkins TR, Heckbert SR, Rea TD. Prediction of critical illness during out-of-hospital emergency care. *JAMA* 2010, 304**:** 747–754.

22 Sterling SA, Miller WR, Pryor J, Puskarich MA, Jones AE. The impact of timing of antibiotics on outcomes in severe sepsis and septic shock: A systematic review and meta-analysis. *Crit Care Med* 2015, 43**:** 1907–1915.

23 Band RA, Gaieski DF, Hylton JH, Shofer FS, Goyal M, Meisel ZF. Arriving by emergency medical services improves time to treatment endpoints for patients with severe sepsis or septic shock. *Academic Emergency Medicine* 2011, 18**:** 934–940.

24 Seymour CW, Gesten F, Prescott HC, Friedrich ME, Iwashyna TJ, Phillips GS et al. Time to treatment and mortality during mandated emergency care for sepsis. New England Journal of Medicine, 21 May, 2017. Available from: http://www.nejm.org/doi/full/10.1056/NEJMoa1703058?query=featured_home#t=articleTop.

25 Shaw J, Fothergill RT, Clark S, Moore F. Can the prehospital National Early Warning Score identify patients most at risk from subsequent deterioration? *EMJ Online First*, 13 May, 2017.

26 Jarvis S, Kovacs C, Briggs J, Meredith P, Schmidt PE, Featherstone PI et al. Aggregate National Early Warning Score (NEWS) values are more important than high scores for a single vital signs parameter for discriminating the risk of adverse outcomes. *Resuscitation* 2015, 87: 75–80.

27 Anderson HA, Young J, Marrelli D, Black R, Lambreghts K, Twa MD. Training students with patient actors improves communication: a pilot study. *Optom Vis Sci* 2014, 91**:** 121–128.

28 Lee BH, Inui D, Suh GY, Kim JY, Kwon JY, Park J, Tada K et al. Association of body temperature and antipyretic treatments with mortality of critically ill patients with and without sepsis: multi-centered prospective observational study. *Crit Care* 2012, 16**:** R33.

SECTION 3 Medical Specific Conditions

29 Janz DR, Bastarache JA, Rice TW, Bernard GR, Warren MA, Wickersham N, Sills G et al. Randomized, placebo-controlled trial of acetaminophen for the reduction of oxidative injury in severe sepsis: the Acetaminophen for the Reduction of Oxidative Injury in Severe Sepsis trial. *Crit Care Med* 2015, **43:** 534–541.

30 Daniels R, Nutbeam T, McNamara G, Galvin C. The sepsis six and the severe sepsis resuscitation bundle: a prospective observational cohort study. *Emerg Med J* 2011, **28:** 507–512.

31 Young P. Acetaminophen to treat fever in intensive care unit patients with likely infection: a response from the author of the HEAT trial. *J Thorac Dis* 2016, **8:** E631–632.

32 Boland LL, Hokanson JS, Fernstrom KM, Kinzy TG, Lick CJ, Satterlee PA, Lacroix BK. Prehospital lactate measurement by emergency medical services in patients meeting sepsis criteria. *West J Emerg Med* 2016, **17:** 648–655.

33 Brown AFT, Cadogan MD. *Emergency Medicine: Diagnosis and Management*. London: Hodder Arnold, 2001.

34 Chamberlain D. Prehospital administered intravenous antimicrobial protocol for septic shock: A prospective randomized clinical trial. *Critical Care* 2009, **13:** S130–S131.

35 Tobias AZ, Guyette FX, Seymour CW, Suffoletto BP, Martin-Gill C, Quintero J, Kristan J, Callaway CW, Yealy DM. Pre-resuscitation lactate and hospital mortality in prehospital patients. *Prehosp Emerg Care* 2014, **18:** 321–327.

Asthma (Adults)

1. Introduction

- Asthma is one of the commonest of all medical conditions. Asthma has varying levels of severity and patients usually present to pre-hospital care with one of four presentations: mild/moderate, severe, life-threatening, and near fatal (refer to Table 3.17).
- Typically in patients requiring hospital admission the symptoms will have developed gradually over a number of hours (>6 hours). Usually patients are known asthmatics and may be on regular inhaler therapy for this. Patients may have used their own treatment inhalers and in some cases will have used a home-based nebuliser.
- Patients may report a history of increased wheezy breathlessness, often worse at night or in the early morning, associated either with infection, allergy or exertion as a trigger.
- Patients over 50 years of age who are long-term smokers with a history of exertional breathlessness and no other known cause of breathlessness should be treated as having COPD (refer to **Chronic Obstructive Pulmonary Disease**).

Table 3.17 – FEATURES OF SEVERITY

Near-fatal asthma

- Raised $PaCO_2$ and/or requiring mechanical ventilation with raised inflation pressures.

Life-threatening asthma

Any one of the following in a patient with severe asthma:

- Altered conscious level.
- Exhaustion.
- Arrhythmia.
- Hypotension.
- Cyanosis.
- Silent chest.
- Poor respiratory effort.
- PEF <33% best or predicted.
- SpO_2 <92%.
- PaO_2 <8 kPa.
- 'Normal' $PaCO_2$ (4.6–6.0 kPa).

Acute severe asthma

Any one of:

- PEF 33–50% best or predicted.
- Respiratory rate ≥25/minute.
- Heart rate >110/minute.
- Inability to complete sentences in one breath.

Moderate asthma exacerbation

- Increasing symptoms.
- PEF >50–75% best or predicted.
- No features of acute severe asthma.

2. Incidence

- Asthma is rare in the older population and practitioners should be aware that many people will describe a range of other respiratory conditions as 'asthma', and therefore other causes of breathlessness need to be considered.
- In adults, asthma may often be complicated and mixed in with a degree of bronchitis, especially in smokers. This can make the condition much more difficult to treat, both routinely and in emergencies. The majority of asthmatic patients take regular 'preventer' and 'reliever' inhalers.

3. Severity and Outcome

- The obstruction in its most severe form can be **TIME CRITICAL** and in the UK some 2,000 people a year die as a result of asthma. Patients with severe asthma and one or more risk factor(s) (refer to Table 3.18) are at risk of death.
- In patients ≤40 years, deaths from asthma peak in July/August in contrast to patients aged >40 years where deaths peak in December/January.

Table 3.18 – RISK FACTORS FOR DEVELOPING NEAR-FATAL ASTHMA

Medical

- Previous near-fatal asthma (e.g. previous ventilation or respiratory acidosis).
- Previous hospital admission for asthma especially if in the last year requiring three or more classes of asthma medication.
- Heavy use of β2 agonist.
- Repeated emergency department attendance for asthma care especially if in the last year.
- Brittle asthma.

Psychological/behavioural

- Non-compliance with treatment or monitoring.
- Failure to attend appointments.
- Fewer GP contacts.
- Frequent home visits.
- Self-discharge from hospital.
- Psychosis, depression, other psychiatric illness or deliberate self-harm.
- Current or recent major tranquilliser use.
- Denial.
- Alcohol or drug abuse.
- Obesity.
- Learning difficulties.
- Employment problems.
- Income problems.
- Social isolation.
- Childhood abuse.
- Severe domestic, marital or legal stress.

4. Pathophysiology

- Asthma is caused by a chronic inflammation of the bronchi, making them narrower. The muscles around the bronchi become irritated and contract, causing sudden worsening of the symptoms. The inflammation can also cause the mucus glands to produce excessive sputum which further blocks the air passages.
- The obstruction and subsequent wheezing are caused by three factors within the bronchial tree:
  1. increased production of bronchial mucus
  2. swelling of the bronchial tube mucosal lining cells
  3. spasm and constriction of bronchial muscles.

These three factors combine to cause blockage and narrowing of the small airways in the lung. Because inspiration is an active process involving the muscles of respiration, the obstruction of the airways is overcome on breathing in. Expiration occurs with muscle relaxation, and is severely delayed by the narrowing of the airways in asthma. This generates the wheezing on expiration that is characteristic of this condition.

- Asthma is managed with a variety of inhaled and tablet medications. Inhalers are divided into two broad categories: preventer and reliever.

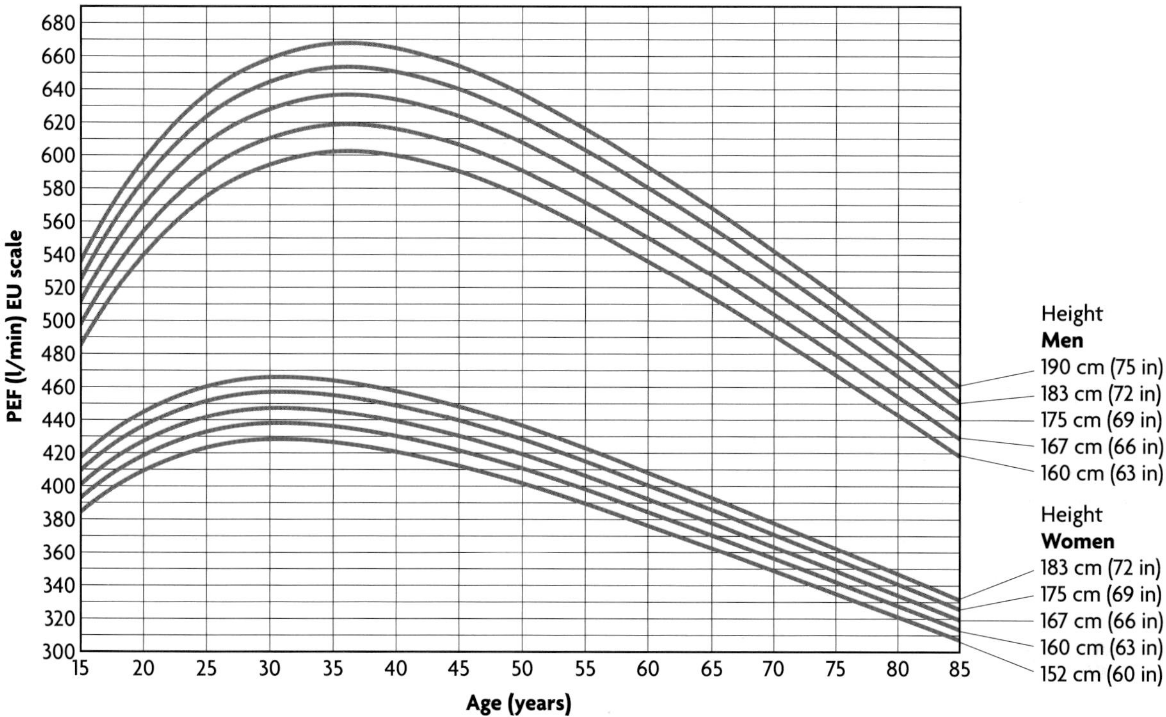

Figure 3.2 – Peak flow charts – Peak expiratory flow rate – normal values. For use with EU/EN13826 scale PEF meters only. Adapted by Clement Clarke for use with EN13826 / EU scale peak flow meters from Nunn AJ Gregg I, Br Med J 1989:298;1068–70.

1. The preventer inhalers are normally anti-inflammatory drugs and these include steroids and other milder anti-inflammatories such as Tilade. The common steroid inhalers are beclomethasone (Becotide), budesonide (Pulmicort), fluticasone (Flixotide) and tiotropium (Spiriva). These drugs act on the lung over a period of time to reduce the inflammatory reaction that causes the asthma. Regular use of these inhalers often eradicates all symptoms of asthma and allows for a normal lifestyle.
2. The reliever inhalers include salbutamol (Ventolin), terbutaline (Bricanyl) and ipratropium bromide (Atrovent). These inhalers work rapidly on the lung to relax the smooth muscle spasm when the patient feels wheezy or tight chested. They are used in conjunction with preventer inhalers. Inhalers are often used through large plastic spacer devices, such as the Volumatic® or Aerochamber®. This allows the drug to spread into a larger volume and allows the patient to inhale it more effectively. In mild and moderate asthma attacks some patients may be treated with high doses of 'relievers' through a spacer device. This has been shown to be as effective as giving a salbutamol nebuliser.

5. Assessment

- Assess **ABCD** (refer to **Medical Emergencies in Adults Overview**), but specifically assess for the severity of the asthma attack (refer to asthma algorithm – Figure 3.3 and Table 3.17).

6. Management

- Refer to the asthma algorithm (Figure 3.3 and Table 3.19) for the management of mild/moderate, severe, life-threatening, and near-fatal.

For less severe attacks:

- Where possible the patient's own β2 agonist should be given (ideally using a spacer) as first line treatment.

Increase the dose by two puffs every 2 minutes according to response up to ten puffs.

- If symptoms are not controlled by ten puffs, then start nebulised salbutamol whilst transferring to the emergency department.
- Patients (or friends/bystanders) who have previously experienced a severe asthma attack may be more likely to call for help early in the development of an attack, and the symptoms may appear mild on arrival of the ambulance.
- Some patients may be appropriate for alternative care pathways, for example, early referral to a general practitioner. However, apparently minor symptoms should not preclude onward referral especially where an alternative pathway is not readily accessible. Local care pathways should be followed where patients are considered for non conveyance. However, caution should be exercised in known severe asthmatics and robust safety netting of patients must be in place.

Peak expiratory flow rate (PEFR)

- Peak flow is a rapid measurement of the degree of obstruction in the patient's lungs. It measures the maximum flow on breathing out, or expiring and therefore can reflect the amount of airway obstruction. Whenever possible, peak flow should be performed before and after nebulised treatment. Many patients now have their own meter at home and know what their normal peak flow is. Clearly, when control is good, their peak flow will be equivalent to a normal patient's measurement, but during an attack it may drop markedly (refer to Figure 3.2).

Table 3.19 – ASSESSMENT and MANAGEMENT of:

Asthma

ASSESSMENT	MANAGEMENT
• Assess **ABCD** Specifically assess for the severity of the asthma attack (refer to Figure 3.3)	• If any of the following **TIME CRITICAL** features present: – major ABCD problems – extreme difficulty in breathing or requirement for assisted ventilations – exhaustion – cyanosis – silent chest – SpO_2 <92% – PEF <33% best or predicted. • Start correcting A and B problems. • Undertake a **TIME CRITICAL** transfer to nearest receiving hospital. • Continue patient management en-route. • Provide an alert/information call.
• Mild/moderate asthma Increasing symptoms, PEF >50–75% best or predicted, no features of acute severe asthma	• Move to a calm quiet environment. • Encourage use of own inhaler, using a spacer if available. Ensure correct technique is used (refer to Figure 3.3). • If unresponsive: – administer high levels of supplementary oxygen – administer nebulised salbutamol (refer to **Salbutamol**).
• Severe asthma Any one of: – PEF 33–50% of best or predicted – Respiratory rate >25/minute – Heart rate >110/minute – Inability to complete sentences in one breath	• Administer high levels of supplementary oxygen. • Administer nebulised salbutamol (refer to **Salbutamol**). • If no improvement administer ipratropium bromide (refer to **Ipratropium Bromide**). • Administer steroids (refer to **relevant steroids guideline**). • Continuous salbutamol nebulisation may be administered unless clinically significant side effects occur (refer to **Salbutamol**).

Asthma *continued*

• Life-threatening asthma Any one of: – Altered conscious level – Exhaustion – Arrhythmia – Hypotension – Cyanosis – Silent chest – Poor respiratory effort – PEF<33% best or predicted – SpO_2 <92%	• Continuous salbutamol nebulisation may be administered unless clinically significant side effects occur (refer to **Salbutamol**). • Administer adrenaline 1 in 1000 IM only (refer to **Adrenaline**).
• Near fatal asthma – Requiring bag-valve-mask ventilation with raised inflation pressures – Transfer	• Assess for bilateral tension pneumothorax. • Transfer rapidly to nearest receiving hospital. • Provide an alert/information call. • Continue patient management en-route. • For cases of mild asthma that respond to treatment consider alternative care pathway where appropriate. Note: exercise caution in known severe asthmatics.

KEY POINTS

Asthma in Adults

- **Asthma is a common life-threatening condition.**
- **Its severity is often not recognised.**
- **Accurate documentation is essential.**
- **A silent chest is a pre-terminal sign.**

Bibliography

1 Soar J, Perkins GD, Abbas G, Alfonzo A, Barelli A, Bierens JJLM, et al. European Resuscitation Council Guidelines for Resuscitation 2010 Section 8: Cardiac arrest in special circumstances: electrolyte abnormalities, poisoning, drowning, accidental hypothermia, hyperthermia, asthma, anaphylaxis, cardiac surgery, trauma, pregnancy, electrocution. *Resuscitation* 2010, 81(10): 1400–1433.

2 The British Thoracic Society, Scottish Intercollegiate Guidelines Network. *British Guideline on the Management of Asthma* (Guideline 101). London/Edinburgh: BTS and SIGN, 2008 (revised May 2012). Available from: https://www.brit-thoracic.org.uk/document-library/clinical-information/asthma/btssign-asthma-guideline-2014/.

3 Rubin BK, Dhand R, Ruppel GL, Branson RD, Hess DR. Respiratory care year in review 2010. Part 1: Asthma, COPD, pulmonary function testing, ventilator-associated pneumonia. *Respiratory Care* 2011, 56(4): 488–502.

4 Nunn AJ, Gregg I. New regression equations for predicting peak expiratory flow in adults. *British Medical Journal* 1989, 298(6680): 1068–70.

Asthma (Adults)

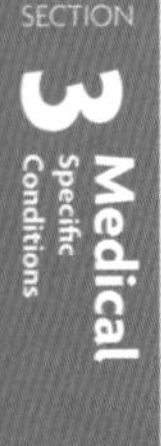

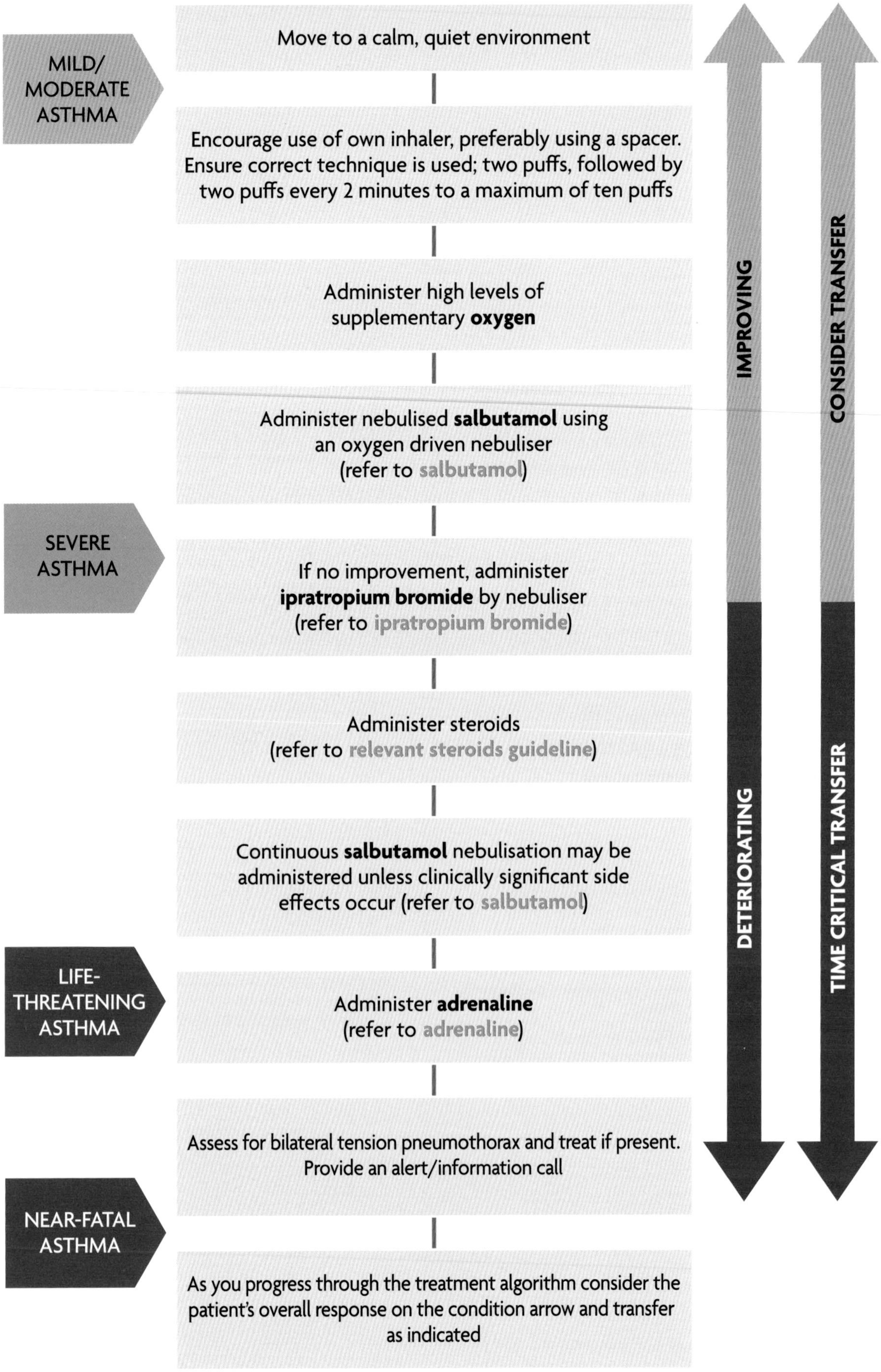

MILD/ MODERATE ASTHMA

Move to a calm, quiet environment

Encourage use of own inhaler, preferably using a spacer. Ensure correct technique is used; two puffs, followed by two puffs every 2 minutes to a maximum of ten puffs

Administer high levels of supplementary **oxygen**

Administer nebulised **salbutamol** using an oxygen driven nebuliser (refer to salbutamol)

SEVERE ASTHMA

If no improvement, administer **ipratropium bromide** by nebuliser (refer to ipratropium bromide)

Administer steroids (refer to relevant steroids guideline)

Continuous **salbutamol** nebulisation may be administered unless clinically significant side effects occur (refer to salbutamol)

LIFE-THREATENING ASTHMA

Administer **adrenaline** (refer to adrenaline)

Assess for bilateral tension pneumothorax and treat if present. Provide an alert/information call

NEAR-FATAL ASTHMA

As you progress through the treatment algorithm consider the patient's overall response on the condition arrow and transfer as indicated

IMPROVING / DETERIORATING

CONSIDER TRANSFER / TIME CRITICAL TRANSFER

Figure 3.3 – Asthma assessment and management algorithm.

Asthma (Children)

1. Introduction

- Asthma is one of the commonest medical conditions requiring hospitalisation.
- The severity of asthma may be subdivided into mild/moderate, severe, or life-threatening (refer to Table 3.21).
- There may be a history of increasing wheeze or breathlessness (often worse at night or early in the morning). Respiratory infections, allergy and physical exertion are common triggers.
- Known asthmatics will be on regular medication, taking inhalers ('preventers' and/or 'relievers') and sometimes oral medications such as Montelukast (Singulair®) and theophyllines.
- Some children with asthma will have an individualised treatment plan with detailed information regarding their daily symptom control as well as what to do in an acute exacerbation.
- **Inhaled foreign body:** Consider an inhaled foreign body in a child experiencing their first wheezy episode, especially if there is a history of playing with small toys and the wheeze was of sudden onset and is unilateral. These children must be transferred for medical assessment. If they are unwell during transport, bronchodilators may provide some clinical benefit.

2. Severity and Outcome

- Children with previous hospital admissions (particularly intensive care admissions), are at risk of future severe or life-threatening episodes (and even death) – so this information should be sought.

Table 3.20 – RISK FACTORS FOR SEVERE ASTHMA

Risk Factors

- Previous severe or life-threatening episodes.
- Previous hospital admission for asthma especially if in the last year.
- Previous admission requiring intensive care.
- Back to back nebulisers with poor or no response.

3. Pathophysiology

- Asthma causes chronic bronchial inflammation which results in narrowing of the airways. In acute attacks, airway irritation causes smooth muscle contraction producing respiratory compromise. Inflammatory processes also cause i) excessive sputum production and ii) swelling of the bronchial mucosal which blocks the small airways.
- Inspiration (an active process) generates sufficient pressures to overcome airway narrowing, but during expiration (a passive process) relaxation of the respiratory muscles causes airway narrowing, producing the characteristic wheeze.
- Various medications are used to treat asthma. In children, these are typically delivered using a spacer device (e.g. a Volumatic® or Aerochamber®). Some children may also have a home nebuliser.

4. Assessment

Following an ABC assessment, the severity of the asthma attack should be established (refer to Table 3.21 and Asthma Algorithm – Figure 3.4).

Table 3.21 – FEATURES OF SEVERITY

Life-threatening asthma

- Silent chest.
- SpO_2 <92%.
- Cyanosis PEFR <33% best or predicted.
- Poor respiratory effort.
- Hypotension.
- Exhaustion.
- Confusion.

Severe asthma

- Can't complete sentences in one breath or too breathless to talk or feed.
- SpO_2 <92%.
- PEFR 33–50% best or predicted.
- Pulse:
  - >140 in children aged 2–5 years
  - >125 in children aged >5 years.
- Respiration:
  - >40 breaths/min aged 2–5 years
  - >30 breaths/min aged >5 years.

Moderate asthma exacerbation

- Able to talk in sentences.
- SpO_2 ≥92%.
- PEFR ≥50% best or predicted.
- Heart rate:
  - ≤140/min in children aged 2–5 years
  - ≤125/min in children >5 years.
- Respiratory rate:
  - ≤40/min in children aged 2–5 years
  - ≤30/min in children >5 years.

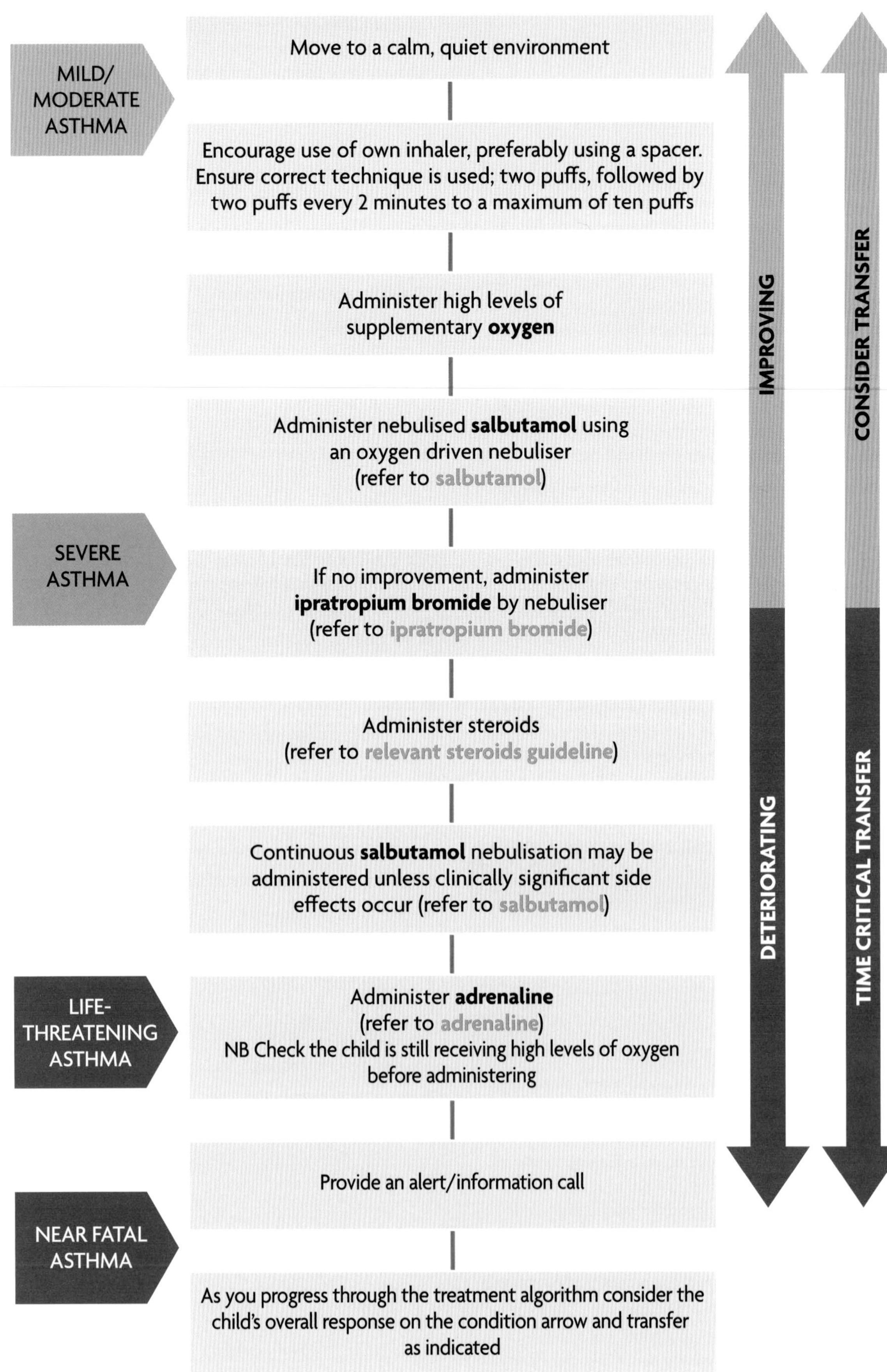

Figure 3.4 – Asthma assessment and management algorithm.

5. Management

The Asthma Algorithm (Figure 3.4) describes the management of mild/moderate, severe and life-threatening asthma. Adrenaline and hydrocortisone are now included in the management of severe/life threatening asthma in children.

Always ask if the child has an individualised asthma treatment plan and follow it, unless clinical circumstances dictate otherwise.

For some children alternative care pathways will already have been created (e.g. early referral to their GP). It is well recognised, however, that children with apparently minor symptoms can subsequently deteriorate and practitioners should therefore have a low threshold for onward referral (especially where an alternative pathway has not already been established).

Peak expiratory flow rate measurements (PEFR): PEFR should be attempted where possible in children before and after nebulised therapy in mild to moderate asthma. However, care should be taken in severe life-threatening attacks as it could exacerbate the attack and the patient may deteriorate. Predicted PEFR are listed in Table 3.22.

Table 3.22 – PEAK EXPIRATORY FLOW CHART

Height (m)	Height (ft)	Predicted EU PEFR (L/min)
0.85	2'9"	87
0.90	2'11"	95
0.95	3'1"	104
1.00	3'3"	115
1.05	3'5"	127
1.10	3'7"	141
1.15	3'9"	157
1.20	3'11"	174
1.25	4'1"	192
1.30	4'3"	212
1.35	4'5"	233
1.40	4'7"	254
1.45	4'9"	276
1.50	4'11"	299
1.55	5'1"	323
1.60	5'3"	346
1.65	5'5"	370
1.70	5'7"	393

Table 3.23 – ASSESSMENT and MANAGEMENT

Asthma	
ASSESSMENT	**MANAGEMENT**
• Assess **ABCD** • Specifically assess for the severity of the asthma attack (refer to Figure 3.4)	• If any of the following **TIME CRITICAL** features present: – major ABCD problems – extreme difficulty in breathing or requirement for assisted ventilations – exhaustion – cyanosis – silent chest – SPO_2 <92% – PEF <33% best or predicted. • Start correcting A and B problems. • Undertake a **TIME CRITICAL** transfer to nearest receiving hospital. • Continue patient management en-route. • Provide an alert/information call.
• Mild/moderate asthma – Able to talk in sentences – SpO_2 >92% – PEFR >50% best or predicted – Pulse <140 in child ages 2–5, <125 in child >5 – Respiration <40 in child ages 2–5 – <30 in child ages >5	• Move to a calm quiet environment. • Encourage use of own inhaler, using a spacer if available. Ensure correct technique is used (refer to Figure 3.4). • If unresponsive: – administer high levels of supplementary oxygen – administer nebulised salbutamol (refer to Salbutamol).

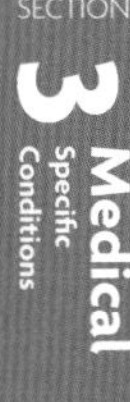

Asthma *continued*	
• Severe asthma – Can't complete sentences in one breath or too breathless to talk or feed – SpO_2 <92% – PEFR 33–50% best or predicted – Pulse >140 in child aged 2–5 years – >125 in child >5 years – Respiration >40 in child ages 2–5 years – >30 in child aged >5 years.	• Administer high levels of supplementary oxygen. • Administer nebulised salbutamol (refer to **Salbutamol**). • If no improvement administer ipratropium bromide (refer to **Ipratropium Bromide**). • Administer steroids (refer to **relevant steroids guideline**). • Continuous salbutamol nebulisation may be administered unless clinically significant side effects occur (refer to **Salbutamol**).
• Life-threatening asthma – Silent chest – SpO_2 <92% – Cyanosis – PEFR <33% best or predicted (exercise caution with PEFR in this patient group) – Poor respiratory effort – Hypotension – Exhaustion – Confusion	• Continuous salbutamol nebulisation may be administered unless clinically significant side effects occur (refer to **Salbutamol**). • Administer adrenaline 1 in 1000 IM only (refer to **Adrenaline**). • Assess for bilateral tension pneumothorax.
• Transfer	• Transfer rapidly to nearest receiving hospital. • Provide an alert/information call. • Continue patient management en-route.
	• For cases of mild asthma that respond to treatment consider alternative care pathway where appropriate. • **Note:** exercise caution in known severe asthmatics.

KEY POINTS

Asthma (Children)

- **Clinical assessment should determine the severity of the attack.**
- **Bronchodilators (e.g. salbutamol) are the mainstay of treatment.**
- **High levels of oxygen may be required during an asthma attack.**
- **Mild/moderate attacks should be managed with inhaled bronchodilators via a spacer device.**
- **Nebulised treatments should be reserved for moderate/severe attacks where oxygen is required.**
- **In addition to β2 agonists, ipratropium is used in severe cases.**

Bibliography

1 Soar J, Perkins GD, Abbas G, Alfonzo A, Barelli A, Bierens JJLM, et al. European Resuscitation Council Guidelines for Resuscitation 2010 Section 8: Cardiac arrest in special circumstances: electrolyte abnormalities, poisoning, drowning, accidental hypothermia, hyperthermia, asthma, anaphylaxis, cardiac surgery, trauma, pregnancy, electrocution. *Resuscitation* 2010, 81(10): 1400–1433.

2 The British Thoracic Society, Scottish Intercollegiate Guidelines Network. *British Guideline on the Management of Asthma* (Guideline 101). London/Edinburgh: BTS and SIGN, 2008 (revised May 2012). Available from: https://www.brit-thoracic.org.uk/document-library/clinical-information/asthma/btssign-asthma-guideline-2014/.

3 Rubin BK, Dhand R, Ruppel GL, Branson RD, Hess DR. Respiratory care year in review 2010. Part 1: Asthma, COPD, pulmonary function testing, ventilator-associated pneumonia. *Respiratory Care* 2011, 56(4): 488–502.

4 O'Driscoll BR, Howard LS, Davison AG, on behalf of the British Thoracic Society. BTS guideline for emergency oxygen use in adult patients. *Thorax* 2008, 63(suppl. 6): vi1–vi68.

5 Resuscitation Council (UK). What is the guidance for emergency oxygen use in children?, 2011.

4

Trauma

Limb Trauma

1. Introduction

- There is one fundamental rule to apply to limb trauma cases and that is NOT to let limb injuries, however dramatic in appearance, distract the clinician from less visible but life-threatening problems, such as airway obstruction, compromised breathing, poor perfusion and spinal injury.
- Patients with limb trauma are likely to be in considerable pain and distress; therefore consider pain management as soon as clinically possible after arriving on scene (refer to **Pain Management in Adults** and **Pain Management in Children**).

2. Pathophysiology

- The pathophysiology differs depending on the nature of the injury (refer to Table 4.1).
- Blood loss from femoral shaft fractures can be considerable, involving loss of 500–2000 millilitres in volume. If the fracture is open, blood loss is increased.
- Nerves and blood vessels are placed at risk from sharp bony fragments, especially in very displaced fractures, hence the need to return fractured limbs to normal alignment as rapidly as possible. Fractures around the elbow and knee are especially likely to injure arteries and nerves.
- The six 'P's of ischaemia are shown in Table 4.2.

Table 4.1 – TYPES OF LIMB INJURY

Compound fracture (open)

A fracture in which the bone protrudes through an open wound.

Closed fracture

A fracture that is contained, the skin is unbroken.

Dislocation

Where the articular surface of the joint is not in continuity. Commonly affecting the digits, elbow, shoulder, patella and occasionally the hip (high energy).

Compartment syndrome

A complication of limb fractures arising from increased pressure in muscular compartments due to contained haemorrhage or swelling. This can lead to ischaemia, with potentially catastrophic consequences for the limb.

Degloving

Degloving can accompany limb fractures and be to the superficial fascia or full depth down to the bone.

Amputations/partial amputations

Amputations most frequently involve digits, but can involve part or whole limbs. Partial amputations may still result in a viable limb, providing there is minimal crushing damage and survival of some vascular and nerve structures.

Neck of femur fractures

Such fractures commonly occur in older people and are one of the most common limb injuries encountered in the pre-hospital environment. Typical patients present with shortening and external rotation of the leg on the injured side, with pain in the hip and referred pain in the knee. The circumstances of the injury must be taken into account – often the older person has been on the floor for some time, which increases the possibility of hypothermia, dehydration, pressure ulcers and chest infection, so careful monitoring of vital signs is essential.

Table 4.2 – SIX 'P's OF ISCHAEMIA

SIGN	SYMPTOM
Pain	Out of proportion to the apparent injury; often in the muscle, which may not ease with splinting/analgesia.
Pallor	Due to compromised blood flow to limb.
Paralysis	Loss of movement.
Paraesthesia	Changes in sensation.
Pulselessness	The loss of peripheral pulses is a grave late sign caused by swelling, which can lead to the complete occlusion of circulation.
Perishing cold	The limb is cold to the touch.

3. Incidence

- Limb trauma is a common injury in high energy impacts. Causes can include but are not limited to falls, sports, traffic accidents, occupational and intentional causes, and can occur at any age.
- In older people injuries can occur from relatively minor trauma (e.g. falls from a standing height can lead to femoral fractures).

4. Severity and Outcome

- Severity and outcome differ depending on the nature of the injury. However, limb trauma can have serious consequences; for example, infection following an open fracture can affect the future viability and long-term function of the limb.

4.1. Splinting

- Splinting will contribute to 'circulation' care by reducing further blood loss and pain en-route to hospital.
- Traction splint – a device for applying longitudinal traction to the femur, using the pelvis and the ankle as static points. Correct splintage technique using a traction splint reduces:
  - pain
  - haemorrhage and damage to blood vessels and nerves
  - bone fragment movement and the risk of a closed fracture becoming an open fracture
  - the risk of fat embolisation (brain and lungs)
  - muscle spasm by pulling the thigh to a natural cylindrical shape
  - blood loss by compression of bleeding sites.
- Traction splints such as the Sager, Trac 3, Donway splints and Kendrick are easy to apply and some now have quantifiable traction, measured on a scale in pounds. The correct amount of traction is best judged by observing that the injured leg is the same length as the uninjured leg.

Table 4.3 – SPLINTING

INJURY	SPLINTAGE TYPE
Fractured neck of femur	Padding between legs. Figure of eight bandage around ankles. Broad bandage: two above, two below the knee.
Fractured shaft of femur	Traction splint or adjacent leg as a splint if the suspected fracture is above the knee. **NB** Fractures of the ankle, tibia, fibula, knee or pelvis on the same side as the femoral fracture may limit use of a traction splint; Trust guidelines should be followed.
Fracture or fracture dislocation around the knee	Vacuum splint. Box splint. Traction splint without the application of traction.
Patella dislocation	Companion strapping (one leg to the other). Support on pillow. Contoured vacuum splint. If the leg is gently straightened, the patella often spontaneously relocates; if resistance is felt, the leg should be splinted in the position of comfort.
Tibia/fibula shaft fracture	Vacuum splint. Box splint.
Ankle fracture	Vacuum splint. Box splint.
Foot fractures	Vacuum splint. Box splint.
Clavicle Humerus Radius Ulna	Self-splintage may be adequate and less painful than a sling. Sling. Vacuum splints may be well suited to immobilising forearm fractures, or a box splint.

5. Assessment and Management

For the assessment and management of limb trauma refer to Table 4.4.

Limb Trauma

Table 4.4 – ASSESSMENT and MANAGEMENT of:

Limb Trauma

ASSESSMENT	MANAGEMENT
● Assess **<C>ABCDE**	● Control any external catastrophic haemorrhage (refer to **Trauma Emergencies Overview**). ● If any of the following **TIME CRITICAL** features are present: – major **ABC** complications – haemodynamic instability (refer to **Intravascular Fluid Management**) – altered level of consciousness (refer to **Altered Level of Consciousness**) – neck and back injuries (refer to **Spinal Injury and Spinal Cord Injury**) – threatened limb – loss of neurovascular function (e.g. resulting from a dislocation that requires prompt realignment), then: ● Correct **ABC** complications. ● Mid shaft femoral fracture – apply a traction splint if this can be done quickly without delaying transfer, otherwise apply manual traction where sufficient personnel are available – once applied it should not be released. ● Undertake a **TIME CRITICAL** transfer to a major trauma centre, unless the patient needs an immediate lifesaving intervention, in which case transfer to nearest trauma unit. ● Provide a pre-alert using ATMIST. ● Continue patient management en-route.
● Specifically assess	● Ascertain the mechanism of injury and any factors indicating the forces involved (e.g. the pattern of fractures may indicate mechanism of injury): – fractures of the heel in a fall from a height may be accompanied by pelvic and spinal crush fractures (refer to **Major Pelvic Trauma** and **Spinal Injury and Spinal Cord Injury**) – 'dashboard' injury to the knee may be accompanied by a fracture or dislocation of the hip – humeral fractures from a side impact are associated with chest injuries (refer to **Thoracic Trauma**) – tibial fractures are rarely isolated injuries and are often associated with high energy trauma and other life-threatening injuries. ● Assess all four limbs for injury to long bones and joints – in suspected fracture, expose site(s) to assess swelling and deformity. ● Assess neurovascular function – MSC × 4: motor, sensation and circulation, distal to the fracture site. Assess foot pulses; palpate dorsalis pedis as capillary refill time can be misleading. ● Assess general skin colour. ● Assess age of patient – consider greenstick fractures in children, and fractures of wrist and hip in older people. ● For accompanying illnesses: – some cancers can involve bones (e.g. breast, lung and prostate) and result in fractures from minor injuries – osteoporosis in older females makes fractures more likely. **NB** Where possible avoid unnecessary pain stimulus.
● Oxygen	● Administer high levels of supplemental oxygen (aim for SpO_2 94–98%) (refer to **Oxygen**).
● Splintage	In pre-hospital care it is difficult to differentiate between ligament sprain and a fracture; therefore ASSUME a fracture and immobilise. ● Remove and document jewellery from the affected limbs before swelling occurs. ● Check and record the presence/absence of pulses, and muscle function distal to injury. ● Consider realignment of grossly deformed limbs to a position as close to normal anatomic alignment as possible. Where deformity is minor and both distal sensation and circulation are intact, then realignment may not be necessary. ● Apply splintage (refer to Table 4.3).

Limb Trauma *continued*	
• Compound fracture	• Gross contamination can be removed from wounds but do not irrigate open fractures of the long bones, hindfoot or midfoot in pre-hospital settings as it may force contamination deeper into the bone or tissue. • Apply a saline-soaked dressing and cover with an occlusive layer. • Any gross displacement from normal alignment must, where possible, be corrected, and splints applied (refer to Table 4.3). **NB** Document the nature of the contamination, as contaminates may be drawn inside following realignment.
• Amputations, partial amputations and degloving	• Do not irrigate grossly contaminated wounds with saline. • Immobilise a partially amputated limb in a position of normal anatomical alignment. • Where possible dress the injured limb to prevent further contamination. • Apply a saline-soaked dressing covered with an occlusive layer. **NB** Reimplantation following amputation or reconstruction following partial amputation may be possible. In order that the amputated parts are maintained and transported in the best condition possible: • remove any gross contamination • cover the part(s) with a moist field dressing • secure in a sealed plastic bag • place the bag on ice – do not place body parts in direct contact with ice as this can cause tissue damage; the aim is to keep the temperature low but not freezing.
• Neck of femur fractures	• Assess for shortening and external rotation of the leg on the injured side, with pain in the hip and referred pain in the knee. • Ascertain whether the patient has been on the floor for some time, assess for signs of hypothermia, dehydration, pressure ulcers and chest infection. • Monitor vital signs. • Immobilise by strapping the injured leg to the normal one with foam padding between the limbs – extra padding with blankets and strapping around the hips and pelvis can be used to provide additional support while moving the patient (refer to Table 4.3).
• Compartment syndrome	• Consider the need for rapid transfer to nearest appropriate hospital as per local trauma care pathway, as the patient may require immediate surgery; elevate limb and consider pain relief en-route.
• Pain management	• Pain management is an important intervention; if indicated, refer to **Pain Management in Adults** and **Pain Management in Children**.
• Fluid	• If fluid resuscitation is indicated, refer to **Intravascular Fluid Therapy (Adults)** and **Intravascular Fluid Therapy (Children)**. • **DO NOT** delay on scene for fluid replacement if peripheral pulses are present.
• Antibiotic	• Administer prophylactic intravenous antibiotic (in line with local guidance) as soon as possible and preferably within 1 hour of injury to patients with open fractures without delaying transport to hospital.
• Non-accidental injury	• When assessing an injury in a child, consider the possibility of non-accidental injury (refer to **Safeguarding Children**).
• Transfer to further care	• Transfer suspected open fractures of the long bone, hindfoot or midfoot directly to a major trauma centre or specialist centre for orthoplastic care. • Transfer suspected open fractures of the hand, wrist or toes to nearest trauma unit, unless there are pre-hospital triage indications for direct transport to a major trauma centre. • Continue patient management en-route. • Provide a pre-alert using ATMIST. • At the hospital, inform staff of: – any skin wound relating to a fracture – any underlying fracture(s) that was initially open. • Complete documentation.

Limb Trauma

KEY POINTS

Limb Trauma

- **Ensure <C>ABCDEs are assessed and managed; consider C-spine immobilisation.**
- **DO NOT become distracted by the appearance of limb trauma from assessing less visible but life-threatening problems, such as airway obstruction, compromised breathing, poor perfusion and spinal injury.**
- **Do not irrigate open fractures of the long bones, hindfoot or midfoot.**
- **Limb trauma can cause life-threatening haemorrhage.**
- **Assess for intact circulation and nerve function distal to the fracture site.**
- **Any dislocation that threatens the neurovascular status of a limb must be treated with urgency.**
- **Splintage is fundamental to prevention of further blood loss and can reduce pain.**
- **Limb trauma can cause considerable pain and distress – consider pain management as soon as clinically possible after arriving on scene.**
- **In cases of life-threatening trauma commence a TIME CRITICAL transfer and perform any splinting en-route if possible.**

Bibliography

1 National Institute for Health and Clinical Excellence. Fractures (Complex): Assessment and Management (NG37). London: NICE, 2016. Available from: https://www.nice.org.uk/guidance/ng37.

2 National Institute for Health and Clinical Excellence. Fractures (Non-complex): Assessment and Management (NG38). London: NICE, 2016. Available from: https://www.nice.org.uk/guidance/ng38.

3 National Institute for Health and Clinical Excellence. Major Trauma: Assessment and Initial Management (NG39). London: NICE, 2016. Available from: https://www.nice.org.uk/guidance/ng39.

4 National Institute for Health and Clinical Excellence. Major Trauma: Service Delivery (NG40). London: NICE, 2016. Available from: https://www.nice.org.uk/guidance/ng40.

5 National Institute for Health and Clinical Excellence. *Spinal Injury: Assessment and Initial Management* (NG41). London: NICE, 2016. Available from: https://www.nice.org.uk/guidance/ng41.

6 National Institute for Health and Clinical Excellence. *When to Suspect Child Maltreatment* (CG89). London: NICE, 2009. Available from: https://www.nice.org.uk/guidance/cg89.

7 Porter A, Snooks H, Youren A, Gaze S, Whitfield R, Rapport F et al. 'Covering our backs': ambulance crews' attitudes towards clinical documentation when emergency (999) patients are not conveyed to hospital. *Emergency Medicine Journal* 2008, 25(5): 292–295.

8 Antoniou D, Kyriakidis A, Zaharopoulos A, Moskoklaidis S. Degloving injury. *European Journal of Trauma* 2005, 31(6): 593–596.

9 Arnez ZM, Khan U, Tyler MPH. Classification of soft-tissue degloving in limb trauma. *Journal of Plastic, Reconstructive and Aesthetic Surgery* 2010, 63(11): 1865–1869.

10 Beekley AC, Sebesta JA, Blackbourne LH, Herbert GS, Kauvar DS, Baer DG, et al. Pre-hospital tourniquet use in Operation Iraqi Freedom: effect on hemorrhage control and outcomes. *Journal of Trauma* 2008, 64 (suppl. 2): S28–37; discussion S37.

11 Burns BJ, Sproule J, Smyth H. Acute compartment syndrome of the anterior thigh following quadriceps strain in a footballer. *British Journal of Sports Medicine* 2004, 38(2): 218–220.

12 Cooper C, Dennison FM, Leufkens HGM, Bishop N, van Staa TP. Epidemiology of childhood fractures in Britain: a study using the General Practice Research Database. *Journal of Bone and Mineral Research* 2004, 19(12): 976–981.

13 Daniels JM, Zook EG, Lynch JM. Hand and wrist injuries. Part II: Emergent evaluation. *American Family Physician* 2004, 69(8): 1949–1956.

14 Griffiths R, Alper J, Beckingsale A, Goldhill D, Heyburn G, Holloway J et al. Management of proximal femoral fractures 2011. *Anaesthesia* 2012, 67(1): 85–98.

15 Hodgetts TJ, Mahoney PF, Russell MQ, Byers M. ABC to <C>ABC: redefining the military trauma paradigm. *Emergency Medical Journal* 2006, 23(10): 745–746.

16 Jagdeep N, Durai N, Umraz K, Christopher M, Stephen B, Frances S et al. *Standards for the Management of Open Fractures of the Lower Limb.* London: British Association of Plastic Reconstructive and Aesthetic Surgeons, British Orthopaedic Association, 2009. Available from: http://www.bapras.org.uk/professionals/clinical-guidance/open-fractures-of-the-lower-limb.

17 Kaye JA, Jick H. Epidemiology of lower limb fractures in general practice in the United Kingdom. *Injury Prevention* 2004, 10(6): 368–374.

18 Klos K, Muckley T, Gras F, Hofmann GO, Schmidt R. Early posttraumatic rotationplasty after severe degloving and soft tissue avulsion injury: a case report. *Journal of Orthopaedic Trauma* 2010, 24(2): el–5.

19 Kragh JF Jr, Walters TJ, Baer DG, Fox CJ, Wade CE, Salinas J et al. Practical use of emergency tourniquets to stop bleeding in major limb trauma. *Journal of Trauma* 2008, 64 (suppl. 2): S38–49; discussion S49–50.

20 Lee C, Porter KM. Pre-hospital management of lower limb fractures. *Emergency Medicine Journal* 2005, 22(9): 660–663.

21 Lee C, Porter KM, Hodgetts TJ. Tourniquet use in the civilian pre-hospital setting. *Emergency Medicine Journal* 2007, 24(8): 584–587.

22 Lisle DA, Shepherd GJ, Cowderoy GA, O'Connell PT. MR imaging of traumatic and overuse injuries of the wrist and hand in athletes. *Magnetic Resonance Imaging Clinics of North America* 2009, 17(4): 639–654.

23 National Library of Medicine. *Fractures.* Available from: http://www.nlm.nih.gov/medlineplus/fractures.html, 2011.

24 Pearse MF, Harry L, Nanchahal J. Acute compartment syndrome of the leg. *British Medical Journal* 2002, 325(7364): 557–558.

25 Taxter AJ, Konstantakos EK, Ames DW. Lateral compartment syndrome of the lower extremity in a recreational athlete: a case report. *American Journal of Emergency Medicine* 2008, 26(8): 973.el–2.

26 van Staa TP, Dennison EM, Leufkens HGM, Cooper C. Epidemiology of fractures in England and Wales. *Bone* 2001, 29(6): 517–522.

27 Weinmann M. Compartment syndrome. *Emergency Medical Services* 2003, 32(9): 36.

28 Wood SP, Vrahas M, Wedel SK. Femur fracture immobilization with traction splints in multisystem trauma patients. *Pre-hospital Emergency Care* 2003, 7(2): 241–243.

29 British Orthopaedic Association, British Association of Plastic Reconstructive and Aesthetic Surgeons. *The Management of Severe Open Lower Limb Fractures.* Available from: http://www.boa.ac.uk, 2009.

30 Melamed E, Blumenfeld A, Kalmovich B, Kosashvili Y, Lin G, Israel Defense Forces Medical Corps Consensus Group on Pre-hospital Care of Orthopedic Injuries. Pre-hospital care of orthopedic injuries. *Pre-hospital Disaster Medicine* 2007, 22(1): 22–25.

31 Bragg S. Avulsion amputation of the hand. *Journal of Emergency Nursing* 2005, 31(3): 282.

32 Bragg S. The boxers' fracture. *Journal of Emergency Nursing* 2005, 31(5): 473.

33 Bragg S. Vertical deceleration: falls from height. *Journal of Emergency Nursing* 2007, 33(4): 377–378.

Spinal Injury and Spinal Cord Injury

1. Introduction

- In the major trauma patient, spinal injuries are common. The majority are stable; some are unstable, risking spinal cord damage, and a small number are associated with spinal cord injury at the outset. Differentiation between stable and unstable injuries requires specific imaging in the ED.
- Effective management from the time of injury is important to ensure optimal outcomes. This guideline provides guidance for the assessment and initial management of cervical spine and spinal trauma, including indicators to guidance for related conditions.

2. Pathophysiology

- The spinal cord runs in the spinal canal down to the level of the second lumbar vertebra in adults.
- The amount of space in the spinal canal in the upper neck is relatively large, and risk of secondary injury in this area can be reduced if adequate immobilisation is applied. In the thoracic area the cord is wide and the spinal canal relatively narrow; injury in this area is more likely to completely disrupt and damage the spinal cord.
- Spinal shock is a state of complete loss of motor function and often sensory function found sometimes after SCI. This immediate reaction may go on for some considerable time, but some recovery may well be possible. Complete and incomplete cord injury cannot be distinguished in the presence of spinal shock.
- Neurogenic shock is the state of poor tissue perfusion caused by sympathetic tone loss after spinal cord injury.

3. Incidence

- Falls are a frequent cause of SCI in the older person. Maintain a high index of suspicion in cases of older people who have had low energy falls.
- SCI affects young and fit people and will continue to affect them to a varying degree for the rest of their lives.
- Road traffic collisions, falls and sporting injuries are the most common causes of SCI – as a group, motorcyclists occupy more spinal injury unit beds than any other group involved in road traffic collisions. Rollover road traffic collisions where occupants are not wearing seatbelts, and the head comes into contact with the vehicle body, and pedestrians struck by vehicles are likely to suffer SCI. Ejection from a vehicle increases the risk of injury significantly.
- UK Trauma Audit Research Network (TARN) data has shown that, in the presence of a cervical bony injury, 13.4% of patients have associated injuries elsewhere in the thoracic and lumbar spine.

3.1. Risk Factors

- Road traffic collisions (RTC):
  - rollover RTC
  - non-wearing of seatbelts
  - ejection from vehicle
  - struck by a vehicle.
- Sporting injuries:
  - diving into shallow water
  - horse riding
  - rugby
  - gymnastics and trampolining.
- Falls:
  - older people.
  - rheumatoid arthritis.
- Violent attacks and domestic incidents
- Certain sporting accidents, especially diving into shallow water, horse riding; rugby, gymnastics and trampolining have a higher than average risk of SCI. Rapid deceleration injury such as gliding and light aircraft accidents also increase the risk of SCI.
- Older people and those with rheumatoid arthritis are prone to odontoid peg fractures that may be difficult to detect clinically. Such injuries can occur from relatively minor trauma (e.g. falls from a standing height).

3.2. Cauda Equina Syndrome (CES)

- Cauda equina syndrome is caused by compression of the nerves in the spinal canal below the end of the spinal cord (at L2 vertebra level). It can occur in patients with trauma, a herniated disc, chronic or acute low back pain, and patients with tumours or infection.
- Clinical diagnosis of CES is not easy. Most cases are of sudden onset and progress rapidly within hours or days. However, CES can evolve slowly and patients do not always complain of pain. Roughly 50–70% of patients have urinary retention on presentation.
- CES is an acute surgical emergency; early diagnosis is essential and the patient requires immediate conveyance to hospital for investigation if CES is suspected. Early surgical decompression is crucial to prevent permanent neurological damage.

Red flag signs and symptoms of CES

- Loss of bladder and/or bowel dysfunction control, causing incontinence.
- Reduced sensation in the saddle (perineal) area.
- New onset sexual dysfunction.
- Neurological deficit in the lower limb (motor/sensory loss, reflex changes).

4. Severity and Outcome

- Injury most frequently occurs at the junctions of mobile and fixed sections of the spine. Hence fractures are more commonly seen in the lower cervical vertebrae, where the cervical and thoracic spine meets (C5, 6, 7/T1 area), and the thoracolumbar junction. Of patients with one identified spinal fracture, 10–15% will be found to have another.

- In the extreme, SCI may prove immediately fatal where the upper cervical cord is damaged, paralysing the diaphragm and respiratory muscles.
- Partial cord damage, however, may solely affect individual sensory or motor nerve tracts producing varying long-term disability. It is important to note that there is an increasing percentage of cases where the cord damage is only partial and quality recovery is possible, providing the condition is recognised and managed appropriately.

5. Immobilisation

- All patients with the possibility of spinal injury should have manual immobilisation commenced at the earliest time, while initial assessment is undertaken.
- If immobilisation is indicated then the whole spine must be immobilised. There are differences between the types of semi-rigid collar; acceptable methods of immobilisation are:
  - manual immobilisation while the spine is supported
  - collar, head blocks and spinal support.

The following techniques may be used:

- Patient lying supine:
  - Use a scoop stretcher and cervical spine immobilisation. To minimise movement of the spine, utilise a 10-degree tilt to the left and right.
  - Patients should be transported on the scoop stretcher unless there is a prolonged journey time, when a vacuum mattress should be utilised.
  - To utilise the vacuum mattress, lift the patient using the scoop stretcher, then insert the mattress underneath and remove the scoop stretcher.
- Patient lying prone:
  - Log roll the patient with manual immobilisation of the cervical spine to enable a scoop stretcher to be used.
  - Perform a 2-stage log roll onto a vacuum mattress.
- Patient requiring extrication:
  - Extrication devices should be used if there is any risk of rotational movement.
  - Rearward extrication on an extrication board.
  - Side extrication invariably involves some rotational component and therefore has higher risks in many circumstances.

NB The longboard should only be used as an extrication device. Do not transport patients to hospital on a longboard.

5.1. Extrication

- Consider asking a patient who is not physically trapped to self-extricate, providing they have none of the following:
  - significant distracting injuries
  - abnormal neurological symptoms (paraesthesia or weakness or numbness)
  - spinal pain or tenderness.
- Explain to a patient who is self-extricating that they should stop moving and wait to be moved if they develop any spinal pain, numbness, tingling or weakness.
- When a patient has self-extricated:
  - ask them to lay supine on a stretcher positioned adjacent to the vehicle or incident
  - assess them further for any signs of spinal injury, spinal tenderness or abnormal neurology in the ambulance.
- **Inviting a patient to self-extricate is not clearing the cervical spine.**
- Any patient who has not had a cervical spine clearance documented in the ambulance clinician's notes should be treated as an uncleared spine whether immobilised or not, and that information must be specifically relayed to staff on handover.

Emergency Extrication

- If there is an immediate threat to a patient's life and rapid extrication is needed, make all efforts to limit spinal movement without delaying treatment.

5.2. Cautions/Precautions

Vomiting

- Vomiting and consequent aspiration are serious consequences of immobilisation. Ambulance clinicians must always have a plan of action in case vomiting should occur.
- The collar will usually need to be removed and manual in-line immobilisation instituted. This may include:
  - suction
  - head-down tilt of the immobilisation device
  - rolling the patient onto one side on the immobilisation device.

Restless/Combative Patients

- There are many reasons for the patient to be restless and it is important to rule out reversible causes (e.g. hypoxia, pain, fear).
- If, despite appropriate measures, the patient remains restless, the use of spinal immobilisation devices may be difficult and could be counterproductive. A struggling patient is more likely to increase any injury, so think about letting them find a position where they are comfortable with manual in-line spinal immobilisation.
- The use of restraint can increase forces on the injured spine and therefore a 'best possible' approach should be adopted.

Head Injury

- Patients with a head injury may have raised intracranial pressure, which restraint can increase; therefore a 'best possible' approach should be adopted.

Special Cases

- Some older patients, and those with known spinal deformities (e.g. ankylosing spondylitis), may not be able to tolerate a collar or breathe adequately when positioned absolutely flat. Therefore a 'best possible' approach should be adopted, which may include manual in-line immobilisation or maintenance of the pre-existing spinal deformity where putting the patient in the in-line neutral position is unsafe.

Immobilisation of Spinal Injuries

- Soft collars do not limit movement and should not be used.
- There is variable difference between the various types of semi-rigid collars.
- The addition of head blocks and tape increases immobilisation.
- The application of devices is more important than the variation of devices.
- To achieve neutral position in an adult, the occupit should be raised by 2cm.
- Extrication devices are better than extrication boards at reducing rotational movement.
- Vacuum mattresses are more comfortable, and give better immobilisation.
- Vacuum mattresses cannot be used for extrication and are vulnerable to damage.
- Long extrication/spinal boards should only be used as an extrication device. Patients should be immobilised using a scoop stretcher. Once on a scoop stretcher they should remain on it unless they are placed on a vacuum mattress when there is a prolonged journey time.

5.3. When Not to Apply Immobilisation

- Not all patients require immobilisation (refer to Figure 4.1). When assessing for spinal injury, it is important to consider whether the patient:
  - is under the influence of drugs or alcohol
  - is uncooperative or confused
  - has any bony spinal pain anywhere along the spine
  - has any significant distracting injuries
  - has a reduced level of consciousness
  - has a priapism (unconscious or exposed male)
  - has any foot or hand weakness (motor assessment)
  - has any absent or altered sensation in the limbs (sensory assessment)
  - has a history of past spinal problems, including previous spinal surgery or conditions that predispose to instability of the spine.
- If the assessment cannot be completed or **any of the above factors are present**, carry out full in-line immobilisation.
- Penetrating injury to the head has not been shown to be an indication for spinal immobilisation, and even penetrating injuries of the neck only rarely need selective immobilisation.
- The few patients missed with SCI are often at the extremes of age. Such criteria can be reproducibly used in the pre-hospital environment. Mechanism of injury was not shown to be an independent predictor of injury.
- Use of such guidelines can significantly reduce the use of unnecessary immobilisation.
- Some patients may sustain thoracic or lumbar injuries in addition to, or in isolation from, cervical spine injuries. If you suspect thoracic or lumbar injuries, whether the cervical spine has been cleared, then full spinal immobilisation should be undertaken whenever possible.

5.4. Hazards of Immobilisation

- The value of routine pre-hospital spinal immobilisation remains uncertain and any benefits may be outweighed by the risks of rigid collar immobilisation, including:
  - compromised airway
  - increased intracranial pressure
  - increased risk of aspiration
  - restricted ventilation
  - dysphagia
  - skin ulceration
  - inducement of pain, even in those with no injury
  - known spinal deformities.

5.5. Sequence for Immobilisation

- All patients should be initially immobilised if the mechanism of injury suggests the possibility of SCI.

Blunt Trauma

- Following assessment, it is possible to remove the immobilisation if ALL the criteria are met (refer to Figure 4.1).
- Spinal pain does not include tenderness isolated to the muscles of the side of the neck.

Penetrating Trauma

- Those with isolated penetrating injuries to limbs or the head do not require immobilisation.
- Those with truncal or neck trauma should be immobilised if there is new neurology and/or the trajectory of the penetrating wound could pass near or through the spinal column.

5.6. Immobilisation of Children

- When carrying out in-line spinal immobilisation in children, manually stabilise the head with the spine in-line and consider the following:
  - If appropriate, involve family members and carers.
  - If possible, keep infants in their car seats.
  - Use a scoop stretcher with blanket rolls, vacuum mattress, vacuum limb splints or Kendrick extrication device.

6. Assessment and Management

For assessment and management of the cervical spine and spine, refer to Table 4.5 and Figure 4.1.

Spinal Injury and Spinal Cord Injury

Table 4.5 – ASSESSMENT and MANAGEMENT of:

Cervical Spine and Spinal Trauma

ASSESSMENT	MANAGEMENT
• Assess **<C>ABCDE** while controlling the spine	• Control any external catastrophic haemorrhage (refer to **Trauma Emergencies Overview (Adults)** and **Trauma Emergencies Overview (Children)**). • At all stages of the assessment protect the patient's cervical spine with manual in-line immobilisation, and avoid moving the remainder of the spine.
• Evaluate whether the patient is **TIME CRITICAL**	• Follow criteria in Trauma Emergencies Overview. • If the patient is **TIME CRITICAL**: – manage the airway – immobilise the spine – transfer to a major trauma centre; unless the patient needs an immediate lifesaving intervention, transfer to nearest trauma unit – provide a pre-alert using ATMIST – continue patient management en-route (see below).
• Assess oxygen saturation (refer to **Oxygen**)	• Adults – administer high levels of supplemental oxygen and aim for target saturation within the range of 94–98% – except for patients with COPD. • Children – administer high levels of supplemental oxygen.
• Determine mechanism of injury	• Forces causing injury include: – hyperflexion – hyperextension – rotation – compression – one or more of these.
• Specific symptoms of SCI	• The patient may complain of: – cervical and/or spinal pain – loss of sensory function in the limbs – loss of motor function in the limbs – sensation of burning in the trunk or limbs – sensation of electric shock in the trunk or limbs.
• Rapidly assess to determine the presence and estimate the level of spinal cord injury	• The following signs may indicate injury: – diaphragmatic or abdominal breathing – hypotension (BP often <80–90 mmHg) with bradycardia – warm peripheries or vasodilatation in the presence of low blood pressure – flaccid (floppy) muscles with absent reflexes – priapism – partial or full erection of the penis. • In a conscious patient – assess sensory and motor function: – use light touch and response to pain – examine upper limbs and hands – examine lower limbs and feet – examine both sides – undertake the examination in the MID-AXILLARY line, NOT the MID-CLAVICULAR line, as C2, C3 and C4 all supply sensation to the nipple line; use the forehead as the reference point to guide what is normal sensation. **NB** Always presume a SCI in the unconscious trauma patient.
• If the patient is non-time critical, perform a more thorough assessment with a brief secondary survey	

Cervical Spine and Spinal Trauma *continued*	
• Assess for neurogenic shock	• Diagnosis is difficult in pre-hospital care – the aim is to: – maintain blood pressure of approximately 90 mmHg systolic – obtain IV access – determine the need for fluid replacement but DO NOT delay on scene (refer to **Intravascular Fluid Therapy (Adults)** and **Intravascular Fluid Therapy (Children)**). • In neurogenic shock, a few degrees of head-down tilt may improve the circulation, but remember that in cases of abdominal breathing, this manoeuvre may further worsen respiration and ventilation. This position is also unsuitable for a patient who has, or may have, a head injury. • If bradycardia is present consider atropine (refer to **Atropine**) – but it is important to rule out other causes (e.g. hypoxia, severe hypovolaemia).
• Assess the need for assisted ventilation	• Refer to **Airway and Breathing Management**.
• Steroids	• Steroids have no part to play in the pre-hospital management of acute spinal cord injuries.
• At hospital	• The patient should be on a scoop stretcher. • Complete documentation and, if possible, record information whether the assessments show that the patient's condition is improving or deteriorating.
• Additional Information	• Transportation of spinal patients: – Driving should balance the advantages of smooth driving and time to arrival at hospital. No immobilisation technique eliminates movement from vehicle swaying and jarring. – There is no evidence to show advantage of direct transport to a spinal injury centre. – Patients should be transported on the scoop stretcher unless there is a prolonged journey time, when a vacuum mattress should be utilised. – As half of all cases of spinal injuries have other serious injuries, any unnecessary delay at the scene or in transit should be avoided.

KEY POINTS

Spinal Injury

- **Immobilise the whole spine until it is positively cleared.**
- **Immobilise the whole spine in all unconscious blunt trauma patients.**
- **If the cervical spine is immobilised, the thoracic and lumbar spine also needs immobilisation.**
- **Asking a patient to self-extricate is acceptable, but does not clear the cervical spine.**
- **Standard immobilisation is by means of collar (unless contra-indicated or counterproductive), head blocks, tape and scoop.**
- **The longboard is solely used as an extrication device, and not for transporting patients to hospital.**
- **Aspiration of vomit, pressure sores and raised intracranial pressure are major complications of immobilisation.**

Bibliography

1 National Institute for Health and Clinical Excellence. Fractures (Complex): Assessment and Management (NG37). London: NICE, 2016. Available from: https://www.nice.org.uk/guidance/ng37.

2 National Institute for Health and Clinical Excellence. Fractures (Non-complex): Assessment and Management (NG38). London: NICE, 2016. Available from: https://www.nice.org.uk/guidance/ng38.

3 National Institute for Health and Clinical Excellence. Major Trauma: Assessment and Initial Management (NG39). London: NICE, 2016. Available from: https://www.nice.org.uk/guidance/ng39.

4 National Institute for Health and Clinical Excellence. Major Trauma: Service Delivery (NG40). London: NICE, 2016. Available from: https://www.nice.org.uk/guidance/ng40.

5 National Institute for Health and Clinical Excellence. *Spinal Injury: Assessment and Initial Management* (NG41). London: NICE, 2016. Available from: https://www.nice.org.uk/guidance/ng41.

6 Hoffman JR, Wolfson AB, Todd K, Mower WR. Selective cervical spine radiography in blunt trauma: methodology of the National Emergency X-Radiography Utilization Study (NEXUS). *Ann Emerg Med*. 1998, 32(4): 461–469.

7 Canadian CT Head and C-Spine (CCC) Study Group. Canadian C-Spine Rule study for alert and stable trauma patients: I. Background and rationale. *CJEM*. 2004, 4(2): 84–90.

8 Trauma Audit and Research Network. *Major Trauma in Older People*. Manchester: University of Manchester, 2017.

Spinal Injury and Spinal Cord Injury

Patients with a history of trauma
Is there a potential for spinal injury in an adult >16 years old?

Yes ↓

- Under the influence of drugs or alcohol?
- Is confused or uncooperative?
- Has a reduced level of consciousness?
- Has any spinal pain (or pain elicited on coughing)?
- Any motor weakness in hands or feet?
- Any history of past spinal problems, including previous spinal surgery, severe osteoarthritis, ankylosing spondylitis?
- Any priapism?

Yes → IMMOBILISE

No ↓

High Risk?

- Dangerous mechanism of injury (fall from a height of >1 metre or five steps, axial load to the head - e.g. diving, high-speed motor vehicle collision, rollover motor accident, ejection from a motor vehicle, accident involving motorised recreational vehicles, bicycle collision, horse riding accidents)

Yes → IMMOBILISE

No ↓

Upon Examination:

- Any abnormal neurology (loss of sensation; numbness; 'pins and needles'; burning pain)?
- Any bony spinal pain anywhere along the spine (at rest or on coughing)?
- Any distracting injury?

Yes → IMMOBILISE

No ↓

Low Risk?

- Was involved in a minor rear-end motor vehicle collision
- Is comfortable in a sitting position
- Has been ambulatory at any time since the injury
- Has no midline cervical spine tenderness (answer 'no' if patient has pain)
- Delayed onset of neck pain

No → IMMOBILISE

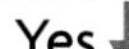

Yes ↓

Is the patient able to actively rotate their head 45° to the left and right?
and
Is the patient able to mobilise without pain or abnormal neurology?

No → IMMOBILISE

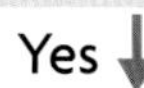

Yes ↓

Spine Cleared

Use of spinal immobilisation devices may be difficult (e.g. in people with short/wide necks, or people with a pre-existing deformity) and could be counterproductive (i.e. increasing pain, worsening neurological signs and symptoms). In uncooperative, agitated or distressed people, think about letting them find a position where they are comfortable with manual in-line spinal immobilisation.

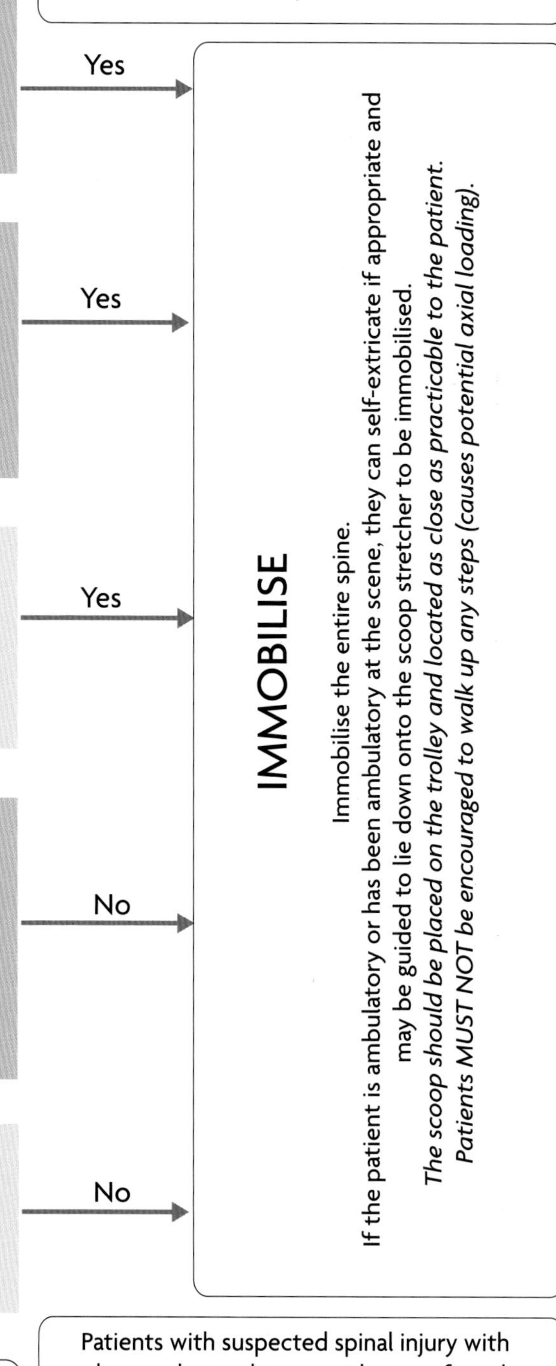

Patients with suspected spinal injury with abnormal neurology must be transferred to a Major Trauma Centre

Figure 4.1 – Immobilisation algorithm
Republished with permission of Yorkshire Ambulance Service.

Major Pelvic Trauma

1. Introduction

- Major pelvic injuries are predominantly observed where there is a high-energy transfer to the patient during road traffic collision, pedestrian accident, fall from height or crush injury.
- Less serious pelvic injuries may also occur in low-energy transfer events, particularly for the older people (for example, in a simple fall), amongst patients with degenerative bone disease or receiving radiotherapy, and rarely as a direct consequence of seizure activity.
- The majority of pelvic injuries do not result in major disruption of the pelvic ring, but rather involve fractures of the pubic ramus or acetabulum. Presentation of these injuries is very similar to neck of femur fractures; therefore refer to **Limb Trauma** for management of these less serious pelvic injuries.

Mechanism of Injury

- Blunt high-energy trauma.
- Fall from height.
- Crush injury.

Risk Factors

- Advancing age.
- Degenerative bone disease.
- Radiotherapy.

2. Incidence

- Pelvic fractures represent 3–6% of all fractures in adults, and occur in up to 20% of all polytrauma cases. They display a bimodal distribution of age with most injuries occurring in the age ranges 15–30 and over 60 years; up to 75% of all pelvic injuries occur in men.
- Unstable pelvic fracture is estimated to occur in up to 20% of pelvic fractures; a further 22% of pelvic fractures will remain stable despite significant damage to the pelvic ring. The remaining 58% of pelvic fractures are less serious retaining both haemodynamic and structural stability.
- The incidence of pelvic fracture resulting from blunt trauma ranges from 5–11.9%, with obese patients more likely to sustain a pelvic fracture from blunt trauma than non-obese patients. Pelvic fracture associated with penetrating trauma is far less frequent. Open pelvic fractures are rare and account for only 2.7–4% of all pelvic fractures.

3. Severity and Outcome

- Major pelvic injuries can be devastating and are often associated with a number of complications that may require extensive rehabilitation. Pelvic trauma deaths frequently occur as a result of associated injuries and complications rather than the pelvic injury itself.
- Haemorrhage is the cause of death in 40% of all pelvic trauma victims and the leading cause of death (60% of fatal cases) in unstable pelvic fracture. Bleeding is usually retroperitoneal; the volume of blood loss correlates with the degree and type of pelvic disruption.
- Reported mortality rates range from 6.4–30% depending on the type of pelvic fracture, haemodynamic status, the nature of concomitant injuries and their complications.
- The mortality rate among haemodynamically stable patients is around 10%, whereas the mortality rate amongst haemodynamically unstable patients approaches 20–30% but has been reported to be as high as 50% in cases of unstable open fracture; combined mortality approaches 16%.

4. Pathophysiology

4.1 Skeletal Anatomy

- Increasing pelvic volume allows for increased haemorrhage; conversely, reducing pelvic volume reduces potential for bleeding by realignment of broken bone ends.

4.2 Classification of Injury

- As with other fractures, pelvic fractures may be classified as open or closed, and benefit from being further described as either haemodynamically stable or unstable. Patients who are haemodynamically unstable are at greater risk of death and would benefit greatly from a pre-hospital alert message.
- Pelvic ring disruptions (as identified by in-hospital imaging) can be subdivided into four classes by mechanism of injury:
  - Antero-posterior compression (APC).
  - Lateral compression (LC).
  - Vertical shear (VS).
  - Combined mechanical injury (CMI), a combination of the aforementioned classes.

4.3 Vascular Injury

- The arteries most frequently injured are the iliolumbar arteries, the superior gluteal and the internal pudendal because of their proximity to the bone, the sacro-iliac joint and the inferior ligaments of the pelvis. Bleeding from the venous network after a pelvic fracture is more frequent than arterial bleeding because the walls of the veins are more fragile than arteries. Blood may pool in the retroperitoneal space and haemostasis may occur spontaneously in closed fractures, especially if there is no concomitant arterial haemorrhage.

4.4 Other Injuries

- The incidence of urogenital injury ranges from 23–57%. Urethral and vaginal injuries are the most common injuries. Vaginal lacerations result from either penetration of a bony fragment or from indirect forces from diastasis of the symphysis pubis. Injuries to the cervix, uterus and ovaries are rare. Bladder rupture occurs in up to 10% of pelvic fractures.

Major Pelvic Trauma

- The incidence of rectal injury ranges from 17–64% dependent upon type of fracture. Bowel entrapment is rare.
- Pelvic injury is commonly associated with concomitant intra-thoracic and/or intra-abdominal injury.

Table 4.6 – ASSESSMENT and MANAGEMENT of:

Major Pelvic Trauma

ASSESSMENT

- Assess <C>ABCDE; <C> catastrophic haemorrhage:
  - Airway
  - Breathing
  - Circulation
  - Disability
  - Exposure and environment
- Evaluate whether patient is **TIME CRITICAL** or **NON-TIME CRITICAL** following criteria as per trauma emergencies guideline. If patient is **TIME CRITICAL**, correct **<C>ABC** problems, stabilise the pelvis on scene and rapidly transport to a major trauma centre, unless the patient needs an immediate lifesaving intervention, in which case transfer to nearest trauma unit. Provide a pre-alert using ATMIST. En-route, continue patient management of pelvic trauma (see below).
- In **NON-TIME CRITICAL** patients perform a more thorough patient assessment with a secondary survey.

Specifically consider:

- Any patient following blunt high-energy trauma and haemodynamic instability must be managed as having a time critical pelvic injury until proven otherwise.
- Clinical assessment of the pelvis includes observation for physical injury such as bruising, bleeding, deformity or swelling to the pelvis. Shortening of a lower limb may be present (refer to **Limb Trauma**)
- Assessment by compression or distraction (e.g. springing) of the pelvis is unreliable and should not be performed, as it may both dislodge clots and exacerbate any injury.

MANAGEMENT

- Control any external catastrophic haemorrhage (refer to **Trauma Emergencies Overview (Adults)** and **Trauma Emergencies Overview (Children)**).

Oxygen Therapy

- Major pelvic injury falls into the category of critical illness and requires high levels of supplemental oxygen regardless of any initial oxygen saturation reading (SpO2). Maintain high flow oxygen (15 litres per minute) until vital signs are normal; thereafter reduce flow rate, titrating to maintain oxygen saturations (SpO2) in the 94–98% range (refer to **Oxygen**).
- Use intravenous tranexamic acid as soon as possible with active or suspected active bleeding from a pelvic fracture.

Pelvic Stabilisation

- If active bleeding is suspected from a pelvic fracture following blunt high-energy trauma:
  - apply a purpose-made pelvic binder, or
  - consider an improvised pelvic binder but only if a purpose-made binder does not fit.
- There is currently no evidence to suggest that any particular pelvic immobilisation device or approach is superior in terms of outcome in pelvic trauma and a number of methods have been reported. Effective stabilisation of the pelvic ring should be instigated at the earliest possible opportunity, preferably before moving the patient, and may be achieved by the following means:
  - Expert consensus suggests the use of an appropriate pelvic splint is preferable to improvised immobilisation techniques. In all methods, circumferential pressure is applied over the greater trochanters and not the iliac crests. Care must be exercised to ensure that the pelvis is not reduced beyond its normal anatomical position.
  - Apply the pelvic splint directly to the skin, if this can be done easily with minimal handling.
  - Reduction and stabilisation of the pelvic ring should occur as soon as is practicable while still on scene, as stabilisation helps to reduce blood loss by realigning fracture surfaces, thereby limiting active bleeding and additionally helping to stabilise clots. Reduction of the pelvis may have a tamponade effect, particularly for venous bleeding; however, there is little evidence to support this belief.
  - Pressure sores and soft tissue injuries may occur when immobilisation devices are incorrectly fitted.
  - Log rolling of the patient with possible pelvic fracture should be avoided as this may exacerbate any pelvic injury; utilise an orthopaedic scoop stretcher to lift patients off the ground and limit movement to a 10-degree tilt.

Fluid therapy

- There is little evidence to support the routine use of IV fluids in adult trauma patients (refer to **Intravascular Fluid Therapy (Adults)** and **Intravascular Fluid Therapy (Children)**).

Pain management

- Patients' pain should be managed appropriately refer to **Pain Management in Adults** and **Pain Management in Children**); analgesia in the form of entonox (refer to **Entonox**) or morphine sulphate may be appropriate (refer to **Morphine**).
- Use IV paracetamol as the first-line analgesic and morphine if further analgesia is required refer to **Pain Management in Adults** and **Pain Management in Children**).

5. Referral Pathway

- The following cases should **ALWAYS** be transferred to further care:
  - Any patient with hypotension and potential pelvic injury MUST be treated as a TIME CRITICAL pelvic injury until proven otherwise.
  - Any patient following blunt high-energy trauma to cause a pelvic injury.
- There are **NO** cases that may be considered suitable/safe to be left at home.

6. Special Considerations for Children

Refer to **Trauma Emergencies Overview (Children)**.

- Pelvic fractures represent 1–3% of all fractures in children, thus there is a lower incidence compared with adults.
- In children, pelvic injuries have a lower mortality accounting for 3.6–5.7% of trauma deaths, with fewer deaths occurring as a direct result of pelvic haemorrhage; blood loss is more likely to be from solid visceral injury than the pelvis.
- Children have different injury patterns – multi-system injuries occur in 60%; there is greater incidence of diaphragmatic injury.
- Principles of management are the same, with the exception of fluid and oxygen therapy (refer to **Intravascular Fluid Therapy** and **Oxygen**).
- Clinical findings in small children can be unreliable.
- Consider an improvised pelvic binder in children with suspected pelvic fractures following blunt high-energy trauma and haemodynamic instability if they are too small to fit a purpose-made pelvic binder.

7. Audit Information

- Incidence of suspected/actual pelvic fracture.
- Incidence of concomitant hypotension.
- Frequency of pelvic immobilisation when pelvic fracture is suspected.
- Method of pelvic immobilisation.

KEY POINTS

Major Pelvic Trauma

- **Always suspect a pelvic fracture in a blunt high-energy trauma.**
- **The majority of pelvic fractures are stable pubic ramus or acetabular fractures.**
- **Any patient with hypotension and a potentially relevant mechanism of injury MUST be considered to have a TIME CRITICAL pelvic injury and rapidly transported to a major trauma centre.**
- **'Springing' or distraction of the pelvis must not be undertaken.**
- **Pelvic stabilisation should be implemented as soon as is practicable while still on scene.**
- **Consider appropriate pain management.**
- **The use of a scoop stretcher is recommended to avoid log rolling the patient unless extrication is required.**

SECTION 4 Trauma

Bibliography

1 National Institute for Health and Clinical Excellence. Fractures (Complex): Assessment and Management (NG37). London: NICE, 2016. Available from: https://www.nice.org.uk/guidance/ng37.

2 National Institute for Health and Clinical Excellence. Fractures (Non-complex): Assessment and Management (NG38). London: NICE, 2016. Available from: https://www.nice.org.uk/guidance/ng38.

3 National Institute for Health and Clinical Excellence. Major Trauma: Assessment and Initial Management (NG39). London: NICE, 2016. Available from: https://www.nice.org.uk/guidance/ng39.

4 National Institute for Health and Clinical Excellence. Major Trauma: Service Delivery (NG40). London: NICE, 2016. Available from: https://www.nice.org.uk/guidance/ng40.

5 National Institute for Health and Clinical Excellence. *Spinal Injury: Assessment and Initial Management* (NG41). London: NICE, 2016. Available from: https://www.nice.org.uk/guidance/ng41.

6 Brown JK, Jing Y, Wang S, Ehrlich PF. Patterns of severe injury in pediatric car crash victims: Crash Injury Research Engineering Network database. *Journal of Pediatric Surgery* 2006, 41(2): 362–367.

7 O'Brien DP, Luchette FA, Pereira SJ, Lim E, Seeskin CS, James L, et al. Pelvic fracture in the elderly is associated with increased mortality. *Surgery* 2002, 132(4): 710–714.

8 Stein DM, O'Connor JV, Kufera JA, Ho SM, Dischinger PC, Copeland CE et al. Risk factors associated with pelvic fractures sustained in motor vehicle collisions involving newer vehicles. *Journal of Trauma* 2006, 61(1): 21–30.

9 Demetriades D, Karaiskakis M, Toutouzas K, Alo K, Velmahos G, Chan L. Pelvic fractures: epidemiology and predictors of associated abdominal injuries and outcomes. *Journal of the American College of Surgeons* 2002, 195(1): 1–10.

10 Demetriades D, Murray J, Brown C, Velmahos G, Salim A, Alo K et al. High-level falls: type and severity of injuries and survival outcome according to age. *Journal of Trauma* 2005, 58(2): 342–345.

11 Gustavo Parreira J, Coimbra R, Rasslan S, Oliveira A, Fregoneze M, Mercadante M. The role of associated injuries on outcome of blunt trauma patients sustaining pelvic fractures. *Injury* 2000, 31(9): 677–682.

12 Inaba K, Sharkey PW, Stephen DJG, Redelmeier DA, Brenneman FD. The increasing incidence of severe pelvic injury in motor vehicle collisions. *Injury* 2004, 35(8): 759–765.

13 Kimbrell BJ, Velmahos GC, Chan LS, Demetriades D. Angiographic embolization for pelvic fractures in older patients. *Archives of Surgery* 2004, 139(7): 728–732.

14 Tarman GJ, Kaplan GW, Lerman SL, McAleer IM, Losasso BE. Lower genitourinary injury and pelvic fractures in pediatric patients. *Urology* 2002, 59(1): 123–126.

15 Demetriades D, Murray J, Martin M, Velmahos G, Salim A, Alo K et al. Pedestrians injured by automobiles: relationship of age to injury type and severity. *Journal of the American College of Surgeons* 2004, 199(3): 382–387.

16 Hill RMF, Robinson CM, Keating JF. Fractures of the pubic rami. *Journal of Bone & Joint Surgery, British Volume* 2001, 83-B(8): 1141–1144.

17 Baxter NN, Habermann EB, Tepper JE, Durham SB, Virnig BA. Risk of pelvic fractures in older women following pelvic irradiation. Journal *of the American Medical Association* 2005, 294(20): 2587–2593.

18 Boufous S, Finch C, Lord S, Close J. The increasing burden of pelvic fractures in older people, New South Wales, Australia. *Injury* 2005, 36(11): 1323–1329.

19 Hauschild O, Strohm PC, Culemann U, Pohlemann T, Suedkamp NP, Koestler W et al. Mortality in patients with pelvic fractures: results from the German pelvic injury register. *Journal of Trauma* 2008, 64(2): 449–455.

20 Croce MA, Magnotti LJ, Savage SA, Wood IGW, Fabian TC. Emergent pelvic fixation in patients with exsanguinating pelvic fractures. *Journal of the American College of Surgeons* 2007, 204(5): 935–939.

21 Duane TM, Tan BB, Golay D, Cole FJ Jr, Weireter LJ Jr, Britt LD. Blunt trauma and the role of routine pelvic radiographs: a prospective analysis. *Journal of Trauma* 2002, 53(3): 463–468.

22 Gonzalez RP, Fried PQ, Bukhalo M. The utility of clinical examination in screening for pelvic fractures in blunt trauma. *Journal of the American College of Surgeons* 2002, 194(2): 121–125.

23 Tien IY, Dufel SE. Does ethanol affect the reliability of pelvic bone examination in blunt trauma? *Annals of Emergency Medicine* 2000, 36(5): 451–455.

24 Heetveld MJ, Harris I, Schlaphoff G, Balogh Z, D'Amours SK, Sugrue M. Hemodynamically unstable pelvic fractures: recent care and new guidelines. *Journal of Surgery* 2004, 28(9): 904–909.

25 Heetveld MJ, Harris I, Schlaphoff G, Sugrue M. Guidelines for the management of haemodynamically unstable pelvic fracture patients. *ANZ Journal of Surgery* 2004, 74(7): 520–529.

26 Grotz MRW, Gummerson NW, Gansslen A, Petrowsky H, Keel M, Allami MK et al. Staged management and outcome of combined pelvic and liver trauma: an international experience of the deadly duo. *Injury* 2006, 37(7): 642–651.

27 Starr AJ, Griffen, MA. Pelvic ring disruptions: mechanisms, fracture pattern, morbidity and mortality. An analysis of 325 patients. OTA Annual Meeting, Texas, USA, 2000.

28 Sriussadaporn S. Abdominopelvic vascular injuries. *Journal of the Medical Association of Thailand* 2000, 83(1): 13–20.

29 Rowe SA, Sochor MS, Staples KS, Wahl WL, Wang SC. Pelvic ring fractures: implications of vehicle design, crash type, and occupant characteristics. *Surgery* 2004, 136(4): 842–847.

30 Dyer GSM, Vrahas MS. Review of the pathophysiology and acute management of haemorrhage in pelvic fracture. *Injury* 2006, 37(7): 602–613.

31 Bottlang M, Simpson T, Sigg J, Krieg JC, Madey SM, Long WB. Noninvasive reduction of open-book pelvic fractures by circumferential compression. *Journal of Orthopaedic Trauma* 2002, 16(6): 367–373.

32 Reiff DA, McGwin G Jr, Metzger J, Windham ST, Doss M, Rue LW III. Identifying injuries and motor vehicle collision characteristics that together are suggestive of diaphragmatic rupture. *Journal of Trauma* 2002, 53(6): 1139–1145.

33 Waydhas C, Nast-Kolb D, Ruchholtz S. Pelvic ring fractures: utility of clinical examination in patients with impaired consciousness or tracheal intubation. *European Journal of Trauma and Emergency Surgery* 2007, 33(2): 170–175.

34 Sauerland S, Bouillon B, Rixen D, Raum MR, Koy T, Neugebauer EAM. The reliability of clinical examination in detecting pelvic fractures in blunt trauma patients: a meta-analysis. *Archives of Orthopaedic and Trauma Surgery* 2004, 124(2): 123–128.

35 Lee C, Porter K. The pre-hospital management of pelvic fractures. *Emergency Medicine Journal* 2007, 24(2): 130–133.

36 Bottlang M, Krieg JC, Mohr M, Simpson TS, Madey SM. Emergent management of pelvic ring fractures with use of circumferential compression. *Journal of Orthopaedic Trauma* 2002, 16(6): 367–373.

37 Friese G, LaMay G. Emergency stabilization of unstable pelvic fractures. *Emergency Medical Services* 2005, 34(5): 65.

38 Jowett AJL, Bowyer GW. Pressure characteristics of pelvic binders. *Injury* 2007, 38(1): 118–121.

39 Katsoulis E, Drakoulakis E, Giannoudis PV. (iii) Management of open pelvic fractures. *Current Orthopaedics* 2005, 19(5): 345–353.

40 Krieg JC, Mohr M, Ellis TJ, Simpson TS, Madey SM, Bottlang M. Emergent stabilization of pelvic ring injuries by controlled circumferential compression: a clinical trial. *Journal of Trauma, Injury, Infection, & Critical Care* 2005, 59(3): 659–664.

41 Salomone JP, Ustin JS, McSwain NE Jr, Feliciano DV. Opinions of trauma practitioners regarding pre-hospital interventions for critically injured patients. *Journal of Trauma* 2005, 58(3): 509–515; discussion 515–517.

42 Simpson T, Krieg JC, Heuer F, Bottlang M. Stabilization of pelvic ring disruptions with a circumferential sheet. *Journal of Trauma, Injury, Infection, & Critical Care* 2002, 52(1): 158–161.

43 Nunn T, Cosker TDA, Bose D, Pallister I. Immediate application of improvised pelvic binder as first step in extended resuscitation from life-threatening hypovolaemic shock in conscious patients with unstable pelvic injuries. *Injury* 2007, 38(1): 125–128.

44 Krieg JC, Mohr M, Mirza AJ, Bottlang M. Pelvic circumferential compression in the presence of soft-tissue injuries: a case report. *Journal of Trauma, Injury, Infection, & Critical Care* 2005, 59(2): 470–472.

45 Junkins EPJ, Nelson DS, Carroll KL, Hansen K, Furnival RA. A prospective evaluation of the clinical presentation of pediatric pelvic fractures. *Journal of Trauma* 2001, 51(1): 64–68.

46 Silber JS, Flynn JM, Koffler KM, Dormans JP, Drummond DS. Analysis of the cause, classification, and associated injuries of 166 consecutive pediatric pelvic fractures. *Journal of Pediatric Orthopaedics* 2001, 21(4): 446–450.

47 Junkins EP, Furnival RA, Bake RG. The clinical presentation of pediatric pelvic fractures. *Pediatric Emergency Care* 2001, 17(1): 15–18.

Thoracic Trauma

1. Introduction

- In pre-hospital care, the most common problem associated with severe thoracic injuries is hypoxia, either from impaired ventilation or secondary to hypovolaemia from massive bleeding into the chest (haemothorax) or major vessel disruption (e.g. ruptured thoracic aorta).

2. Incidence

- Severe thoracic injuries are one of the most common causes of death from trauma, accounting for approximately 25% of such deaths.

3. Severity and Outcome

- Despite the very high percentage of serious thoracic injuries, the vast majority of them can be managed in hospital with chest drainage and resuscitation, and only 10–15% require surgical intervention.

4. Pathophysiology

- The mechanism of injury is an important guide to the likelihood of significant thoracic injuries. Injuries to the chest wall usually arise from direct contact, for example, intrusion of wreckage in a road traffic collision or blunt trauma arising from direct blow. Seat belt injuries fall into this category and may cause fractures of the sternum, ribs and clavicle.
- If the force is sufficient, the deformity and the damage to the chest wall structures may induce tearing and contusion to the underlying lung and other structures. This may produce a combination of severe pain on breathing (pleuritic pain) and a damaged lung, both of which will significantly reduce the ability to ventilate adequately. This combination is a common cause of hypoxia.
- Blunt trauma to the sternum may cause myocardial contusion, which may result in cardiac rhythm disturbances.
- Penetrating trauma may well damage the heart, the lungs and great vessels both in isolation or combination. It must be remembered that penetrating wounds to the upper abdomen and neck may well have caused injuries within the chest remote from the entry wound. Conversely, penetrating wounds to the chest may well involve the liver, kidneys and spleen.
- The lung may be damaged with bleeding causing a haemothorax or an air-leak causing a pneumothorax. Penetrating or occasionally a blunt injury may result in cardiac injuries. Blood can leak into the non-elastic surrounding pericardial sac and build up pressure to an extent that the heart is incapable of refilling to pump blood into circulation. This is known as cardiac tamponade and can be fatal if not rapidly relieved at hospital (see additional information in Table 4.8).
- Rapid deceleration injuries may result in sheering forces sufficient to rupture great vessels such as the aorta, caused by compressing the vessels between the sternum and spine.
- The five major thoracic injuries encountered in the pre-hospital setting include:
    1. tension pneumothorax
    2. massive haemothorax (following uncontrolled haemorrhage into the chest cavity)
    3. open chest wounds
    4. flail chest
    5. cardiac tamponade.

5. Assessment and Management

For the assessment and management of thoracic trauma refer to Table 4.7 and Table 4.8.

Thoracic Trauma

Table 4.7 – ASSESSMENT and MANAGEMENT of:

Thoracic Trauma	
ASSESSMENT	**MANAGEMENT**
• Assess **<C>ABCDE**	• Control any external catastrophic haemorrhage (refer to **Trauma Emergencies Overview (Adults)** and **Trauma Emergencies Overview (Children)**). • If any of the following **TIME CRITICAL** features are present: – major **ABCD** complications – penetrating chest injury – flail chest – tension pneumothorax – cardiac tamponade – surgical emphysema – blast injury to the lungs. • Correct **ABC** problems. • Undertake a **TIME CRITICAL** transfer to a major trauma centre.[a] • Major unmanageable **A** and **B** problems should be transferred to nearest trauma unit. • Provide a pre-alert using ATMIST. • Continue patient management en-route.
• Specifically consider: – tension pneumothorax – open chest wounds – flail chest – surgical emphysema – cardiac tamponade – impaling objects	• Refer to Table 4.8 for the assessment and management of these conditions/ situations.
• If the patient is **NON-TIME CRITICAL**, undertake a secondary survey	
• Monitor SpO_2 and assess for signs of hypoxia	• Administer high levels of supplemental oxygen until the vital signs are normal, then aim for a target saturation within the range of 94–98% (refer to **Oxygen**).
• Assess breathing adequacy, respiratory rate, effort and volume, and equality of air entry	• Consider assisted ventilation at a rate of 12–20 respirations per minute, if any of the following are present: – SpO_2 $<90\%$ on high levels of supplemental oxygen. – Respiratory rate is <10 or >30 breaths per minute. – Inadequate chest expansion. **NB** Exercise caution, as any positive pressure ventilation may increase the size of a pneumothorax.
• Monitor nasal $EtC0_2$	• $EtC0_2$ presents an immediate picture of the patient's condition. • Normal ranges are between 4.5 and 6 kPa (35 and 45 mmHg).
• Monitor heart rate and rhythm	• Attach ECG monitor.
• Consider the need for IV fluids	• Obtain IV access. • Refer to **Intravascular Fluid Therapy (Adults)** and **Intravascular Fluid Therapy (Children)** – **DO NOT** delay on scene.
• Assess patient's level of pain	• Refer to **Pain Management in Adults** and **Pain Management in Children**. **NB** Avoid Entonox in a patient with a chest injury as there is a significant risk of enlarging a pneumothorax. **NB** Adequate morphine analgesia may improve ventilation by allowing better chest wall movement, but high doses may induce respiratory depression. Careful titration of doses is therefore required (refer to **Morphine**).

a Patients should normally be transported in a semi-recumbent or upright posture; however, this may often not be possible due to other injuries present or suspected.

Thoracic Trauma *continued*	
● Assessment (children) ● Assess as above	**Management (children)** Manage as above but consider: ● Children can have severe internal chest injuries with minimal or no external evidence of chest injuries. ● Children show signs of shock late due to good compensatory mechanisms. ● Always consider multiple injuries in children with rib fractures, as this suggests a significant mechanism of injury and isolated chest injuries are rare in children. ● Consider non-accidental injury.
● Additional Information	● Chest trauma is treated with difficulty in the field, and prolonged treatment before transportation is **NOT** indicated if significant chest injury is suspected. ● Open chest wounds – seal the wound with a proprietary dressing with a valve, but if none are available use a three-sided dressing. ● Specifically consider the need for thoracic surgery intervention. ● Impaling objects – handle carefully, secure the object with a dressing and if the object is pulsating do not completely immobilise it but allow the object to pulsate. **NB** Be vigilant – the patient may try to remove the object and this could be used as a weapon. ● Remember any stab or bullet wound to the chest, abdomen or back may penetrate the heart. ● Patients with significant chest trauma may often insist on sitting upright and this is especially common in patients with diaphragmatic injury who may get extremely breathless when lying down. In this instance, the patient is best managed sitting upright or at 30–45 degrees, and it must be documented that the spine has not been cleared. ● In the rare incident of gunshot/stab injury to personnel wearing protection vests (e.g. ballistic and stab), these may protect from penetrating injury. However, serious underlying blunt trauma (e.g. pulmonary contusion) may be caused to the thorax. ● **NEVER UNDERESTIMATE THESE INJURIES.** There is a strong link between serious blunt chest wall injury and thoracic spine injury. Maintain a high index of suspicion.

Table 4.8 – ASSESSMENT and MANAGEMENT of:

Specific Thoracic Trauma

Flail Chest

Flail chest is usually the result of a significant blunt chest injury, causing two or more rib fractures in two or more places. A sternal flail can also occur where the ribs or costal cartilages are fractured on both sides of the chest. This results in a flail segment that moves independently of the rest of the chest during respiration leading to inadequate ventilation. The ensuing pulmonary insufficiency is caused by three pathophysiological processes:

1. The negative pressure required for effective ventilation is disrupted due to the paradoxical motion of the flail segment.
2. The underlying pulmonary contusion, which causes haemorrhage and oedema of the lung.
3. The pain associated with the multiple rib fractures will result in a degree of hypoventilation.

- Small flail segments may not be detectable.
- Large flail segments may impair ventilation considerably as a result of pain.

ASSESSMENT	MANAGEMENT
● Assess for signs of a flail chest	● Flail segments should not be immobilised and efforts to maintain ventilation are the priority. ● Allow the patient to sit supported at 30–45 degrees rather than try to make them stay on a scoop stretcher. **NB** Traditionally, the patient has been turned onto the affected side for transportation, but this CANNOT be achieved on a scoop stretcher.
● Assess the patient's level of pain	● Consider the need for analgesia (if indicated refer to **Pain Management in Adults** and **Pain Management in Children**).

Specific Thoracic Trauma *continued*

• Transfer	• Undertake a **TIME CRITICAL** transfer to a major trauma centre, unless the patient needs an immediate lifesaving intervention, in which case transfer to nearest trauma unit. • Provide a pre-alert using ATMIST. • Continue patient management en-route.

Tension Pneumothorax

- This is a rare respiratory emergency, which may require immediate action at the scene or en-route to further care. A tension pneumothorax occurs when a damaged area of lung leaks air out into the pleural space on each inspiration, but does not permit the air to exit from the chest via the lung on expiration.
- This progressively builds up air under tension on the affected side collapsing that lung and putting increasing pressure on the heart and great vessels and the opposite lung. Decreased venous return is significantly affected by the kinking of the vessels, especially the inferior vena cava, as the mediastinum is pushed towards the contralateral side. Coughing and shouting can make a situation worse. If this air is not released externally, the heart will be unable to fill and the other lung will no longer be able to ventilate, inducing cardiac arrest.
- Tension pneumothorax is most often related to penetrating trauma, but can arise spontaneously from blunt or crushing injuries to the chest and as the result of a blast wave. This will present rapidly with an increase in breathlessness and extreme respiratory distress (respiratory rate often >30 breaths per minute). Subsequently the patient may deteriorate and the breathing rate may rapidly slow to <10 breaths per minute before the patient arrests.
- Signs and symptoms:
  - The chest on the affected side may appear to be moving poorly or not at all.
  - At the same time, the affected chest wall may appear to be over-expanded (hyperexpansion).
  - Air entry will be greatly reduced or absent on the affected side.
  - In the absence of shock, the neck veins may become distended.
  - Later, the trachea and apex beat of the heart may become displaced away from the side of the pneumothorax, and cyanosis and breathlessness may appear.
  - Hyperresonance may be present.
  - Occasionally, the patient will only present with rapidly deteriorating respiratory distress.
  - The patient may appear shocked as a result of decreased cardiac output.
  - Patients are usually tachycardic and hypotensive.
- Ventilation of a patient with a chest injury is a common cause of tension pneumothorax in the pre-hospital setting. Forcing oxygenated air down into the lung under positive pressure will progressively expand a small, undetected simple pneumothorax into a tension pneumothorax. This will take some minutes and may well be several minutes after ventilation has commenced. It is usually noticed by increasing back pressure during ventilation; either by the bag becoming harder to squeeze or the ventilator alarms sounding.

ASSESSMENT	MANAGEMENT
• Assess breathing adequacy, respiratory rate, volume, and equality of air entry. FEEL, LOOK, AUSCULTATE and PERCUSS • View both sides of the chest and check they are moving; auscultate to ensure air entry is present and percuss on both sides	• **Only perform needle thoracocentesis in a patient if there is haemodynamic instability, hypotension, or increasing respiratory compromise.** • If a tension pneumothorax is likely, decompress rapidly by needle thoracocentesis. • If the patient requires positive pressure ventilation, an open thoracostomy should be performed if an appropriately skilled practitioner is available (**Caution** - performing a thoracostomy on a spontaneously breathing patient will leave a simple pneumothorax with a poorly ventilated lung. Bilateral thoracostomies on a spontaneously breathing patient should only be done one at a time, and appropriate chest seal dressings should be applied).
• Observe the patient for signs of recurrence of the tension pneumothorax	• If the procedure was unsuccessful, repeat the thoracocentesis. • Consider the use of a thicker needle in patients with a thicker chest wall, following your organisation's guidelines.
• Transfer	• Undertake a **TIME CRITICAL** transfer to a major trauma centre, unless the patient needs an immediate lifesaving intervention, in which case transfer to nearest trauma unit. • Provide a pre-alert using ATMIST. **NB** Needle thoracocentesis may not always decompress pneumothoraces in large patients. In such cases, a thoracostomy with or without a chest drain may need to be performed. This needs to be done either in hospital or by appropriately skilled practitioners (e.g. BASICS or HEMS doctors on scene or in hospital).

Specific Thoracic Trauma *continued*

Cardiac Tamponade

The heart is enclosed in a tough, non-elastic membrane, called the pericardium. A potential space exists between the pericardium and the heart itself. If a penetrating wound injures the heart, the blood may flow under pressure into the pericardial space. As the pericardium cannot expand, a leak of as little as 20–30 ml of blood can cause compression of the heart. This decreases cardiac output and causes tachycardia and hypotension. Further compression reduces cardiac output and cardiac arrest may occur.

ASSESSMENT	MANAGEMENT
• Assess for signs of cardiac tamponade • Signs of hypovolaemic shock, tachycardia and hypotension, accompanied by blunt or penetrating chest trauma may be an indication of cardiac tamponade • Note the presence of distended neck veins and muffled heart sounds when listening with a stethoscope	• Cardiac tamponade is a **TIME CRITICAL**, **LIFE-THREATENING** condition that requires rapid surgical intervention, resulting in an open chest operation to evacuate the compressing blood. • **DO NOT** delay on scene inserting cannulae or commencing fluid therapy.
• Transfer	• Undertake a **TIME CRITICAL** transfer to a major trauma centre, unless the patient needs an immediate lifesaving intervention, in which case transfer to nearest trauma unit. • Provide a pre-alert using ATMIST.
• Re-assess **ABC** en-route to hospital	**NB** Pericardiocentesis is not recommended in the pre-hospital setting, as it is rarely successful, has significant complications and delays definitive care.

Surgical Emphysema

- Surgical emphysema produces swelling of the chest wall, neck and face with a cracking feeling under the fingers when the skin is pressed. This indicates an air leak from within the chest, either from a pneumothorax, a ruptured large airway or a fractured larynx.
- Normally it requires no specific treatment, but it does indicate potentially SERIOUS underlying chest trauma. Sometimes the surgical emphysema might be extensive and cause the patient to swell up. Where the emphysema is progressively increasing, look for a possible underlying tension pneumothorax.
- In some cases, surgical emphysema may become so severe as to tighten the overlying skin and restrict chest movement. A tension pneumothorax must be excluded as above. If there is no improvement, the patient must be transferred to hospital as soon as possible.

ASSESSMENT	MANAGEMENT
• Assess for signs of surgical emphysema, swelling of the chest wall, neck and face with a cracking feeling under the fingers when the skin is pressed	
• Consider possible underlying tension pneumothorax	• Refer to tension pneumothorax guidance above.

Blast Injury

Blast injury is caused by three mechanisms:

1. Rupture of air-filled organs.
2. Missiled debris.
3. Contact injury.

Although rare in survivors, strongly suspect a blast lung injury if the patient is suffering from tympanic injury. However, the absence of a tympanic injury DOES NOT exclude lung injury.

NB Being shielded from blast debris DOES NOT exclude lung injury.

ASSESSMENT	MANAGEMENT
• Assess for blast injury	• Pre-hospital management is supportive.

Thoracic Trauma

KEY POINTS

Thoracic Trauma

- **Thoracic injury is commonly associated with hypoxia, either from impaired ventilation or secondary to hypovolaemia from massive bleeding into the chest (haemathorax) or major vessel disruption.**
- **Count the respiratory rate and look for asymmetrical chest movement.**
- **Pulse oximetry must be used as this will assist in recognising hypoxia.**
- **The mechanism of injury is an important guide to the likelihood of significant thoracic injury.**
- **Blunt trauma to the sternum may induce myocardial contusion, which may result in ECG rhythm disturbances.**
- **ECG monitoring.**
- **Impaling objects should be adequately secured. If the object is pulsating do not completely immobilise, but allow the object to pulsate.**
- **Do not probe or explore penetrating injuries.**

Bibliography

1 National Institute for Health and Clinical Excellence. Fractures (Complex): Assessment and Management (NG37). London: NICE, 2016. Available from: https://www.nice.org.uk/guidance/ng37.

2 National Institute for Health and Clinical Excellence. Fractures (Non-complex): Assessment and Management (NG38). London: NICE, 2016. Available from: https://www.nice.org.uk/guidance/ng38.

3 National Institute for Health and Clinical Excellence. Major Trauma: Assessment and Initial Management (NG39). London: NICE, 2016. Available from: https://www.nice.org.uk/guidance/ng39.

4 National Institute for Health and Clinical Excellence. Major Trauma: Service Delivery (NG40). London: NICE, 2016. Available from: https://www.nice.org.uk/guidance/ng40.

5 National Institute for Health and Clinical Excellence. *Spinal Injury: Assessment and Initial Management* (NG41). London: NICE, 2016. Available from: https://www.nice.org.uk/guidance/ng41.

6 National Institute for Health and Clinical Excellence. *When to Suspect Child Maltreatment* (CG89). London: NICE, 2009. Available from: https://www.nice.org.uk/guidance/cg89.

7 Revell M, Porter K, Greaves I. Fluid resuscitation in pre-hospital trauma care: a consensus view. *Emergency Medicine Journal* 2002, 19(6): 494–498.

8 Lee C, Revell M, Porter K, Steyn R. The pre-hospital management of chest injuries: a consensus statement. Faculty of Pre-hospital Care, Royal College of Surgeons of Edinburgh. *Emergency Medicine Journal* 2007, 24(3): 220–224.

9 Warner KJ, Copass MK, Bulger EM. Paramedic use of needle thoracostomy in the pre-hospital environment. *Prehospital Emergency Care* 2008, 12(2): 162–168.

10 Waydhas C, Sauerland S. Pre-hospital pleural decompression and chest tube placement after blunt trauma: a systematic review. *Resuscitation* 2007, 72(1): 11–25.

11 Dretzke J, Sandercock J, Bayliss S, Burls A. Clinical effectiveness and cost effectiveness of pre-hospital intravenous fluids in trauma patients. *Health Technology Assessment* 2004, 8(23).

12 Turner J, Nicholl J, Webber L, Cox H, Dixon S, Yates D. A randomised controlled trial of prehospital intravenous fluid replacement therapy in serious trauma. *Health Technology Assessment* 2000, 4(31).

13 Stern SA. Low-volume fluid resuscitation for presumed hemorrhagic shock: helpful or harmful? *Current Opinion in Critical Care* 2001, 7(6): 422–430.

14 Pepe PE, Mosesso VNJ, Falk JL. Pre-hospital fluid resuscitation of the patient with major trauma. *Prehospital Emergency Care* 2002, 6(1): 81–91.

15 Borman JB, Aharonson-Daniel L, Savitsky B, Peleg K. Unilateral flail chest is seldom a lethal injury. *Emergency Medicine Journal* 2006, 23(12): 903–905.

16 BMJ Evidence Centre. Best Practice: Cardiac tamponade. Available from: http://bestpractice.bmj.com/best-practice/monograph/459.html, 2012.

17 Fitzgerald M, Spencer J, Johnson F, Marasco S, Atkin C, Kossmann T. Definitive management of acute cardiac tamponade secondary to blunt trauma. *Emergency Medicine Australasia* 2005, 17(5–6): 494–499.

18 Friend KD. Prehospital recognition of tension pneumothorax. *Prehospital Emergency Care* 2000, 4(1): 75–77.

19 Massarutti D, Trillo G, Berlot G, Tomasini A, Bacer B, D'Orlando L et al. Simple thoracostomy in pre-hospital trauma management is safe and effective: a 2-year experience by helicopter emergency medical crews. *European Journal of Emergency Medicine* 2006, 13(5): 276–280.

20 Wanek S, Mayberry JC. Blunt thoracic trauma: flail chest, pulmonary contusion, and blast injury. *Critical Care Clinics* 2004, 20(1): 71–81.

21 Blaivas M. Inadequate needle thoracostomy rate in the pre-hospital setting for presumed pneumothorax. *Journal of Ultrasound in Medicine* 2010, 29(9): 1285–1289.

Falls in Older Adults

1. Introduction

- Falls are defined as an unintentional or unexpected loss of balance resulting in coming to rest on the floor, the ground or an object below knee level. The impact of a fall on the individual and their family is not to be underestimated, with falls often leading to a fear of falling and potentially having psychological, as well as physical effects. A fall is distinguished from a collapse, which occurs as a result of an acute medical problem such as an acute arrhythmia, a transient ischaemic attack or vertigo.[1] A fall can be precipitated by an acute medical condition, and the actual cause of the fall can be very difficult to establish on initial presentation. This guideline covers falls from a standing height. Falls from above standing height or 2 metres above the ground, are not covered in this guideline (refer to **Trauma guidelines**).
- The term 'mechanical fall' is **not** an appropriate term to use when describing a fall; it implies that a benign aetiology for an older person's fall exists and it is inaccurate, inconsistently used, is not associated with a discrete fall evaluation and does not predict outcomes.[2]
- Older people in contact with healthcare professionals for any reason should be asked routinely whether they have fallen in the past year, asked about the frequency, context and characteristics of the falls and referred to appropriate falls prevention pathways as per local arrangements. Recently the SAFER 2 study (a large multi-centre cluster randomised controlled trial) has shown that a paramedic protocol for assessment of older patients (aged ≥65) who have fallen, with an option to refer direct to a community-based falls service (in place of conveyance to the ED), is safe, inexpensive and reduced subsequent 999 calls in those patients. There was no overall difference in outcomes (whether taken to hospital or managed at home) between the trial arms.

2. Incidence

- Falls are the leading cause of emergency calls in the over 65s and account for 10–25% of emergency ambulance responses each year for adults aged over 65 years.[3] In the London Ambulance Service alone, there were 70,380 incidents of people aged 65 and over who were coded as presenting with a fall in the period for 2015–16.
- Falls represent the second leading cause of accidental injury death worldwide and the leading cause of injury-related mortality in the UK.[4] Every year 1 in 3 people aged over 65 and up to 1 in 2 aged over 80 will fall at least once.[5] By 2025 it is estimated that this will account for over 3.2 million falls in people over the age of 65 in England alone.[6] Up to 14,000 people will die each year as a result of a fall and a subsequent fractured neck of femur.[7]
- A fall of <2 metres is the commonest mechanism of injury in older patients.[8]

3. Severity and Outcome

- As part of the normal ageing process there is a loss of bone density, muscle tone, skin changes and often increased poly-pharmacy. A simple fall in an older person may result in a much more significant injury than would be seen in a younger person. Clinicians should have a higher index of suspicion of injury in older people. However, falls are not a part of normal ageing and are typically due to pathological changes described earlier.
- The Silver Book[9] recommends ways in which emergency admissions for older people can be reduced and emphasises that health and social care services must adapt to meet older people's urgent care needs, including ambulance services.
- Falls can be a marker of frailty, which is associated with common syndromes of ageing including immobility, incontinence, susceptibility to the side effects of medication, delirium and dementia, all of which increase the complexity of the presentation and may indicate a change in normal health status. Frail older people typically suffer falls indoors. For a person with frailty a relatively small event (e.g. a minor infection, a new medication or constipation) may trigger a sudden and dramatic functional decline. Frailty is a clinically recognised state of increased vulnerability. It results from ageing associated with a decline in the body's physical and psychological reserves. This can cause the person to fall and also to struggle to recover following a fall. It is important to recognise the presence of frailty in weighing the benefits and risks of any intervention or treatment plan. Even if no injury has been sustained, further assessment and support post-fall will enable the provision of the right care and support for the person.

4. Risk Factors for Falls

Refer to Table 4.9.

- Risk factors for falls can be broadly classified into three categories:
  - intrinsic factors – relating to the person
  - extrinsic factors – relating to the person's environment
  - exposure to risk.
- However, it is recognised that falls often result from the dynamic interactions of risks in all categories.
- Intrinsic risk factors include changes in the body caused by the normal ageing process, certain medical conditions, excessive alcohol, being physically inactive or a combination of these.
- It is important to consider dementia and cognitive impairment in the assessment of a patient who has fallen. As many as 11–26% of patients presenting with a fall will have cognitive impairment, some of which will be undiagnosed.[10, 11] Patients with dementia are more likely to fall, have more falls and are more likely to sustain an injury (such as a hip fracture or head injury) from the fall. If sustaining an injury, the outcomes are

worse for the patient, their family, the health service and society at large. It is therefore vital to recognise this as a high-risk group.

- It is important that the cause of the fall is considered so that the correct pathways are chosen or excluded; red flags should always be excluded and modifiable factors considered.

Table 4.9 – INTRINSIC AND EXTRINSIC FALLS RISK FACTORS[12]

Common intrinsic risks of falls[13]	Common extrinsic risk factors of falls
• lower extremity weakness • previous falls • gait and balance disorders • visual impairment • depression • functional and cognitive impairment • dizziness • low body mass index • urinary incontinence • postural hypotension • female sex • being over age 80. **Other intrinsic causes of falls** • sensory deficit (poor vision, peripheral neuropathy) • musculoskeletal disease (osteoarthritis, proximal muscle weakness, previous joint replacement) • other neurodegenerative conditions • central nervous system disease (cognitive dysfunction, vestibular hypofunction, cerebrovascular disease, cerebral hypoperfusion) • Parkinson's disease and Parkinsonism.	• polypharmacy (use of multiple medications) • psychotropic medications • poor lighting (especially on stairs), glare and shadows • low ambient temperature • wet, slippery or uneven floor surfaces • thresholds at room entrances • obstacles and tripping hazards, including clutter • chairs, toilets or beds being too high, low or unstable • inappropriate or unsafe walking aids • inadequately maintained wheelchairs, for example, brakes not locking • improper use of wheelchairs, for example, failing to clear foot plates • unsafe or absent equipment, such as handrails • pets, such as cats and dogs • loose fitting footwear and clothing, such as trailing dressing gowns • access to the property, wheelie bins, the garden, uneven ground.

Many medicines cause postural hypotension and may contribute to over 20% of extrinsic falls. Common causes are:

- cardiac drugs:
  - antiarrhythmics (e.g. digoxin)
  - alpha-blockers (e.g. doxazosin)
  - beta-blockers (e.g. bisoprolol, atenolol)
  - ACE inhibitors (e.g. ramipril, lisinopril)
  - angiotensin 2 blockers (e.g. losartan, candesartan)
  - diuretics (e.g. furosemide, bumetanide, spironolactone, bendroflumethiazide)
  - calcium channel blockers (e.g. amlodipine, diltiazem)
- urological drugs (e.g. oxybutynin)
- neuropsychiatric drugs:
  - Parkinson's drugs (e.g. madopar, sinemet, ropinirole)
  - tricyclic antidepressants (e.g. amitriptyline)
  - antipsychotics (e.g. haloperidol, risperidone)
  - painkillers (e.g. opioids)
- In these patients a formal medicines optimisation review may be indicated by the GP practice or another clinical lead (following local guidance).

Certain activities can be 'high risk' because of the specific interaction of risk factors involved, for example, poor balance combined with standing on a stool to change a light bulb or reach a high shelf. To understand falls risk in the environment fully, it is important to observe a person moving around in their environment; referral for a falls assessment in line with local pathways/guidelines will facilitate this.

4.1 Risks Related to a 'Long Lie'

- A 'long lie' is usually defined as someone who has been on the floor for over one hour and has been unable to get up. However, the estimated time on the floor, and mobility while there, may vary greatly and will influence clinical decision making, i.e. a patient who has been completely immobile on the floor for several hours will be at higher risk than someone who can move across the floor, but cannot pull themselves up onto a chair or bed or into a standing position.
- Anyone who has experienced a long lie is at a higher risk of complications, such as pneumonia, pressure areas, rhabdomyolysis, dehydration and hypothermia.
- Increasing age and other co-morbidities will increase the risk of complications from a long lie; each patient will need to be assessed on an individual basis, to plan ongoing management.

5. Psychology of Falling

- Depression, fear of falling and other psychological problems are common effects of falls. Loss of confidence as well as social withdrawal and loneliness can occur, even when there is no injury. A person who is fearful about falls will often avoid physical activity, become weaker and may fall more as a result. Social isolation can also result if the person stops going out.
- Some older people are fearful that a fall may lead to a loss of independence, being admitted to hospital, loss of control over their life, or being rehoused. These well documented fears can lead to patients not reporting falls, masking symptoms, or being reluctant to attend an emergency department or be referred to their GP. Clinicians should be aware of these issues and help to promote independence. Positive conversations should emphasise the simple things that can be done to reduce falls risk, regain confidence and maintain independence through referral to other services for further assessment and support.

6. Assessment and Management

6.1 Specific History and Examination Considerations

- A thorough and careful physical examination is required along with a high index of suspicion, to exclude common but easily missed injuries, such as rib fractures, spinal fractures and delayed presentation of a previous head injury.
- A perceived minor injury, such as a fractured rib, may have more serious long term consequences for an older person, e.g. pulmonary contusions. Minor injuries can also lead to a temporary loss of independence, which, for a person with frailty, can become permanent without aggressive management and rehabilitation. Every rib fracture increases the risk of dying by 15% in frail older people.
- The history taken on scene needs to be thorough and well documented in the patient record; where possible it should be corroborated with relatives, carers or associated health care professionals.
- Initial assessment should exclude the possibility of syncope. Transient loss of consciousness should be assumed to have occurred unless proven otherwise (refer to **Altered Level of Consciousness**).
- Clinical history should include:
  - details of any previous altered level of consciousness, including number and frequency
  - the person's medical history and family history of cardiac disease (for example, personal history of heart disease and family history of sudden cardiac death)
  - current medication that may have contributed to altered level of consciousness (for example, diuretics)
  - vital signs and NEWS score (for example, pulse rate, respiratory rate and temperature) – repeat if clinically indicated
  - lying and standing blood pressure if clinically appropriate
  - other cardiovascular and neurological signs.
- It is important to consider that medications prescribed for co-morbidities may complicate the clinical picture and presentation.

6.2 12-Lead ECG

- Older people who fall should have a 12-lead ECG (with auto interpretation) recorded. This must be interpreted by the assessing clinician unless they are confident the patient has complete recall of the event and clearly describes an extrinsic factor that caused the fall. Transient loss of consciousness (TLoC) should be assumed unless proven otherwise, refer to TLOC and NICE guidance.

'Red Flags' for syncope seen in a 12-lead ECG include:

- conduction abnormality (for example, complete right or left bundle branch block, atrial fibrillation or any degree of heart block)
- evidence of a long or short QT interval
- any ST segment or T wave abnormalities.

6.3 Atrial Fibrillation (AF) and Falls

- Ensure that a 12-lead ECG is performed on any patient with an irregular pulse felt on palpation to identify the underlying rhythm.
- It may be difficult to determine if AF is new or not. The patient may know themselves or have been told that they have an irregular heartbeat/AF, or you may be able to contact the patient's health professional/GP or review care plans/medical notes.
- If the patient is asymptomatic and has a heart rate below 120/minute, and an extrinsic cause of the fall has been identified, consider contacting a GP to have a clinical discussion and agree a care plan.
- Consider conveyance to hospital as a priority if the patient is found to be in atrial fibrillation (AF) after a fall and has symptoms such as:
  - altered mental status
  - dizziness
  - chest pain
  - heart rate above 120/minute
  - dyspnoea
  - palpitations
  - hypotension.
- If the patient has atrial fibrillation and has had a potential syncope, refer to local syncope pathways or follow local guidance.

6.4 Postural Hypotension

- Postural hypotension should be checked for if there is no clear extrinsic cause of the fall, no features to suggest an alternative cause, symptoms are typical such as light-headedness, dizziness or feeling weak and faint on standing **and the patient is being considered for management at home**.

- First, record the blood pressure with the patient lying supine, the result is at its most accurate when the patient has been in this position for 10 minutes or longer. Then ask the patient to stand, and record the blood pressure again once they have been standing for 3 minutes.
- Clinically significant postural hypotension is defined as:
  - ≥20 mmHg reduction in systolic BP
  - ≥10 mmHg reduction in diastolic BP
  - the original symptoms are reproduced on standing.
- If the patient is unable to stand, a sitting reading may be taken; however, the sensitivity of the test is reduced in this case.
- Symptomatic postural hypotension is a significant finding that requires further investigation and medication review but rarely requires admission (refer to local guidance for further assessment). Asymptomatic postural hypotension may be managed through primary care.

6.5 Confusion/Delirium

- Confusion is routinely encountered with older adults who have fallen. Often associated with dementia, confusion can also be an indication of an acute pathology presenting as delirium. The patient may be either more (hyperactive delirium) or less (hypoactive delirium) active than normal, although the mixed type is the commonest. However, dementia is characterised by a gradual onset and is not reversible, whereas delirium typically is described as having a rapid onset and is attributed to a reversible cause.
- Be mindful that the confusion may pre-exist and even contribute to the fall, or may occur as a consequence of the fall. This makes gaining a comprehensive and corroborated history very important.
- Where a patient presents with confusion, apply the principles of assessing capacity to consent and be prepared to modify your communication to the needs of the patient. Look for documents such as 'This is me'.[14] Listening to the family, carers or friends who know the patient best may provide clear indications regarding the onset, severity or any changes to the confusion, as this is the most reliable single indicator of delirium, especially in patients who cannot communicate. Where concerns are expressed, you should have a high index of suspicion that the confusion is new and requires further investigation or referral.
- New onset confusion can be due to physiological changes resulting from head injury, hypoxia, infection, stroke or TIA, hypoglycaemia, ketoacidosis, side effects of medications or drugs and the effects of withdrawal from drugs or alcohol. In addition, other causes could include carbon monoxide poisoning, encephalitis or meningitis, electrolyte imbalance, post-seizure and, more rarely, an underactive thyroid gland, tumour, thiamine deficiency, hypo/hyperparathyroidism and Cushing's disease.

6.6 Skin Assessment for Adults

- Consider performing an assessment of the patient's skin after a fall to ensure that the skin is intact. Gain the patient's consent or act in their best interests. Consider patient dignity and body temperature as you examine them. Pay attention to areas of bony prominence that are subject to pressure when lying on a hard surface, such as the back of head and ears, shoulders, elbows, lower back and buttocks, hips, inner knees and heels.
- A skin assessment in adults should take into account:
  - any pain or discomfort reported by the patient
  - skin integrity in areas of pressure
  - colour changes or discoloration
  - variations in heat, firmness and moisture (due to incontinence, oedema, dry or inflamed skin).
- If any concerns are identified, consider referral to community nursing teams in line with local pathways/ guidance.
- Refer to Figure 4.2 for an aid to assessing skin breakdown.

6.7 Continence

- Confirm the patient's usual toileting/continence regime. Consider new symptoms, including dysuria, increased frequency of urination, suprapubic tenderness, urgency and polyuria, but do not carry out a urine dipstick in the absence of symptoms of UTI.[15]
- If continent/partially continent; consider if they are likely to be able to locate and physically get to the toilet/commode, rearrange clothes and clean the genital area and hands.
- If incontinent/partially continent; consider if the patient/carer is able to manage pads/catheter care, rearrange clothes, clean the genital area and hands and dispose of waste safety. Community nursing services may be available to provide rapid continence assessment including recatheterisation.

6.8 How to Decide If the Patient Could Be Managed in the Community?

- Decisions on whether to manage a patient at home/ in the community can be challenging and should be made following a comprehensive history, clinical assessment and examination. Decisions on the best management of an older person who has fallen are made on a risk/benefit basis and may benefit from discussion with locally agreed clinical contacts. These could include ambulance service clinical advice lines, or other healthcare professionals clinical advice lines using a shared decision making approach, and should always consider the views of the patient and relatives/ carers. The final referral decision will also depend on the availability and responsiveness of local community health and social care services. Well-structured advice on how to assess and make decisions related to choosing an appropriate clinical pathway, improves patient safety and outcomes.[16]

Early warning sign - blanching erythema

Areas of discoloured tissue that blanch when fingertip pressure is applied and the colour recovers when pressure is released, indicating damage is starting to occur but can be reversed.

On darkly pigmented skin, blanching does not occur and changes to colour, temperature and texture of skin are the main indicators.

Grade 1	Grade 2	Grade 3	Grade 4
Non-blanchable erythema	**Partial thickness skin loss**	**Full thickness skin loss**	**Full thickness tissue loss**
Intact skin with non-blanchable redness, usually over a bony prominence. Darker skin tones may not have visible blanching but the colour may differ from the surrounding area. The affected area may be painful, firmer, softer, warmer or cooler than the surrounding tissue.	Loss of the epidermis/dermis presenting as a shallow open ulcer with a red/pink wound bed without slough or bruising.[1] May also present as an intact or open/ruptured blister.	Subcutaneous fat may be visible but bone, tendon or muscle is not visible or palpable. Slough may be present but does not obscure the depth of tissue loss. May include undermining or tunnelling.[2]	Extensive destruction with exposed or palpable bone, tendon or muscle. Slough may be present but does not obscure the depth of tissue loss. Often includes undermining or tunnelling.[2]

Moisture lesions

Moisture lesions are skin damage due to exposure to urine, faeces or other body fluids.

a) Location:
Located in peri-anal, gluteal, cleft, groin or buttock area. Not usually over a bony prominence.

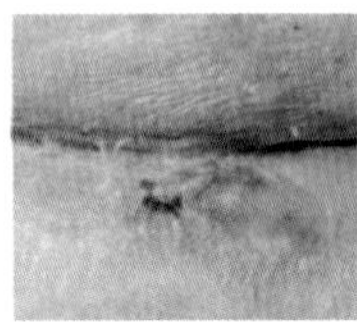

b) Shape:
Diffuse often multiple lesions. May be 'copy', 'mirror' or 'kissing' lesion on adjacent buttock or anal cleft. Linear.

c) Edges:
Diffuse irregular edges.

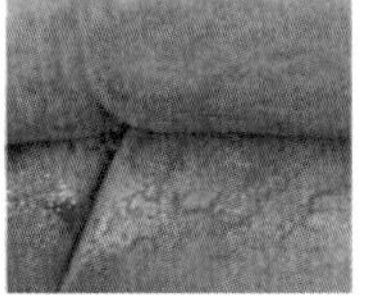

d) Necrosis:
No necrosis or slough. May develop slough if infection present.

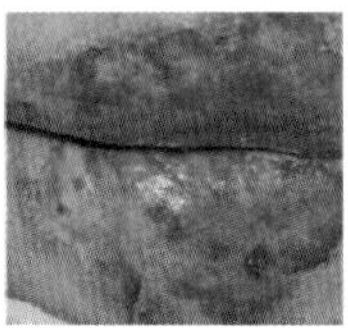

e) Depth:
Superficial partial thickness skin loss. Can enlarge or deepen if infection present.

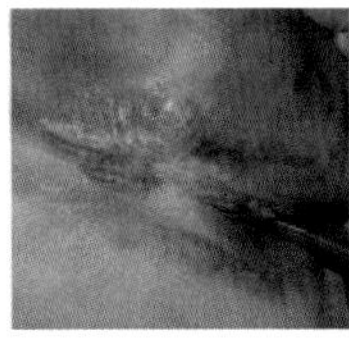

f) Colour:
Colour of redness may not be uniform. May have pink or white surrounding skin (maceration). Peri-anal redness may be present.

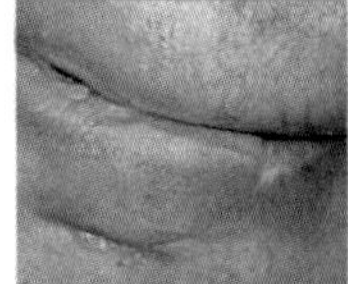

Where pressure ulcers commonly occur

The shaded points indicate vulnerable areas of the body with regards to pressure ulcers

Head, Back, Elbows, Base of Spine, Bottom, Knees, Toes, Heels

[1] Bruising can indicate deep tissue injury

[2] The depth of a Grade 3 or 4 pressure ulcer varies by anatomical location. Areas such as the bridge of the nose, ears, occiput and malleolus do not have fatty tissue so the depth of these ulcers may be shallow. In contrast areas which have excess fatty tissue can develop deep Grade 3 pressure ulcers where bone, tendon, muscle is not directly visible or palpable.

Figure 4.2 – Grading tool for assessing skin breakdown. Reproduced with kind permission of Healthcare Improvement Scotland.

- There are also risks in taking an older person to hospital, including institutionalisation and/or deconditioning (the consequence of prolonged bed-rest, leading to loss of functional status through reduced muscle mass and strength). The decline in muscle mass and strength has been linked to falls, functional decline, increased frailty, immobility and healthcare-associated infection.[17]
- Some older people who fall may prefer to be managed in the community or at home, and where possible this should be supported, particularly where family/carers can also provide support. Following a comprehensive patient assessment and wider review of the circumstances of the fall (having excluded injuries/ acute illness), ambulance clinicians should provide the referral for this to occur in line with local pathways and guidance.

6.9 Ongoing Referral

- All older people who have fallen resulting in an ambulance call/attendance, but are then managed at home, should be offered referral pathways as per local guidelines. The purpose of referral/re-referral is to prevent further falls and injury.
- Referrals should take into account current care plans and other health and social care organisations already involved in the patient's care.
- Decision making should be a shared process, including the patient and their family/carers/other health and social care professionals/any person holding their lasting power of attorney for health and welfare.
- Referral to services via locally agreed pathways may result in:
  - multifactorial falls risk assessment
  - frailty assessment
  - assessment of care needs, including telecare.

6.10 Falls Prevention[4]

- Ambulance clinicians have a role to play in having conversations with people who are at risk of falling, or who have fallen, to try and prevent further falls. The evidence-based Making Every Contact Count (MECC) approach[18] can be applied or other locally agreed methods of ensuring health prevention messages can be given. A MECC interaction takes a matter of minutes and is not intended to add to busy workloads, but should be part of the conversations after a fall or with patients who have been identified as at risk of falling. Evidence suggests that the broad adoption of the MECC approach could potentially have a significant impact on the health of the population.
- Support can be given to older people at risk of falling by routinely asking them about falls and encouraging them to stay active, connected, eat well and reduce alcohol intake, to reduce the risk of falling and to improve outcomes if a fall happens. Consider discussing the measures a person can take to reduce their risk factors for falling, doing exercises recommended by falls teams or other health care professionals, the preventable nature of some falls and where they can seek further advice and assistance.
- Consider leaving the patient with an information leaflet about falls prevention and suggesting telecare options, such as a pendant type alarm so help can be summoned for any further falls, or simple solutions to providing a safer physical environment. Conversations can take place with carers/family members if the person has cognitive impairment.
- Older people in contact with healthcare professionals for any reason should be asked **routinely** whether they have fallen in the past year and asked about the frequency, context and characteristics of the falls. Referrals should be made in line with local guidance.

Falls in Older Adults

Table 4.10 – ASSESSMENT and MANAGEMENT of:

Falls in Older People

ASSESSMENT	MANAGEMENT
IMMEDIATE PRIORITY	
Primary Survey ● Assess **<C>ABCD** ● Are any of the following **TIME CRITICAL** features present? – major **CABC** problems – altered level of consciousness – neck and back injuries	● Refer to: – Airway and Breathing Management – **Trauma Emergencies Overview (Adults)**
SECONDARY ASSESSMENT – TRAUMA	
Assess for trauma/injuries ● Make a careful physical assessment, as relatively minor injury can have significant consequences in older people; all should include a pain assessment **Caution:** ● Older adults can present with major trauma with seemingly minor mechanism of injury and kinetic energy transfer ● Assess specifically for evidence or risk of occult bleeding (intracranial, intrathoracic and intra-abdominal) ● Be mindful of apparently minor head injuries in the context of concurrent anticoagulant, clopidogrel or combination anti-platelet therapy and other coagulopathies. Refer to local policies around minor head injuries **Consider spinal injuries**[19, 20, 21, 22, 23, 24] ● Falls are a more frequent cause of spinal 'cord' injury in the older patient ● Central Cord Syndrome (CCS) may occur in susceptible older individuals with degenerative spinal disease who sustain hyperextension of the cervical spine during trauma ● CCS can result from ground height/level surface falls and is also associated with flexion and compression trauma mechanisms **Specifically assess for:** ● Motor weakness in the upper and lower extremities, any impairment will usually be greater in the upper extremities than that in the lower extremities, especially in the muscle of the hands ● Sensory impairment may be variable and limited to mild sensory impairment in the hands or feet **Note:** ● In trauma, CCS may present with/without bony spinal injury. ● Assess carefully for fragility fractures.	● Refer to: – **Head Injury** – **Spinal Injury and Spinal Cord Injury** – **Thoracic Trauma** – **Abdominal Trauma** – **Limb Trauma**. ● Also consider: – skin integrity/turgor (long lies) – chest injuries, including thorough palpation of the chest to exclude rib fractures – osteoporosis.

Falls in Older People *continued*

SECONDARY ASSESSMENT – MEDICAL

Intrinsic factors

- Take a detailed history of how the fall is described
- Can the history be corroborated by a reliable third party?
- Document a NEWS score[25, 26]

- Refer to:
  - **Altered Level of Consciousness** (in particular transient loss of consciousness (TLoC))
  - **Glycaemic Emergencies (Adults)**
  - **Cardiac Rhythm Disturbance**
  - **Convulsions (Adults)**
  - **Sepsis** (check for pyrexia or hypothermia as markers of possible infection)
  - **Stroke/Transient Ischaemic Attack (TIA)**
  - **Overdose and Poisoning (Adults)** (intentional or unintentional).

Also consider:
  - possible bleeding – intracranial, intrathoracic, intra-abdominal
  - acute kidney injury
  - delirium
  - frailty, in line with local guidance
  - polypharmacy – use of multiple medicines.

REVIEW OF SYSTEMS

- Cardiovascular (include postural hypotension assessment and consider 12-lead ECG)
- Respiratory system
- Gastrointestinal (bowels, bladder, eating/drinking)
- Genitourinary (if a urinary infection is suspected clinically with signs such as increased frequency/dysuria and suprapubic tenderness, follow local guidelines)
- Neurological (stroke/TIA)
- Musculoskeletal
- Hair, skin (look for pressure areas) and nails
- Mental health (anxiety, depression, fear of falling)

HISTORY OF THE FALL

- Consider using a mnemonic such as SPLAT:[27]
  - **Symptoms** prior to and at the time of the fall
  - **Previous** falls, near falls, and/or fear of falling
  - **Location** to identify contributing environmental factors (for example, was there poor lighting, was footing poor, did they trip, or were they in a crowd?)
  - **Activity** the person was participating in when they fell (for example, were they turning, changing position, or transferring?)
  - **Time** of day the fall occurred (falls in the morning could be due to postural hypotension and later in the day could be due to fatigue)

- Ascertain how the fall happened, considering the following:
  - Intrinsic factors (including pathological factors, e.g. collapse).
  - Extrinsic factors (including environment, trips and hazards).
  - Can the patient recall the fall in detail? Words such as 'I must have tripped' suggest no recollection (refer to **Altered Level of Consciousness**, especially transient loss of consciousness (TLoC)).
  - Can the history of the fall be corroborated by a reliable third party?
  - Is there a history of previous falls? When did these occur, with what frequency, were any injurious?
  - Is this fall consistent with previous falls or different?
  - Is there a new onset of confusion?
  - Are alcohol/drugs/medication involved?

Falls in Older People *continued*

FUNCTIONAL ASSESSMENT – MOBILITY

- Mobility must be considered to:
  - help exclude injury
  - determine if mobility is a factor contributing to falls risk
  - ascertain a person's ability to function safely at home following the fall
- Observe the person getting up from their chair, balancing on standing, walking round their home (including turning) and sitting down again – using their usual walking aid if applicable)
- A formal test may be used as per local guidance, such as the 'get up and go' test or the 'turn 180 degrees' test[28, 29, 30]
- A mobility assessment should also take into account the use and the state of repair of walking aids
- While the person is moving around, check they can weight-bear and consider how steady, safe and confident they are
- Where possible, find out the person's normal mobility status; it may be that a person has limited mobility normally but is managing well with regular visits from family or carers and/or with equipment such as a commode

- Consider whether the person is able to:
  - get to the toilet/commode and transfer on and off it safely
  - access a drink or simple snack
  - manage on the stairs if this is essential to get to the toilet/bed or other rooms
  - take essential medications as prescribed
  - summon help.
- If the person receives care, consider the timing of the next visit. Contact the agency if possible. Information may be found in a care plan.
- Consider local services that may be available to respond to support the person in remaining at home and avoiding hospital admission.

OTHER CONSIDERATIONS

• General	• Look/ask for other information about the patient, such as anticipatory care plans that may detail preferences for place of care, clinical management, home care input, nursing/therapy input, including access to electronic care records. • Ask about lasting power of attorney/end of life and DNACPR/ReSPECT decisions. • In cases of worsening chronic confusion, consider referral back to GP/local pathway. • Consider frailty in line with local guidance. • Consider the need for senior clinical advice/support.
• Extrinsic factors	• Walking aids (consider correct use, state of repair, suitability for the patient). • Footwear (good fit, not worn out, adequate grip and support). • Floor surfaces (clear of obstructions, carpets and rugs not frayed or lifted, not slippery or wet/greasy). • Lighting. • Temperature. • Spectacles and hearing aids, telecare alarm (worn, clean and working, regular check-ups). • Home safety, smoke alarms, clutter and other trip hazards, exit routes, crime risks, ability to self-evacuate, home adaptations. • Shared decision making with patients and families/carers/other health and social care professionals. • Respect the autonomy of the individual.
• Safeguarding	• Ask the patient if they feel safe. • Consider the need for additional support, protection or referral for safeguarding. • Refer to **Safeguarding Adults at Risk**.

Falls in Older People *continued*	
• Social context	• Housing type. • Living alone or with spouse/family/partner. – What is the level of support offered by the above? – Does the patient have caring responsibilities? What are they and are they affected by the fall? – What are the existing support/care packages in place? When is the next planned visit of carers? – Are the patient/relatives and carers coping or in denial? • Is support/care assessment required? • Does the family and carer burden/need require assessment? • Does the patient suffer social isolation/loneliness?
• Referral and safety-netting	• Follow local policies or guidelines. • Patients who have fallen should be offered referral to a community-based falls service to enable secondary prevention as per local policies.[16]
• Prevention	• Self-care and links to the voluntary sector. • Signposting. • Local leaflets, contacts and information. • Written advice for non-injury falls. • Advice for the patient, their relatives and carers. • Make every contact count (MECC) opportunities.

KEY POINTS

Falls in Older Adults

- **The term 'mechanical fall' is not an appropriate term to use when describing a fall.**
- **Initial assessment should exclude the possibility of syncope.**
- **A thorough and careful physical examination is required along with a high index of suspicion, to exclude common but easily missed injuries.**
- **Some older people who fall may prefer to be managed in the community or at home, and where possible this should be supported, particularly where family/carers can also provide support.**
- **All older people who have fallen resulting in an ambulance call/attendance, but are then managed at home, should be offered referral pathways as per local guidelines.**
- **Ambulance clinicians have a role to play in talking with people who are at risk of falling, or who have fallen, to try and prevent further falls.**

Further Reading

Further important information and evidence in support of this guideline can be found in the Bibliography.[31]

Other useful resources include:

http://www.sciencedirect.com/science/article/pii/S096663621400705X

Bibliography

1 National Institute for Health and Clinical Excellence. *Falls in Older People* (QS86). London: NICE, 2017. Available from: https://www.nice.org.uk/guidance/qs86/chapter/Quality-statement-6-Medical-examination-after-an-inpatient-fall.

2 Tirrell GP, Lipsitz LA, Liru SW. Is there such a thing as a mechanical fall? *American Journal of Emergency Medicine* 2016, 34(3): 582–585. doi: 10.1016/j.ajem.2015.12.009.

3 Ambulance Service Network Community Health Services Forum. Falls prevention: new approaches to integrated falls prevention services. *Briefing* 2012: 234. NHS Confederation. Available from: http://www.nhsconfed.org/-/media/Confederation/Files/Publications/Documents/Falls_prevention_briefing_final_for_website_30_April.pdf.

4 National Institute for Health and Clinical Excellence. *Falls in Older People: Assessing Risk and Prevention* (CG161). London: NICE, 2013.

5 Department of Health. *National Service Framework for Older People*. London: The Stationery Office, 2001.

6 Projecting Older People Population Information Systems. Available from: http://www.poppi.org.uk/index.php?pageNo=315&PHPSESSID=eujokv2jii3d1vj7q70s8eh5c4&sc=1&loc=8640&np=1.

7 Age UK. *Stop Falling: Start Saving Lives and Money*. London: Age UK, 2012.

8 Trauma Audit and Research Network. *Major Trauma in Older People*. Manchester: University of Manchester, 2017.

9 British Geriatrics Society. *Quality Care for Older People with Urgent and Emergency Care Needs: The 'Silver Book'*. London: British Geriatric Society, 2012.

10 Davies AJ, Kenny RA. Falls presenting to the accident and emergency department: types of presentation and risk factor profile. *Age and Ageing*. 1996, 25(5): 362–366.

11 Bloch F, Jegou D, Dhainaut J-F et al. Do ED staffs have a role to play in the prevention of repeat falls in elderly patients? *American Journal of Emergency Medicine* 2009, 27(3): 303–307.

12 College of Occupational Therapists. *Occupational Therapy in the Prevention and Management of Falls in Adults* (Practice Guideline). London: COT, 2015.

13 American Geriatrics Society. *AGS/BGS Clinical Practice Guideline: Prevention of Falls in Older Persons*. 2010. Available from: http://www.medcats.com/FALLS/frameset.htm.

14 Alzheimer's Society. *This Is Me*. Available from: https://www.alzheimers.org.uk/download/downloads/id/3423/this_is_me.pdf.

15 Scottish Intercollegiate Guidelines Network. *Management of Suspected Bacterial Urinary Tract Infection in Adults* (SIGN Guideline 88). Edinburgh: Healthcare Improvement Scotland, 2012.

16 Snooks HA et al. Support and assessment for fall emergency referrals (SAFER) 2. *Health Technol Assess* 2017, 21(13): 1–218. Available from: https://www.ncbi.nlm.nih.gov/pubmed/28397649.

17 Gillis A, McDonald B. Deconditioning in the hospitalised elderly. *Canadian Nurse* 2005, 101(6): 16–20. Available from: https://www.ncbi.nlm.nih.gov/pubmed/16121472.

18 Health Education England. *Making Every Contact Count*. Available from: http://www.makingeverycontactcount.co.uk/.

19 Shadler P, Shue J, Giradi F. Central Cord Syndrome, A review of epidemiology, treatment and prognostic factors. *JSM Neurosurg Spine* 2016, 4(3): 1075.

20 National Association of Emergency Medical Technicians. *Prehospital Trauma Life Support*. Spinal Trauma, Chapter 17 Geriatric Trauma, St Louis, MO: Mosby JEMs Elsevier, 2016. Especially Ch. 11, Spinal trauma and Ch. 17 Geriatric trauma.

21 McKinley M, Santos K, Meade M et al. Incidence and outcomes of spinal cord injury clinical syndromes, *J Spinal Cord Med* 2007, 30: 215–224.

22 Ryan M, Henderson J. The epidemiology of fractures and fracture-dislocations of the cervical spine. *Injury* 1992, 23: 38–40.

23 Mandavia D, Newton K. Geriatric trauma. *Emerg Med Clin North Am* 1998, 16: 257–274.

24 Wagner R, Jagoda A. Spinal cord syndromes. *Emerg Med Clin North Am* 1997, 15: 699–711.

25 Cei M et al. In-hospital mortality and morbidity of elderly medical patients can be predicted at admission by the modified early warning score: a prospective study. *Int J Clin Pract* 2009, 63(4): 591–595.

26 Romero-Ortunoa R, Wallisa S, Birama R, Keevila V, Clinical frailty adds to acute illness severity in predicting mortality in hospitalized older adults: an observational study. *European Journal of Internal Medicine* 2016, 35: 24–34.

27 Bauman CA, Milligan JD, Patel T et al. Community-based falls prevention: lessons from an Inter-professional Mobility Clinic, *J Can Chiropr* 2014, 58(3): 300–311

28 Mathias S, Nayak USL, Isaacs B. Balance in elderly patients: the 'get-up and go' test. *Arch Phys Med Rehabil*. 1986, 67: 387–389.

29 Nevitt MC, Cummings SR, Kidd S, Black D. Risk factors for recurrent nonsyncopal falls. A prospective study. *Journal of the American Medical Association* 1989, 261(18): 2663–2668.

30 Simpson JM, Worsfold C, Reilly E, Nye N. A standard procedure for using TURN180: testing dynamic postural stability among elderly people. *Physiotherapy* 2002, 88(6): 342–353.

31 Murdoch I, Turpin S, Johnson B, MacLullich A, Losman E. *Geriatric Emergencies*. London: Wiley-Blackwell, 2015.

5

Maternity Care

1. Introduction

- Any woman of childbearing age may be pregnant and, unless there is a history of hysterectomy, there must be a high index of suspicion that any abdominal pain or vaginal bleeding may be pregnancy related.
- There are three fundamental rules which must be followed at all times when dealing with a pregnant woman:
  a. Resuscitation of the mother must always be the priority.
  b. Manual uterine displacement must be employed to support resuscitation measures beyond 20 weeks gestation, refer to Figure 5.1.
  c. Hypotension is a late sign of shock. Any signs of hypovolaemia during pregnancy are likely to indicate a 35% (class III) blood loss and must be treated aggressively.
- In cases of maternal cardiac arrest requiring ongoing cardiopulmonary resuscitation, pre-alert the nearest emergency department with an obstetric unit when transferring a pregnant woman in order to ensure preparedness for an emergency perimortem caesarean section (resuscitative hysterotomy), as delivering the fetus may be required to help facilitate maternal resuscitation. **NB Effective resuscitation of the mother will provide effective resuscitation of the fetus.**
- When ambulance clinicians attend an obstetric emergency, they should work as a team, with the paramedics responsible and accountable for the care of the woman or newborn baby and delegating tasks accordingly.
- When a midwife is present, paramedics and midwife must work together to act in the best interests of the woman and the newborn baby. If both mother and newborn baby are clinically well, the midwife is the responsible and accountable clinician. The midwife can either discharge the ambulance clinicians, and arrange for ongoing community midwifery care, or arrange conveyance of the mother and baby together to the most appropriate facility.
- In the event of a newborn requiring conveyance to hospital ahead of the mother, it may be preferable that the midwife remains on scene with the mother to manage the third stage of labour, assess for perineal trauma, and manage any ongoing post-partum bleeding. Ambulance clinicians can manage ongoing care of the newborn, utilise the established communication channels, and pre-alert the nearest ED where the baby can be assessed. The mother should be repatriated with the baby as soon as reasonably possible at the same location.
- The MBRRACE-UK annual report, Saving Lives, Improving Mothers' Care, reviews maternal deaths in the UK and produces recommendations relating to care provision. The report continues to show an overall decrease in the maternal death rate, which is currently 8.5 women per 100,000 maternities.
  - Maternal deaths from direct causes – complication from the pregnancy itself such as bleeding, blood clots, pre-eclampsia or infection – continue to decrease.
  - Maternal deaths from indirect causes – pre-existing conditions that are not direct pregnancy complications such as heart disease, epilepsy, mental health problems or cancer – remain high.
  - Deaths from mental health problems contribute to around a quarter of maternal deaths occurring between six weeks and one year after the end of pregnancy.
  - The focus of care must be upon establishing appropriate resuscitative measures, placing a pre-alert to the nearest emergency department with an obstetric unit attached, conveying the woman, with manual uterine displacement in place, and preparation for further assessment and treatment, including a perimortem caesarean section if necessary.
  - Effective communication is therefore essential to ensure clinical information being passed on is complete and relevant, utilising a structured communication tool.

2. Communication, Information Sharing and Consent

All women who are booked for maternity care should have access to their handheld maternity records. These will provide key information regarding medical history, previous and current pregnancies, obstetric problems as well as emergency contact details for care providers, including next of kin. Information within these notes may aid assessment during the primary and/or secondary survey. Maternity units may also have their own unique set of handheld records or, in some cases, these may be electronic.

2.1 Human Factors and 'SBAR'

- Clinical performance and safe practice can be enhanced through an understanding of the effects of teamwork, tasks, equipment, workspace, culture and organisation on human behaviour and abilities, and application of that knowledge within a clinical setting.
- Increasing situational awareness and the utilisation of communication tools (such as SBAR) help to promote a safer environment and enhance clinical outcome. Awareness of what is happening around us can be reduced during emergency situations, and this can lead to near misses and/or adverse outcomes. It is therefore essential that enhanced communication skills, and an environment in which open and honest lines of communication is encouraged, are maintained.
- The use of the Situation, Background, Assessment, Recommendation (SBAR) communication tool is recommended in order to optimise transfer of information between members of the multi-disciplinary team. The purpose of SBAR is to promote the accurate and unambiguous handover of clinically

SECTION 5 Maternity Care

relevant information regarding care of the mother from one healthcare professional to another. The use of SBAR has the potential to improve the speed at which care is delivered and the quality of care that is ultimately provided.

2.2 Consent

- Consent to treatment is the principle that a person must give permission before they receive any type of medical treatment, investigation or examination. Consent from a woman is needed regardless of the procedure. For consent to be valid it must be voluntary and informed, and the person consenting must have the capacity to make the decision. If an adult has the capacity to make a voluntary and informed decision to consent to or refuse a particular treatment, their decision must be respected. This is still the case even if refusing treatment would result in their death, or the death of their unborn child.
- The provision of adequate information should include the benefits and risks of the proposed treatments, and alternative treatments. If the woman is not offered as much information as they reasonably need to make their decision, and in a format that they can understand, their consent will not be valid.
- Consent can be given verbally or in writing and should be given to the health care professional directly responsible for the person's current treatment.
- Consent may not be necessary if a person requires emergency treatment that is believed to be in their best interests or to save their life and they are unable to give consent due to a lack of capacity caused by either mental or physical complications.
- During obstetrics emergencies, it may be necessary to perform intimate examination in order to perform lifesaving treatment. Practitioners must, where possible, obtain informed consent and offer the woman a chaperone. All examinations must be carried out sensitively, with respect for the woman's dignity, cultural beliefs and confidentiality.

3. Physiological Changes in Pregnancy

Pregnancy is timed from the FIRST day of the last period and may last up to or in excess of 42 weeks. The pregnancy is divided into three trimesters (1–12 weeks +6 days, 13–25 weeks +6 days and 26 weeks+). These terms are used with the maternity handheld records, they will also detail the lead clinician, i.e. the midwife or the obstetrician who is responsible for the provision of maternity care with the woman.

There are a multitude of physiological and anatomical changes during pregnancy that may influence the management of the pregnant woman. These changes include:

- Cardiovascular system:
  - An increase in cardiac output by 20–30% in the first 10 weeks of pregnancy.
  - An increase in average maternal heart rate by 10–15 beats per minute.
  - A decrease in systolic and diastolic blood pressure by an average of 10–15 mmHg due to a reduction in peripheral resistance caused by an increase in the release of the progesterone hormone.
  - The weight of the gravid uterus, from 20 weeks gestation onwards, may cause compression of the inferior vena cava (IVC), reducing venous return, and lowering cardiac output, by up to 40%, for women in the supine position; this in turn can reduce blood pressure. The combined effects of the gravid uterus on the IVC and a reduction in peripheral vascular resistance can result in the woman feeling faint or having an episode of syncope, resolved by repositioning her onto her side or into the lateral position.
  - An increase in blood volume through haemodilution (increasing by 45%) occurs together with a small increase in the numbers of red blood cells. The disproportionate increase of plasma volume relative to the increase in red cell mass can lead to a 'physiological' anaemia in the mother from around 27 weeks gestation. Due to the increase in blood volume, a pregnant woman is able to tolerate greater blood loss before showing signs of hypovolaemia. This compensation is at the expense of shunting blood away from the uterus and placenta, and therefore fetus.
- Respiratory system:
  - An increase in breathing rate and effort and a decrease in vital capacity, as the gravid uterus enlarges and the diaphragm becomes splinted. Some shortness of breath is common during pregnancy but early consideration should be given to the need for increased oxygen requirements.
  - Oedema of the larynx may compromise airway management and a collapsed pregnant woman requires the airway to be secured as soon as possible.
  - Placement of an advanced airway (supraglottic airway or endotracheal intubation) should be secured in all maternal cardiac arrests (refer to **Maternal Resuscitation**).
- Gastrointestinal system:
  - An increase in the acidity of the stomach contents, due to a delay in gastric emptying, caused by progesterone-like effects of the placental hormones.
  - Relaxation of the cardiac sphincter makes regurgitation of the stomach contents more likely (refer to **Maternal Resuscitation**).
  - Nausea and vomiting can occur around 4–8 weeks gestation and continue until around 14–16 weeks. Some severe cases may continue for a longer period of time and can result in rapid dehydration (hyperemesis gravidarum) requiring hospital assessment/admission.

4. Appropriate Destination for Conveyance

- The choice of destination to convey mother and baby should be carefully considered and in line with local procedures. Ideally mother and baby should be conveyed to the same destination. There are units, commonly called birth/birthing centres (or 'standalone' maternity units), that are solely midwifery-led. Be aware that there are no resident obstetricians, anaesthetists or neonatologists with the capability of performing advanced obstetric or neonatal interventions at these sites. There are no specialist neonatal facilities.
- The mother may choose to book for delivery at a particular unit and request to be conveyed there; however, in an emergency situation this may have to be overridden:
  - The nearest ED will be the appropriate destination when there is cardiac arrest, major airway problems, ongoing eclamptic convulsions and severe uncontrollable bleeding.
  - In other obstetric emergencies (e.g. shoulder dystocia, mild to moderate bleeding etc.) transfer to the nearest full obstetric unit (i.e. not a birthing centre or 'standalone' midwifery unit) will be appropriate. Remember, that in many cases, a full obstetric unit will be co-located with an ED but this may not always be the case.
- Careful consideration should always be given to the most appropriate destination in each case. Also consider carefully the accessibility of a unit (e.g. out-of-hours, locked doors, corridors and lifts). In line with local procedures, pre-alert arrangements and telephone numbers should be agreed and readily available to clinicians.

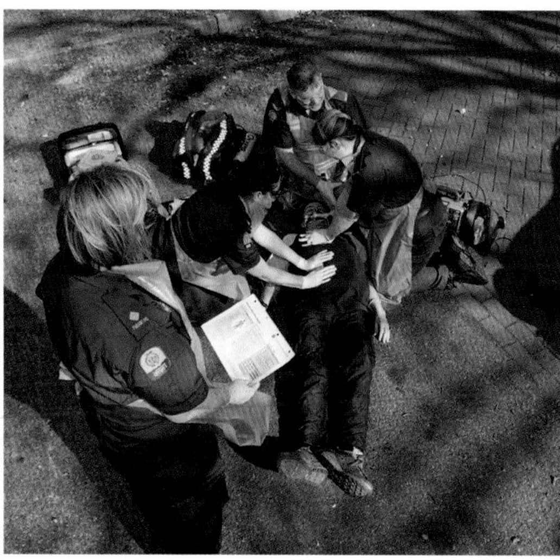

Figure 5.1 – Manual uterine displacement.

5. Assessment

- Critical assessment of the mother is vital in all situations, while fetal assessment may be indirect based on reported movements etc. Refer to Table 5.1
- Neonatal assessment is also important, with particular reference to respiratory effort and maintaining body temperature. Refer to Table 5.5.

Table 5.1 – ASSESSMENT

• Quickly assess the woman and scene as you approach	
• Primary survey	• It is important to remember that a woman and, if born, a newborn baby will require assessment. • The aim of the primary survey is to identify any life-threatening problems, to enable management to be commenced as rapidly as possible, and to reach an early determination of the priority for transportation. The primary survey should be modified in the presence of actual or suspected trauma (refer to **Trauma in Pregnancy**).
• Massive external haemorrhage	• Is there a significant volume of blood visible without the need to disturb the woman's clothing? – Is the woman's clothing soaked? – Is there blood on the floor? – Are there a number of blood-soaked sanitary pads visible?
• Airway	• Is the woman able to talk? (Yes = airway open.) If the woman is unresponsive, refer to **Maternal Resuscitation**. • Is the woman making unusual sounds? (Gurgling = fluid in the airway.) • Is suction required? (Snoring = tongue/swelling/foreign body obstruction.) • If the woman is unresponsive, open the airway and look in – suction for fluids, manually remove solid obstructions.

Table 5.1 – ASSESSMENT *continued*

• Breathing	• Document respiratory rate and effort. (Are accessory muscles being used?) • Obtain oxygen saturations as soon as possible. • Auscultate for added sounds. (Wheeze = bronchospasm; coarse sounds = pulmonary oedema.) • Assess for the presence of cyanosis. • Give oxygen based on clinical findings (not routinely).
• Circulation	• Document radial pulse rate and volume. (Capillary refill time (CRT) may be used if neither the radial nor carotid pulses can be palpated.) • Assess skin colour and temperature (to touch). (Pallor, or cold or damp skin = an adrenergic reaction to shock.) • Record blood pressure – the systolic is most valuable if you suspect shock. • Visually inspect the abdominal area and gently palpate for evidence of internal bleeding (indicated by tenderness, guarding, firm woody uterus).
• Disability	• Perform an AVPU assessment of consciousness level (is the woman Alert, responding only to Voice, responding only to Pain or Unresponsive?). • Document the woman's posture (normal, convulsing (state whether focal or generalised), abnormal flexion, abnormal extension). • Document pupil size and reaction (PEaRL – pupils equal and reacting to light).
• Expose/environment/evaluate	• Ensuring consent is obtained, expose and visually inspect the vaginal opening: – Is there any evidence of bleeding? – Can you see a presenting part of the baby? – Is there a prolapsed loop of cord? – Have the waters broken (and if so, is the amniotic fluid clear, blood stained or meconium stained)? – Does the perineum bulge with each contraction? – If the baby has been born, is there a significant perineal tear? Can you see any part of the uterus? • Assess the environment: – Is the woman or baby at risk of hypothermia? – Are the surroundings as clean as you can make them if the birth is imminent? – Are there other children present (this may indicate a previous pregnancy with live birth)? • Evaluate how time critical the woman's condition is. – If it is time critical, decide immediately whether you need to transport the woman urgently to the nearest hospital with an obstetric unit, placing a pre-alert as early as reasonably possible. (The nearest hospital with an obstetric unit may not be the booked unit; however, it is critical the woman has rapid obstetric or appropriate assessment at the nearest facility.) – If the birth is imminent, remember to call for additional clinical resource. This may include midwifery assistance, which may be deployed from the nearest maternity unit to the location of the woman (follow local guidelines).
• Fundus	• Make a quick assessment of fundal height: a fundus at the level of the umbilicus equates to a gestation of approximately 22 weeks. By definition, if fundal height is below the umbilicus, this suggests that if the fetus is delivered, it is unlikely to survive.
• Fetal activity	• Ask the mother when she last felt her baby move.
• Secondary survey	• If any critical problems are identified during the primary survey, the secondary survey should only be undertaken when any **ABCDE** problems have been addressed and transportation to definitive care has commenced (if this is possible). In many cases where critical problems are identified, it will not be possible or appropriate to undertake a secondary survey in the pre-hospital phase of care.

6. Special Cases

6.1 Concealment, Denial and Unknown Pregnancy

Occasionally pregnancy may be concealed or denied until labour commences. In both situations there may have been no antenatal care. There may be mental health, drug and alcohol abuse issues and safeguarding concerns (refer to **Safeguarding Adults at Risk** and **Safeguarding Children**). Some concealed pregnancies may result in the birth occurring in secret. Ambulance clinicians must be aware that the consequences of concealment and denial can have a fatal outcome for both mother and baby.

- Always consider the possibility of pregnancy in any woman of reproductive age. Ask the woman if she could be pregnant. Be aware that a young teenage girl may not want to answer such a question in the presence of a parent or carer.
- It may be necessary to visually inspect and palpate the abdomen for evidence of a pregnant uterus.
- If labour is confirmed and birth is not imminent, determine if there is any relevant medical history. Transfer the woman to the nearest obstetric unit.
- Determine how many weeks pregnant the woman is if known, or by visual inspection of the abdomen; where the uterine fundus is at the level of the umbilicus the pregnancy may be more than 22 weeks.
- If birth is in progress or occurs en-route, request a midwife from the nearest maternity unit, if this service is available, and additional resources and prepare for birth (see Table 5.1).
- Once the baby has been born and assessed, transfer mother and baby to the nearest obstetric unit.
- If the woman is unaware of pregnancy, consider birth/miscarriage in any significant PV bleed that cannot be explained.
- Pre-alert the nearest obstetric unit or nearest ED with an obstetric unit, dependent upon considered gestation.
- Discuss at handover any safeguarding concerns identified when attending the home environment (refer to **Safeguarding Adults at Risk** and **Safeguarding Children**).

6.2 Female Genital Mutilation (FGM)

These women should have had their delivery planned with a consultant obstetrician and a midwife who have received special training in the management of FGM. If de-infibulation (reversal of FGM) is required, it may have been undertaken antenatally or may have been planned to be undertaken in labour or after a planned caesarean section.

- Some women with previous pregnancies may have had an illegal re-infibulation operation after childbirth.
- Unless the mother has had a previous normal vaginal delivery and has not had a de-infibulation, she must be regarded as having a high risk of perineal trauma and haemorrhage.
- If de-infibulation is planned, when in labour, the woman must be transferred immediately to her booked obstetric unit. However, if this is likely to incur a delay, the woman must be conveyed to the nearest obstetric unit.
- If a woman has not received antenatal care and evidence of FGM is noted upon arrival of ambulance clinicians at a birth, further resources should be requested and an early attempt at conveying the woman to the nearest obstetric unit made.
- An information call should be placed to the identified obstetric unit informing them of the additional indications of transfer.

7. Glossary of Terms

Table 5.2 provides a glossary of abbreviations specific to maternity and commonly used in handheld maternity records.

Table 5.2 – GLOSSARY

ABBREVIATION	TERM
LMP	Last menstrual period.
EDD	Estimated date of delivery – the timing of the pregnancy is written in the notes in the format 12/40, i.e. 12 weeks have elapsed out of the 40-week pregnancy.
T or D	Term or expected date of delivery/pregnancy, therefore T+3 or D+3 in the notes is 3 days over the EDD.
CEPH	Cephalic (head).
BR	Breech.
G	Gravida, the number of times a woman has been pregnant (including the present pregnancy), e.g. G3.
P	Parity, the number of times a woman has given birth to a liveborn or stillborn baby, e.g. P3. A second figure implies previous miscarriages or terminations, e.g. P3+2.

Maternity Care (including Obstetric Emergencies Overview)

KEY POINTS

Maternity Care (including Obstetric Emergencies Overview)

- **Any woman of childbearing age MAY be pregnant.**
- **Due to the increase in blood volume, the pregnant woman is able to tolerate greater blood or plasma loss before showing signs of hypovolaemia, establish large bore (16G) IV cannulation early.**
- **A pregnant woman in cardiac arrest must ideally be conveyed with left manual uterine displacement after 20 weeks gestation. (Maintaining left lateral tilt is an alternative but may be more difficult to use effectively in the pre-hospital care environment.)**
- **The use of SBAR to communicate between ambulance clinicians and maternity clinicians can optimise transfer of information.**

Further Reading

Further important information and evidence in support of this guideline can be found in the Bibliography.

Bibliography

1 Knight M, Tuffnell D, Kenyon S, Shakespeare J, Gray R, Kurinczuk JJ (eds) on behalf of MBRRACE-UK. *Saving Lives, Improving Mothers' Care – Surveillance of maternal deaths in the UK 2011–13 and lessons learned to inform maternity care from the UK and Ireland Confidential Enquiries into Maternal Deaths and Morbidity 2009–13.* Oxford: National Perinatal Epidemiology Unit, University of Oxford, 2015.

2 Catchpole (2010), cited in Department of Health. *Human Factors Reference Group Interim Report, 1 March 2012.* National Quality Board. Available from: http://www.england.nhs.uk/ourwork/part-rel/nqb/ag-min/, 2012.

3 Woollard M, Hinshaw K, Simpson H, Wieteska S, (eds). *Pre-hospital Obstetric Emergency Training.* Oxford: Wiley-Blackwell, 2009.

4 Centre for Maternal and Child Enquiries. Saving mothers' lives: reviewing maternal deaths to make motherhood safer: 2006–2008. *BJOG: An International Journal of Obstetrics & Gynaecology* 2011, 118 (suppl. 1).

5 Bourjeily G, Paidas M, Khalil H, Rosene-Montella K, Rodger M. Pulmonary embolism in pregnancy. *The Lancet* 2010, 375(9713): 500–12.

UNDERTAKE PRIMARY SURVEY
Establish gestation and frequency of contractions

BIRTH IMMINENT

↓

Request midwife if available
Prepare for newborn life support
Reassure the woman and support her in a comfortable position, avoiding the supine position
Provide Entonox for pain relief

↓

Support the birth of the baby's head by applying gentle pressure as head advances

↓

Support the baby during the birth and place on the maternal abdomen

↓

Thoroughly dry the baby with a warm towel and wrap with a dry towel

↓

If the baby is crying provide 'skin-to-skin' contact with the mother

→ If the baby is not crying refer to **Newborn Life Support**

↓

Allow the umbilical cord to stop pulsating prior to clamping and cutting

↓

The placenta may take 15–20 mins to birth – **DO NOT** pull on the cord – encourage the mother to pass urine

Deliver the placenta into a plastic bag for the midwife to inspect and check for completeness

Assess and record estimated blood loss

If the placenta remains undelivered with minimal bleeding, plan to transfer to the nearest appropriate destination as agreed locally

Maternal safety is the prime consideration

Consider the specific clinical situation **and which interventions may be required for the woman and baby on arrival**

Refer to 'Appropriate Destination for Conveyance' in **Maternity Care**

If the placenta remains undelivered and bleeding refer to Figure 5.5

BIRTH NOT IMMINENT

↓

Contact booked unit for advice if no time critical features present
(The woman may travel by car or taxi to booked unit if ambulance is not required)

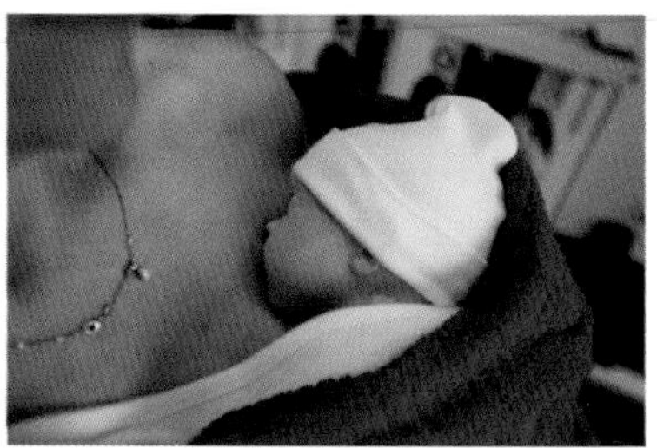

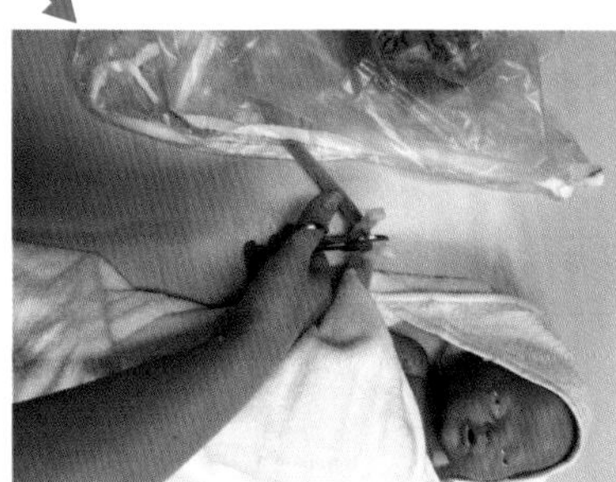

Figure 5.2 Pre-hospital maternity emergency management – normal birth.

Birth Imminent: Normal Birth and Birth Complications

1. Introduction

The best clinical management for a woman who is experiencing an abnormal labour or complications with the birth is to be transferred to the NEAREST appropriate unit without delay. This will usually be the nearest obstetric unit but in certain circumstances may involve transfer to the nearest ED (refer to 'Appropriate Destination for Conveyance' in Maternity Care).

When there is a midwife on scene it is their responsibility to manage the labour and birth, and ambulance clinicians should work under their direction, while working together as a team. If the midwife is not present, the decision on whether to convey the woman should be based on the principle that any situation that deviates from a normal uncomplicated labour should result in the woman being transported immediately to the nearest hospital with an obstetric unit once the appropriate number of conveying resources are available.

In this situation the ambulance clinicians must alert the hospital either directly or via the emergency operations centre (EOC). An early assessment of the need for additional resources may be necessary, including the request for a second ambulance where a newborn baby is required to be conveyed separately from the woman. Ensure that the request is made as soon as possible.

The most important feature of attending a pregnant woman is to complete a rapid assessment, to ascertain whether there is anything abnormal taking place.

The maternal assessment process outlined in Table 5.3 MUST be followed in order to decide whether to:

- STAY ON SCENE AND REQUEST A MIDWIFE (if not already present and available within the locality).
- TRANSFER TO FURTHER CARE IMMEDIATELY.

In maternity cases where birth is not imminent and there are no complications, it may be appropriate to contact the midwife in the booked maternity unit for advice regarding the transport arrangements. This may involve the woman making her own way to her planned place of birth if there are no immediately time critical features, or conveying her to the nearest maternity unit for assessment.

The assessment should be repeated en-route and, if any complications occur, the condition should be treated appropriately and destination changed if a nearer facility is available. If the woman is booked into a unit that is not within a reasonable distance or travelling time, ambulance clinicians should base their judgements on the maternal assessment, and take her to the nearest appropriate unit.

Table 5.3 – ASSESSMENT and MANAGEMENT of:

Normal Birth

ASSESSMENT	MANAGEMENT
• Quickly assess the woman and scene as you approach • Undertake a primary survey **<C>ABCDEF**	• If any time critical features are present, correct **<C>ABC** problems and transport to the nearest ED with an obstetric unit (refer to **Medical Emergencies in Adults – Overview** and **Medical Emergencies in Children – Overview**). • Provide a pre-alert.
• Ascertain the period of gestation • Ask the woman, and also review the woman's maternity records. Refer to antenatal pages for assessment of any obstetric risk factors or complications	
Assess for: • operculum (show) • ruptured amniotic fluid sac (waters broken) • contractions • and/or bleeding (See Figure 5.2. For additional information, refer to **Maternity Care**)	If **NONE** of these indications is present **AND** there is no other medical/traumatic condition, discuss the woman's management with the **BOOKED OBSTETRIC UNIT**, informing of: • woman's name • woman's age and date of birth • woman's hospital registration number • name of lead clinician (midwifery or obstetric led care) • history of this pregnancy • estimated date of delivery (EDD) • period of gestation (number of weeks pregnant) • previous obstetric history.

Normal Birth *continued*

If ANY of the above indications are present, assess: • contraction interval • the urge to push or bear down • crowning/top of the baby's head/breech presentation visible at the vulva	• Undertake a visual inspection of the vaginal entrance if there are regular contractions (1–2 minute intervals) and an urge to push or bear down.
• If birth is imminent, that is regular contractions (1–2 minute intervals) and an urge to push or bear down and or crowning/top of the baby's head/breech presentation visible at the vulva	• Remain on scene, request a midwife if available in the locality and an additional ambulance with a paramedic if not already present, and prepare for the birth of the baby (see below).
• Second stage of labour (from full dilatation of the cervix until complete birth of the baby) • Continue assessing the woman's level of pain	• Reassure the woman, tell her what you are doing and include her birth partner if present. • Ensure the environment is safe and secure for the birth of the baby with particular attention to the temperature of the room: – incontinence pads – cover the ambulance stretcher or birthing area – maternity pack – open and set out – towels (warm towels if possible) – enough to dry and wrap the baby – blanket(s) – cover the mother for warmth and modesty – heat – turn the heat up in the birth area (aim for 25°C). 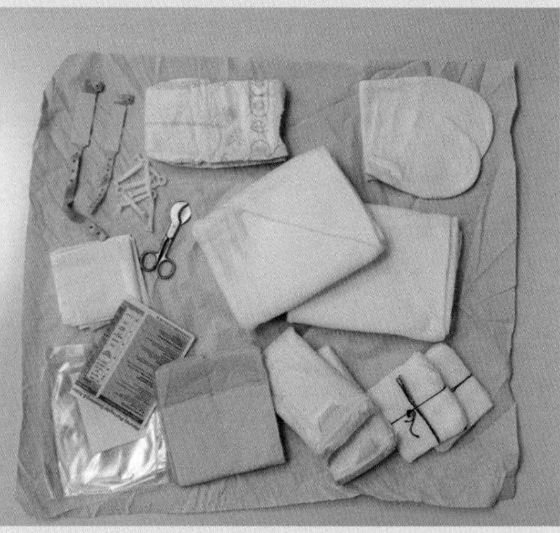 Contents of the maternity pack. • Support the woman in any position she finds comfortable – discourage her from lying flat on her back because of the risk of supine hypotension.

Normal Birth *continued*	
	• Encourage the woman to continue taking Entonox to relieve pain/discomfort if necessary. • **CAUTION** – at this stage, morphine should only be administered in exceptional circumstances due to the risk of neonatal respiratory depression. • To allow for the baby's head to be born slowly, encourage the woman to concentrate on panting or breathing out during the birth. The use of Entonox can assist here. • Consider applying gentle pressure to the top of the baby's head as it advances through the vaginal entrance to prevent very rapid birth of the head. Pressure may also assist in keeping the head flexed to allow the smallest diameter of the fetal skull to be born. This may reduce perineal trauma. • The umbilical cord may be around the baby's neck and does not require removal, as the baby can be born with the cord left in place. • Hold the baby as it is born and lift it towards the woman's abdomen. • Wipe any obvious large collections of mucous from the baby's mouth and nose.
• Undertake an initial **ABCD** assessment of the baby – include head, trunk, axilla and groin	• Newborns are at risk of hypothermia. • **CAUTION** – premature babies lose heat faster than full term babies (refer to **Care of the Newborn**). • Quickly and thoroughly dry the baby using a warm towel while you make your initial assessment. • Remove the now wet towel and wrap the baby in a dry towel to minimise heat losses.
• Assess the baby's airway	• If the baby is crying, it has a clear airway. • If the baby is not breathing, confirm that the airway is open – the head is ideally placed in the 'neutral' position, i.e. not the extended 'sniffing position'. 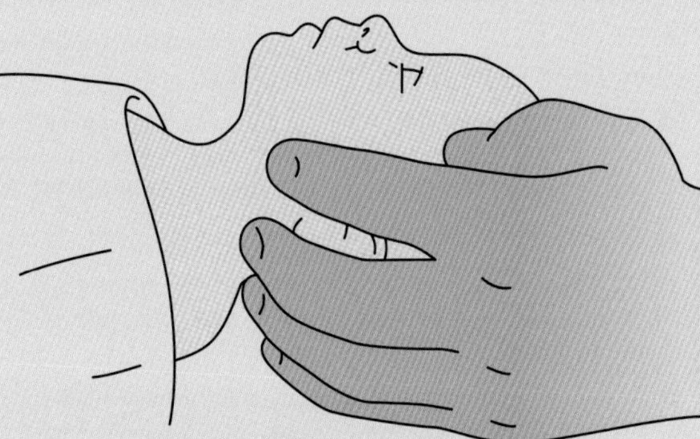 Figure reproduced with the kind permission of the Resuscitation Council (UK). • **SUCTION IS NOT USUALLY NECESSARY** – if required, use the suction unit on low power (around 75 mmHg) with a CH12–14 catheter and then only within the oral cavity. **ONLY** use suction to remove **VISIBLE** thick particulate lumps of meconium. During suctioning, the tip of the catheter should be visible to the operator. **DO NOT** probe blindly with the catheter as this can cause a vagal response and depress respiration. • If the baby is not breathing refer to **Newborn Life Support**. • Once the baby is breathing adequately, cyanosis will gradually improve over several minutes – if the cyanosis is not clearing, enrich the atmosphere near the baby's face with a low flow of oxygen at 2 litres. • Where available, oxygen saturation probes should be used. Refer to **Care of the Newborn**.

Normal Birth *continued*

Cutting the cord ● Assess whether the cord has stopped pulsating	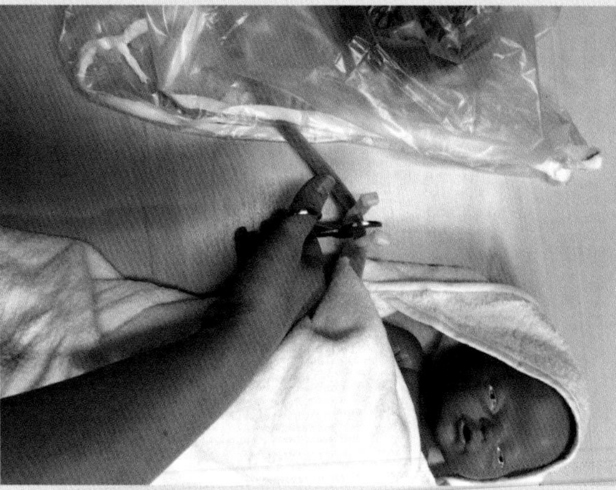
	● Wait until the cord has stopped pulsating; apply two cord clamps securely 3 cm apart and about 15 cm from the umbilicus. Cut the cord between the two clamps. **CAUTION** – ensure the newborn's fingers and genitals are clear of the scissors. ● Ensure the baby remains warm; keep the baby wrapped and ensure the head is covered. ● Place the baby with its mother in a position where the mother can breastfeed if she wants to (breastfeeding will also encourage birth of the placenta). ● Reassure the mother, and birth partner if present. ● Await the midwife and third stage (birth of the placenta and membranes). ● If birth has occurred en-route, proceed to the nearest obstetric unit. It is not necessary to await birth of the placenta before continuing with the transfer. ● Provide an alert/information call, including the detail of whether mother and baby are being conveyed together or not.
● Third stage of labour (birth of the placenta and membranes) – may take 15–20 minutes	● Assist the mother in expelling the placenta naturally by encouraging her to adopt a squatting, upright position, but only if there has been no delay in delivery of the placenta and **NOT IF THERE IS ANY SIGNIFICANT BLEEDING**. ● Encourage the woman to empty her bladder to facilitate uterine contraction. ● Do not pull the cord during birth of the placenta as this could rupture the cord, making birth of the placenta difficult and cause excessive bleeding or inversion of the uterus. ● Allow the placenta to be born straight into a bowl or plastic bag. Keep it, together with any blood and membranes, for inspection by a midwife. ● **NB** If the placenta has not been born within 20 minutes following birth insert a LARGE BORE (16G) cannula, as there is an increased risk of haemorrhage and may require intravenous fluid and further intervention (oxytoxics).
● Assess how much blood has accompanied the delivery of the placenta and membranes – this should not exceed 200–300 ml	● If bleeding continues after birth of the placenta, palpate the mother's abdomen and feel for the top of the uterus (fundus) usually at the level of the umbilicus and massage firmly with a cupped hand in a circular motion. ● The fundus will become firm as massage is applied and this may be quite uncomfortable, so Entonox should be offered (refer to Entonox for administration and information). ● Be aware that the uterus may relax again and bleeding recommence. 'Rubbing up a contraction' may need to be repeated.
● Assess blood loss – if bleeding is severe	● Obtain IV access – insert two LARGE BORE (16G) cannulae. ● Administer an oxytocic drug (refer to **Intravascular Fluid Therapy (Adults)** and **Intravascular Fluid Therapy (Children)**). ● Administer Syntometrine intramuscularly if available (refer to **Syntometrine**). ● If Syntometrine is **NOT** available or the woman is hypertensive (≥140/90), administer misoprostol 800 micrograms (4 tablets) sublingually (refer to **Misoprostol**). ● Tranexamic acid (1g slow IV over 10 minutes) can be given additionally. ● Refer to post-partum haemorrhage section within this guideline.

Normal Birth *continued*	
• Assess and monitor respiration rate, pulse and blood pressure	• Administer O_2 to aim for target saturation within the range of 94–98% (refer to **Oxygen**).
	A number of complications may arise during pregnancy and/or labour. Refer to Table 5.4 for the assessment and management of: 1 pre-term birth 2 maternal convulsions (eclampsia) 3 prolapsed umbilical cord 4 post-partum haemorrhage 5 continuous severe/sudden abdominal/back pain/placental abruption 6 multiple births – delayed birth of second or subsequent baby 7 malpresentation 8 shoulder dystocia.

Table 5.4 – ASSESSMENT and MANAGEMENT of:

Birth Complications	
1. Pre-term birth – birth before the completion of 37 weeks	
ASSESSMENT	**MANAGEMENT**
• Ascertain the period of gestation	• Less than 20 weeks gestation – transfer the woman to the nearest ED with an obstetric unit. • 20–37 weeks gestation – transfer the woman to the nearest obstetric unit or ED with an obstetric unit dependent on local policy, as the baby will require specialist assessment by the neonatal team once born.
• Re-assess the mother constantly en-route	• Should birth take place en-route assess both the mother and the baby and take appropriate action. • Keeping the baby warm is a priority in the preterm newborn (refer to **Newborn Life Support**). • Convey mother and baby to the **NEAREST** obstetric unit or ED with an obstetric unit dependent on local policy. • Provide a pre-alert to enable a midwifery and neonatal team to receive the mother and newborn baby upon your arrival. • In some circumstances, it may be necessary to convey the baby separately from the mother, dependent upon the clinical condition of either newborn or mother. In this instance, mother and baby should be conveyed to the same ED with an ID bracelet placed on each of them.
	• If transfer to further care is not possible because the birth is imminent, request a midwife plus an additional ambulance and inform the EOC. • Once the baby is born, utilise the additional ambulance to transport the baby **IMMEDIATELY** to the **NEAREST** appropriate destination as agreed locally. • The baby should be transported once appropriate resource is available even if the midwife has not yet arrived. • Provide a pre-alert to the hospital (it will be necessary to identify the nearest, most appropriate ED with an obstetric unit, with the necessary neonatal facilities). • The mother should be transferred to the same location as the baby; where no complications are identified, a courtesy call should be placed ahead of her arrival.
2. Maternal convulsions (eclampsia) (see Figure 5.3)	
ASSESSMENT	**MANAGEMENT**
• Quickly assess the woman and scene as you approach	• Refer to **Pregnancy-induced Hypertension**. • **ALL** generalised tonic/clonic type convulsions after 24th week of pregnancy should be regarded as eclampsia until proved otherwise, **EVEN IF THERE IS A HISTORY OF EPILEPSY**. • If the woman is convulsing, refer to **Convulsions (Adults)** and **Convulsions (Children)**.

Birth Complications *continued*	
Undertake a primary survey **<C>ABCDEF** Assess for **TIME CRITICAL** features	• Correct A and B problems and transfer to the nearest ED with an obstetric unit.
3. Prolapsed umbilical cord (see **Figure 5.4**)	
ASSESSMENT The descent of the umbilical cord into the lower uterine segment. This is a **TIME CRITICAL EMERGENCY** requiring immediate intervention, rapid removal and transfer to the nearest obstetric unit	**MANAGEMENT** Avoid handling the umbilical cord. Using a dry pad, replace the cord GENTLY within the opening of the vulva to keep it warm and prevent spasm, and use the pad to prevent further prolapse. (Do not use moist/wet pads as this will make the cord cold). If available, use underwear to hold the pad in position. If attending as a solo responding clinician, position the woman in the knee/chest position while awaiting an ambulance. 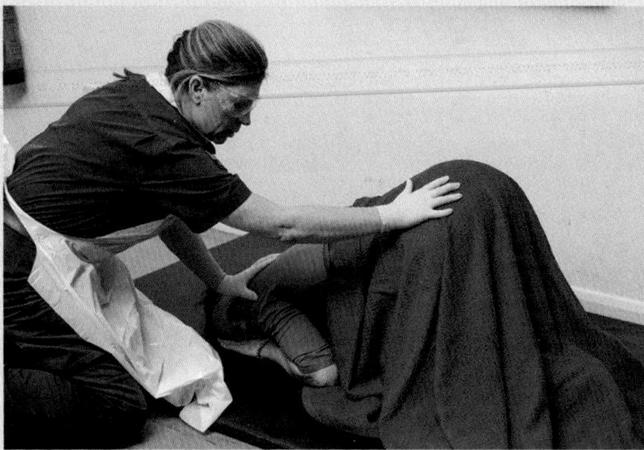 To enable rapid transfer to the ambulance, the woman can be walked, avoiding the use of the carry chair where possible. Once in the ambulance, position the mother on her side with padding placed under her hips to raise the pelvis and reduce pressure on the cord. 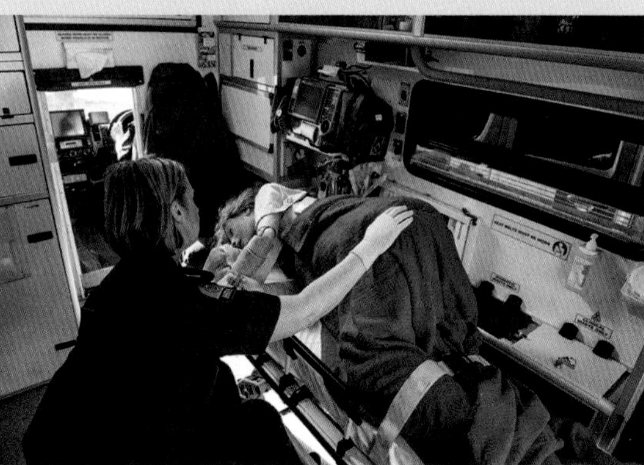 Administer Entonox if the mother experiences pain or the urge to push. Provide ongoing assessment of the woman to ensure that birth is not imminent (if birth is imminent, refer to the **normal birth** section of this guideline.) It is not safe to convey the woman in the all fours position in the ambulance.
	• Transfer to the nearest obstetric unit. • Place an early pre-alert stating the obstetric emergency of cord prolapse. • It may be necessary to request maternity staff to meet the ambulance clinicians at a suitable entrance to avoid any delays due to accessing lifts or entry to buildings.

Birth Complications *continued*

4. Post-partum haemorrhage (PPH)The commonest cause of severe haemorrhage immediately after delivery is uterine atony (i.e. poor uterine contraction) (see **Figure 5.5**).

ASSESSMENT

Primary PPH: blood loss of 500 ml or more within 24 hours of birth

Massive PPH: blood loss of 50% of the blood volume within 3 hours of birth

MANAGEMENT

NOTE – If severe haemorrhage occurs following birth of the baby (post-partum) follow one of the two treatment regimens below en-route to further care if possible.

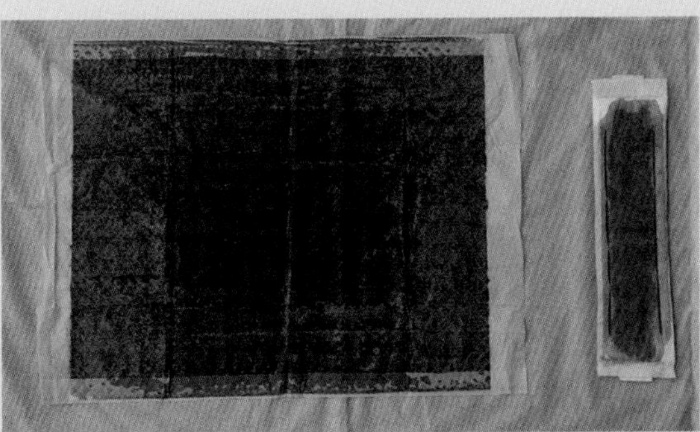

Maternity pad with 500 ml blood and sanitary pad with 50 ml blood.

1. IF THE PLACENTA HAS DELIVERED:

- Palpate the abdomen and feel for the top of the uterus (fundus), usually at the level of the umbilicus, and massage with a cupped hand in a circular motion.
- The fundus will become firm as massage is applied. This may be quite uncomfortable and Entonox can be offered (refer to Entonox for administration and information).
- Administer **Syntometrine intramuscularly** (refer to Syntometrine).
- If Syntometrine or other oxytocics are unavailable, have been ineffective at reducing haemorrhage after 15 minutes, or the woman is hypertensive (BP >140/90), administer misoprostol 800 micrograms sublingually (refer to Misoprostol).
- Administer **tranexamic acid** (1g slow IV over 10 minutes en-route to hospital).
- Establish IV access (ideally with two large bore (16G) cannulae).
- Convey to the nearest obstetric unit or, where there is on-going bleeding with evidence of maternal collapse, convey to the nearest appropriate destination as agreed locally.
- In the presence of catastrophic haemorrhage, the first line of management in the pre-hospital setting should be to apply *fundal massage* (known as 'rubbing up' a uterine contraction) and administer first line drugs such as Syntometrine or Syntocinon.
- The use of 'bimanual uterine compression' is an invasive procedure requiring intimate internal manoeuvres and may be considered only by those paramedics that have received appropriate training to undertake this life saving intervention.

2. IF THE PLACENTA HAS NOT DELIVERED:

- In the presence of haemorrhage, **DO NOT** massage the top of the uterus (fundus) when the placenta is undelivered. This may provoke partial separation of the placenta and cause further haemorrhage. (However, in the event of life-threatening haemorrhage, massaging the uterus while transferring to hospital may be considered).
- Administer a bolus of Syntometrine intramuscularly (refer to Syntometrine) – if Syntometrine or other oxytocics are unavailable, have been ineffective at reducing haemorrhage after 15 minutes, or if the woman is hypertensive (BP >140/90), administer misoprostol (refer to Misoprostol).
- **Administer tranexamic acid** (1g slow IV over 10 minutes).

NB Administration of Syntometrine or misoprostol may cause the placenta to separate and deliver. If the placenta delivers, ensure there is no further bleeding. If bleeding continues after the placenta is delivered – commence massage of uterine fundus.

Birth Complications *continued*

● Assess blood loss – if bleeding is >500 ml ● Re-assess prior to further fluid replacement ● If bleeding continues, check for bleeding from tears at the vaginal entrance	● Obtain IV access – insert a **LARGE BORE (16G)** cannula. ● Administer fluid replacement (refer to **Intravascular Fluid Therapy (Adults)** and **Intravascular Fluid Therapy (Children)**) ● Apply external pressure to a tear using a gauze or maternity pad. ● Transfer the mother and baby to the **NEAREST OBSTETRIC UNIT** immediately. ● Provide a pre-alert stating an obstetric emergency of post-partum haemorrhage. ● During conveyance provide ongoing assessment and, where necessary, uterine massage. ● Administer **tranexamic acid** (1g slow IV over 10 minutes) can be given.

5. Multiple births – delayed birth of second or subsequent baby

ASSESSMENT	MANAGEMENT
NOTE – with a twin birth, the mother is at increased risk of immediate post-partum haemorrhage due to poor uterine tone (refer to 4 above). It is now very unusual for a mother expecting a multiple birth to give birth outside hospital. However, twin pregnancies are at much higher risk of delivering pre-term (i.e. before 37 weeks) – the babies may therefore need resuscitation	If birth is **NOT** in progress: ● Transfer mother to the nearest obstetric unit without delay. ● Constantly re-assess en-route and take appropriate action if the circumstances change. ● Place an information call informing the hospital of a woman expecting a twin birth.
	If birth is in progress or occurs en-route: ● Request a second ambulance and, where available, midwifery support. ● Follow normal birth guidance and refer to **Care of the Newborn**.
	● When the first baby has been born and assessed, if birth of the second baby is not imminent, transfer the mother and baby to the **NEAREST OBSTETRIC UNIT IMMEDIATELY** (it is not necessary to await the arrival of the midwife). ● Provide a pre-alert to the hospital. It may be necessary to request maternity staff meet the ambulance clinicians at a suitable entrance to avoid any delays due to accessing lifts or entry to buildings.
	● If the birth of the second baby occurs en-route, request via the EOC an **ADDITIONAL AMBULANCE**. ● When the second baby is born, utilise both vehicles to transfer mother and babies to the nearest obstetric unit. ● Provide a pre-alert including the number of babies due to arrive with one mother (this is particularly relevant with higher birth multiples, although uncommon).
● Assess if any/either baby requires resuscitation	● Refer to **Newborn Life Support**.

6. Malpresentation – including vaginal breech birth (see **Figure 5.6**)

ASSESSMENT	MANAGEMENT
● Vaginal breech birth is where the feet or buttocks of the baby present first rather than the baby's head ● NB Cord prolapse is more common with a breech presentation (refer to 3 above); follow local guidelines	**Vaginal breech birth** – if birth is **NOT** in progress: ● Recognise breech presentation (may be documented in the woman's antenatal notes, thick meconium may be seen at vaginal opening, fetal buttocks or feet visible at vaginal opening). ● Transfer mother to the nearest obstetric unit without delay. ● Constantly re-assess en-route and take appropriate action if the circumstances change.

Birth Complications *continued*

Vaginal breech birth – if birth **IS** in progress:

- Request a midwife (if available locally) and additional resources.
- Prepare for newborn resuscitation (refer to **Newborn Life Support**).
- Encourage the woman to adopt a position to enable gravity to help the birth of the baby, for example the edge of the bed, the edge of a sofa or the 'all fours' position.

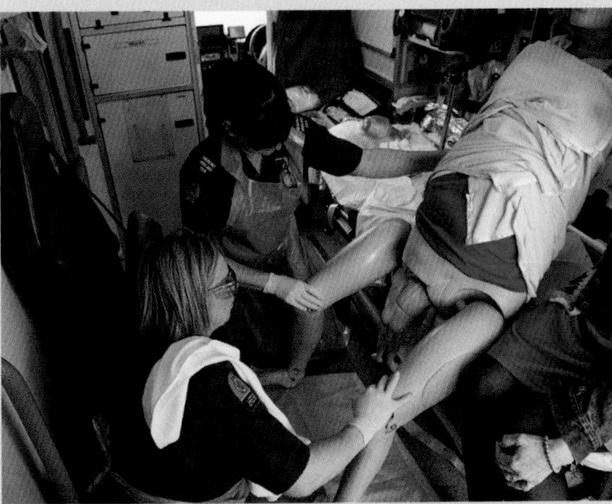

Breech delivery with mother semi-recumbent. Note – the fetal back should be upwards.

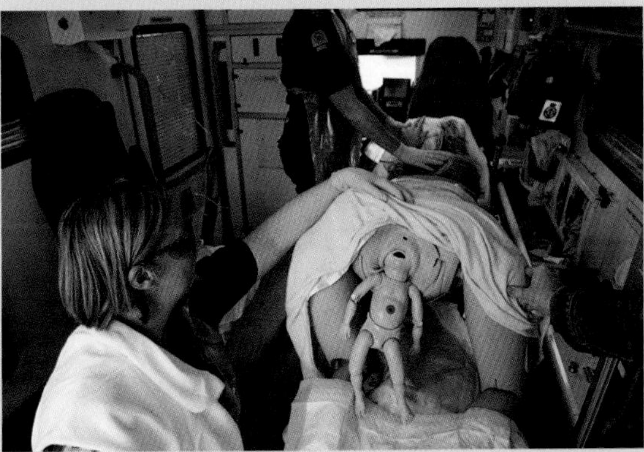

Breech delivery in 'all fours' position. Note – the fetal abdomen should face upwards (i.e. the fetal back faces the maternal abdomen).

- Allow breech to descend spontaneously with maternal pushing, and maintain a 'hands off' position. It is not necessary to touch the baby or handle the umbilical cord during the birth.
- The baby's legs and arms will spontaneously birth and do not require any assistance.
- Only assist to ensure the baby's back remains facing towards the woman's abdomen.
- If the baby's back rotates away from the woman's abdomen, handle the baby over the hips (the bony pelvis) and gently rotate the baby's back to face towards the woman's abdomen.
- In the semi-recumbent position, once the baby's body is born to the nape of the neck, allow slow spontaneous birth of the head by supporting the baby's body on your forearm and gently lift the baby to facilitate birth of the baby's head. In the all fours position, as the head delivers the baby's body will deliver onto the bed/trolley.
- Once the birth is complete, if the baby does not require any resuscitation, management of the umbilical cord should be as per normal birth guidelines, and should be left to stop pulsating.
- Breech babies are more likely to be covered in meconium and may require resuscitation (refer to **Newborn Life Support**).

Birth Complications *continued*

- If delays occur during the birth:
  - **Legs.** If the legs delay birth of the body, apply gentle pressure to the back of the baby's knee (popliteal fossa) enabling birth of each individual leg.
  - **Arms.** If the arms are extended, gently rotate baby's pelvis 90 degrees and aid delivery of the first (uppermost) arm, then rotate the baby in the opposite direction 180 degrees and release the other arm.
  - **Head.** If the head delays birth, refer to Burn's Marshall Technique - support the baby with one arm and use the other hand to aid flexion of the back of the baby's head while delivering baby.
- Where ambulance clinicians have received appropriate training in management of breech birth, additional manoeuvres can be undertaken as detailed above for management of the legs, arms and head where delays in birth are identified.
- Where the ambulance clinician has not received appropriate training, the nearest obstetric unit can be contacted to provide guidance on the ongoing management of the birth.

Any presenting body part other than the head, buttocks or feet (e.g. one foot or a hand/arm).

- Transfer the mother immediately to the nearest obstetric unit.
- Provide a pre-alert. It may be necessary to request maternity staff meet the ambulance clinicians at a suitable entrance to avoid any delays due to accessing lifts.

7. Shoulder dystocia (see **Figure 5.7**)

ASSESSMENT

- An arrest of spontaneous birth; when birth of the baby's shoulders is delayed because the baby's anterior shoulder is stuck behind the symphysis pubis

MANAGEMENT

- Request a midwife (if available locally) and additional resources.
- Prepare for newborn resuscitation (refer to **Newborn Life Support**).
- An attempt must be made to deliver the shoulders using the McRoberts manoeuvre if:
  - the shoulders are not born within two contractions following the birth of the head
  - there is difficulty with delivery of the face and chin
  - the head remains tightly applied to the vulva or retracts ('turtle-neck' sign)
  - there is failure of the fetal head to fully rotate to face toward the mother's inner thigh once born.

McRoberts manoeuvre (alters the angle of the pelvis)

- Ask the woman to lie flat and bring her bottom to the end of the bed.
- Bring the woman's knees up onto her abdomen (the legs will naturally abduct due to the pregnant uterus). If available, use an assistant to support each leg or ask the woman to hold them. Ask the woman to push with the next contraction, as the shoulders may now be released.

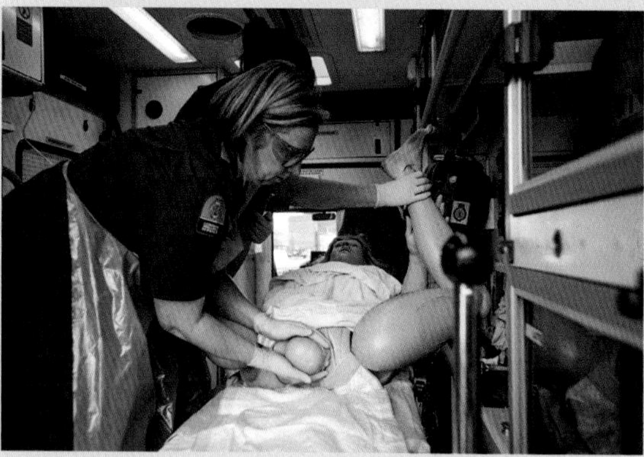

- If the shoulders do not release, attempt to deliver the baby's shoulders with gentle 'axial' traction applied to the baby's head (this is outward traction keeping the baby's head in line with its own spine, and is angled just below the horizontal); the mother is encouraged to push. **AVOID** pulling on the baby's head downwards or laterally

Birth Complications *continued*

towards the floor and avoid twisting the baby's neck at any time (this can damage the brachial plexus nerves).

- If undelivered after 30 seconds move on to applying suprapubic pressure while maintaining the McRoberts position.

Suprapubic pressure

- Identify where the fetal back is facing.
- With the mother still in McRoberts position, ask the assistant to:
  a Stand on the maternal side where the baby's back is (if the baby's back is facing left, stand on the woman's left or vice versa).
  b Place hands in CPR grip with the heel of the hand two finger breadths above the maternal symphysis pubis.
  c Apply moderate pressure in a downwards and lateral direction **continuously** for 30 seconds.
  d Encourage the mother to push or attempt gentle **AXIAL** traction to deliver the baby.

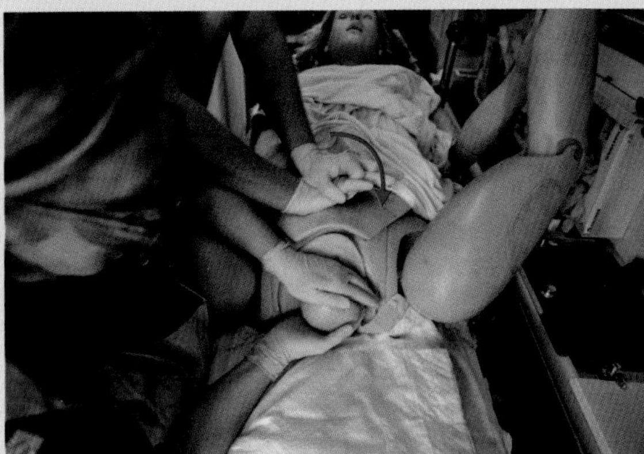

- If the shoulders do not release, attempt **intermittent pressure** on the shoulder for 30 seconds:
  a Ask the assistant to apply intermittent pressure on the shoulder by rocking gently backwards and forwards.
  b Encourage the mother to push or attempt gentle **AXIAL** traction to deliver the baby.
  c If unsuccessful change the woman's position to 'all fours'.

'All fours' position

(For the lone clinician this is an ideal first position to use as it provides a very effective McRoberts manoeuvre.)

- Position the woman on her hands and knees with her hips well flexed, (any movement of the pelvis may help release the shoulders).

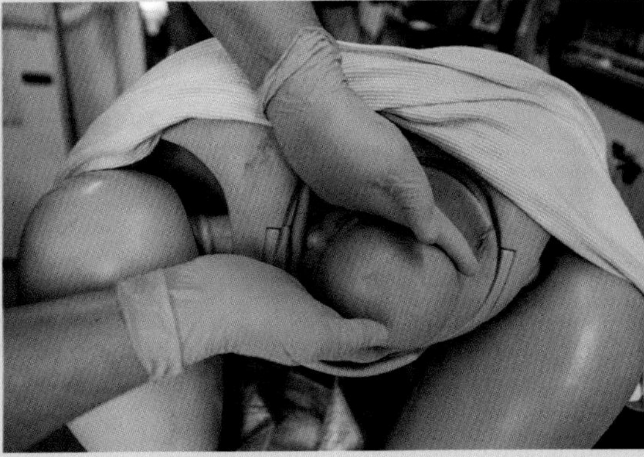

- Encourage the woman to push to release shoulders or apply gentle **AXIAL** traction to release the shoulder nearest to the maternal back first.

Birth Complications *continued*

- If unsuccessful, transfer the woman to the ambulance; she may be walked as this may also encourage the birth. Ambulance clinicians should be prepared to anticipate the birth during transfer and/or conveyance.

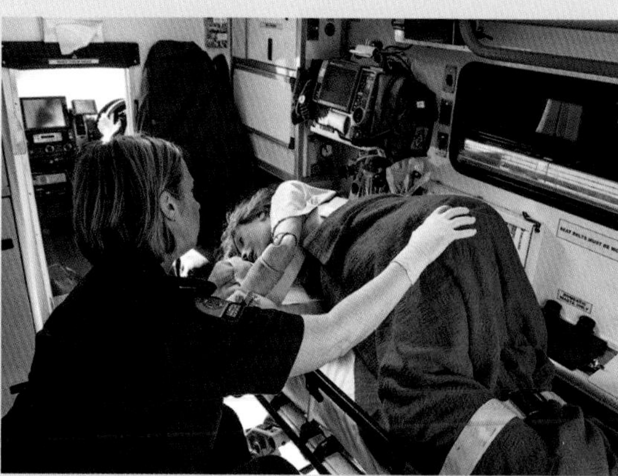

- Convey the woman to the nearest obstetric unit positioned in a lateral position using a pillow to seperate the woman's legs and avoid pressure on the baby's head. Offer Entonox to provide analgesia if required. Do not delay to await arrival of the midwife.
- Place a pre-alert stating the obstetric emergency of shoulder dystocia. It may be necessary to request maternity staff meet the ambulance clinicians at a suitable entrance to avoid any delays due to accessing lifts or access to buildings.

The use of internal manoeuvres by ambulance clinicians

- Where McRoberts manoeuvre, suprapubic pressure and all fours position have been attempted to expedite the birth, the use of specific internal manoeuvres may be appropriate where a registered paramedic has received additional training to undertake them.
- In a pre-hospital setting where a lone attending clinician is first on scene, the use of all fours position may facilitate the removal of the posterior arm, notably when awaiting an ambulance to the scene.

KEY POINTS

Birth Imminent: Normal Birth and Birth Complications

- **For a woman experiencing an abnormal labour or birth, transfer immediately to the nearest obstetric unit. This includes:**
  - **severe vaginal bleeding**
  - **preterm or multiple births**
  - **prolapsed umbilical cord**
  - **continuous severe abdominal/epigastric pain**
  - **maternal convulsions (eclampsia)**
  - **presentation of the baby other than the head (e.g. arm or leg or buttocks)**
  - **shoulder dystocia.**
- **If the woman presents with an obvious medical or traumatic condition that puts her life in imminent danger, transfer to the nearest ED with an obstetric unit.**
- **The period of gestation is important in informing the appropriate course of action, including the most appropriate location for conveyance, namely an ED, an early pregnancy unit or an obstetric unit.**
- **In the event of an obstetric emergency, detailing the exact emergency via a pre-alert call will assist the ED or maternity unit to summon the appropriate staff.**
- **Maintaining normothermia in the newborn is critical while on scene and during conveyance. The optimum body temperature of the baby should be between 36.5 and 37.5 degrees.**

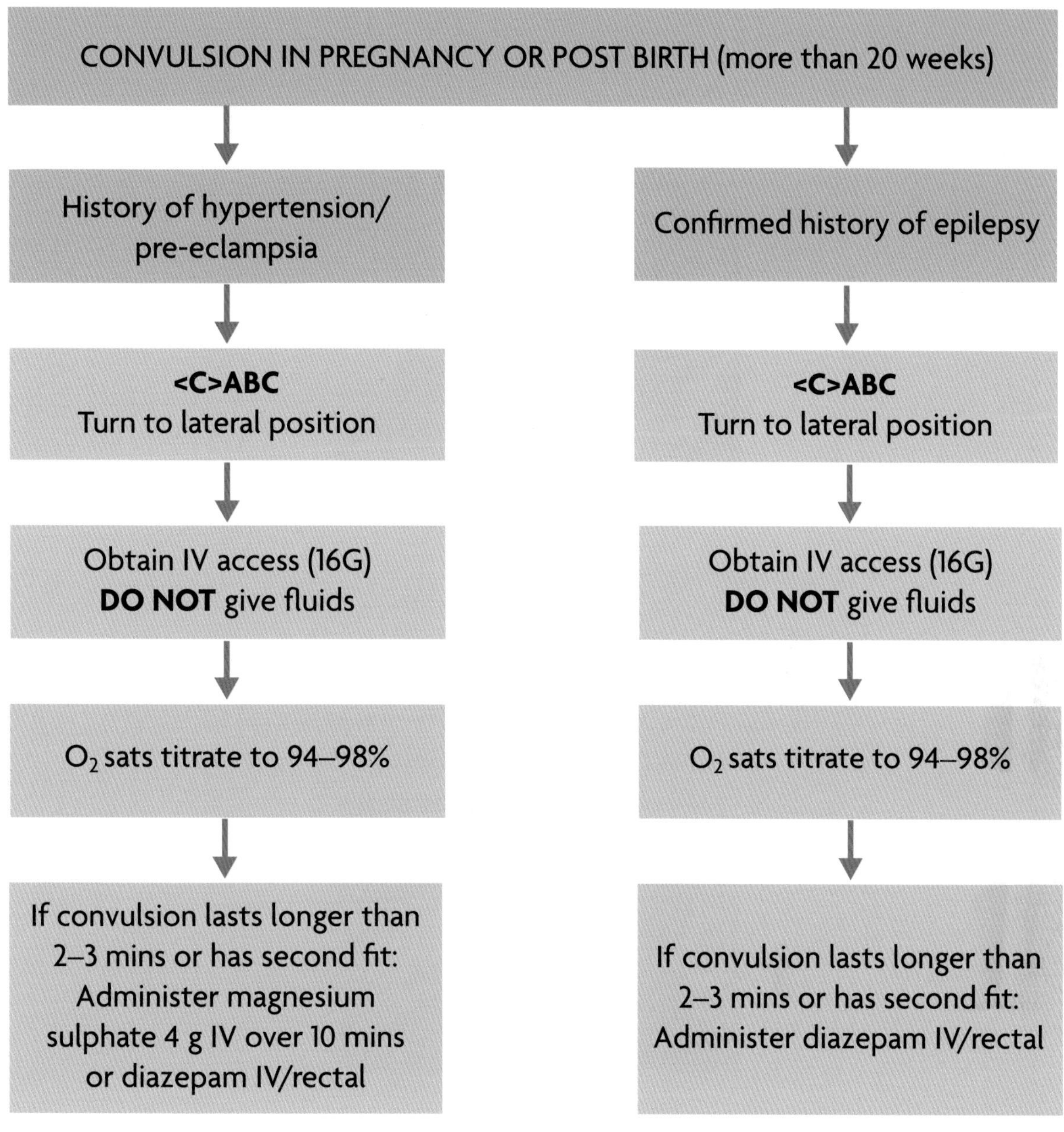

Transfer to nearest appropriate destination as agreed locally
Maternal safety is the prime consideration
Consider the specific clinical situation **and which interventions may be required for the woman and baby on arrival**
Refer to 'Appropriate Destination for Conveyance' in **Maternity Care**
Pre-alert stating obstetric emergency eclampsia
Take maternity notes if available

Figure 5.3 – Pre-hospital maternity emergency – management of eclampsia.

Gently replace the umbilical cord within the opening of the vagina using a dry pad

↓

Position the woman in the knee chest position while awaiting the ambulance

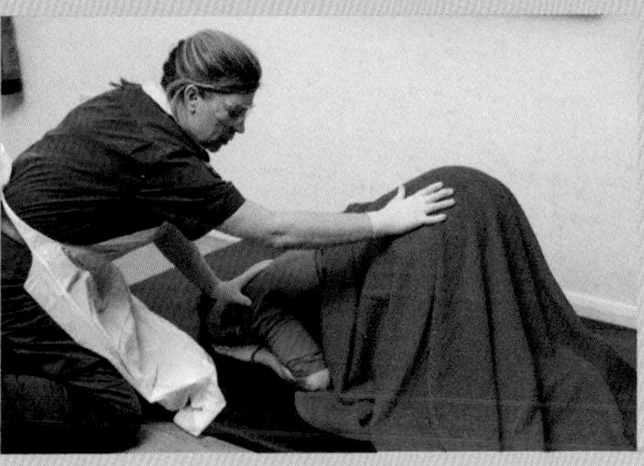

↓

Walk the woman to the ambulance

Position the woman in the lateral position
Elevate the pelvis using a blanket below the right hip

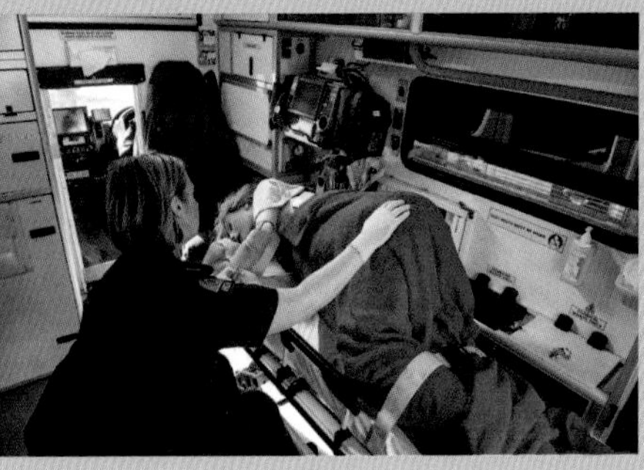

↓

Assess for imminent birth en-route
Administer Entonox if required

Transfer to nearest appropriate destination as agreed locally
Maternal safety is the prime consideration
Consider the specific clinical situation **and which interventions may be required for the woman and baby on arrival**
Refer to 'Appropriate Destination for Conveyance' in **Maternity Care**
Pre-alert stating obstetric emergency of cord prolapse
Take maternity notes if available

Figure 5.4 – Pre-hospital maternity emergency – management of cord prolapse.

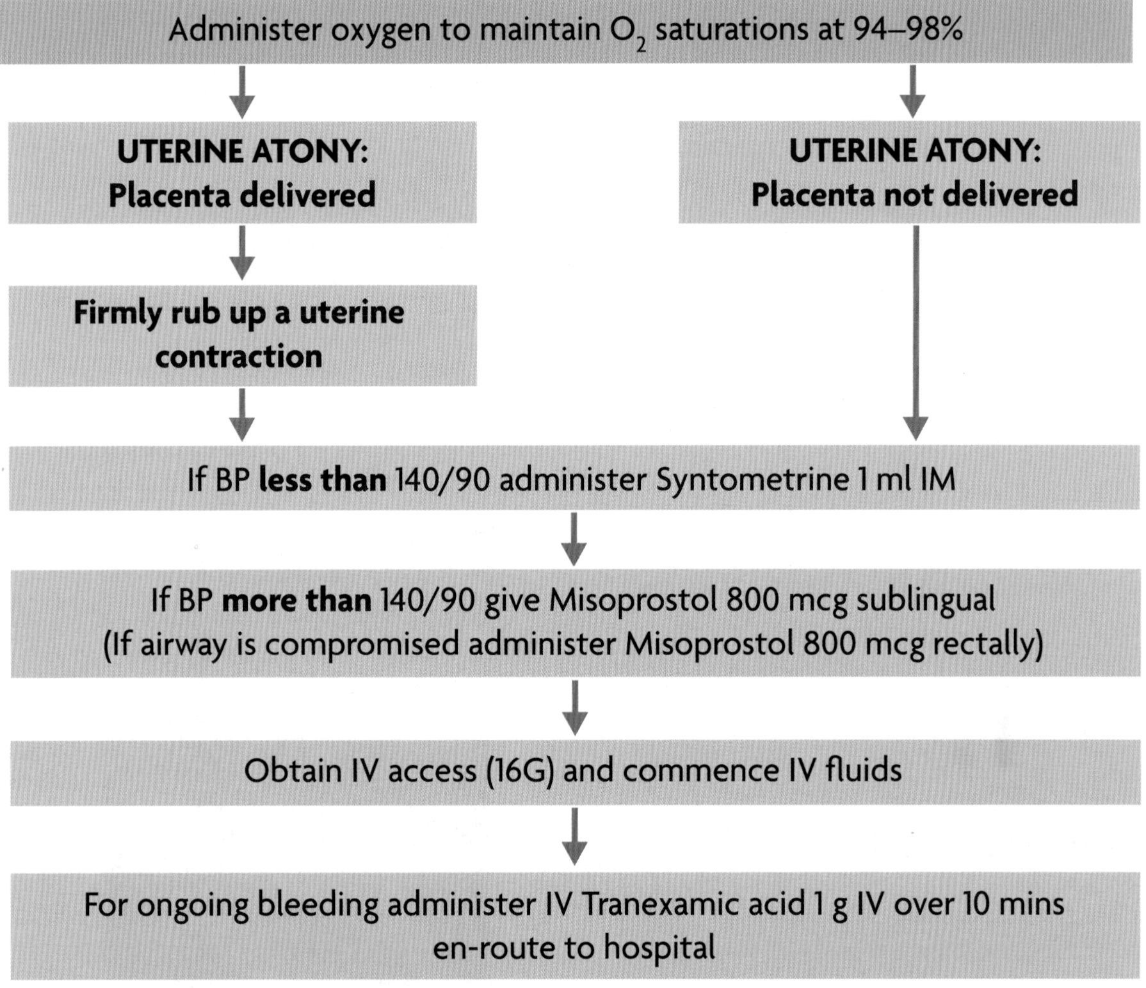

If uterus is well contracted, check for perineal trauma:
Apply external direct pressure gauze/maternity pad
Obtain IV access (16G) and commence IV fluids
For ongoing bleeding administer IV Tranexamic acid 1 g IV over 10 mins en-route to hospital

Transfer to nearest appropriate destination as agreed locally
Maternal safety is the prime consideration
Consider the specific clinical situation **and which interventions may be required for the woman and baby on arrival**
Refer to 'Appropriate Destination for Conveyance' in **Maternity Care**
Pre-alert stating obstetric emergency PPH
Perform ongoing assessment of uterine contraction and/or perineal trauma/maternal observations

Figure 5.5 – Pre-hospital maternity emergency – management of post-partum haemorrhage.

Breech position noted in maternal notes or thick meconium seen at vaginal opening

↓

BREECH BIRTH IMMINENT

↓

Request midwife if available
Prepare for newborn life support

↓

Position on edge of bed/trolley or on all fours

↓

HANDS OFF
Allow breech to descend spontaneously with maternal pushing
DO NOT touch baby or handle umbilical cord

↓

In either position, ensure the baby's back is always facing towards the maternal abdomen

↓

Support baby as head births

↓

Treat as normal birth or
refer to Newborn Life Support

↓

BREECH BIRTH NOT IMMINENT OR ANY OTHER PRESENTING PART (i.e. hand/arm)

↓

Transfer to nearest appropriate destination as agreed locally

Maternal safety is the prime consideration

Consider the specific clinical situation **and which interventions may be required for the woman and baby on arrival**

Refer to 'Appropriate Destination for Conveyance' in **Maternity Care**

Continuously assess for birth imminent en-route

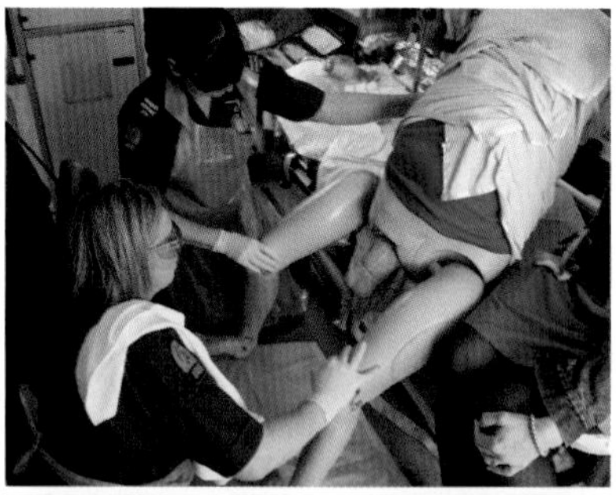

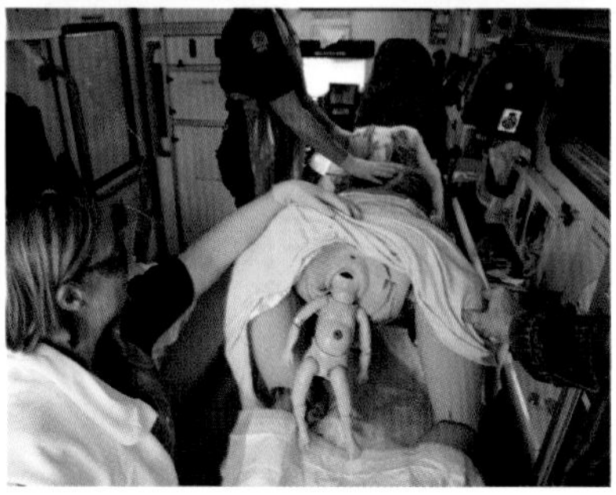

IF DELAY OCCURS DURING THE BIRTH:

LEGS: apply gentle pressure behind the baby's knee
ARMS: gently rotate the baby's pelvis 90 degrees to aid birth of the first arm – rotate the baby's body in the opposite direction if required to birth the second arm – allow the baby's body to hang unassisted
HEAD: support the baby with one arm and use the other hand to aid flexion of the back of the baby's head while delivering baby

DO NOT PULL ON THE BABY
DO NOT CLAMP AND CUT THE UMBILICAL CORD DURING THE BIRTH

Figure 5.6 – Pre-hospital maternity emergency – management of breech birth.

REQUEST A MIDWIFE IF AVAILABLE AND PREPARE FOR NEWBORN LIFE SUPPORT
Position the woman in the McRoberts position
For a solo clinician – ask the woman to hold her legs and push with her next contraction

If shoulders do not release:
Attempt to deliver the baby
- With your hands on the baby's head apply gentle 'axial' traction, keeping the baby's head in line with its spine for up to 30 seconds

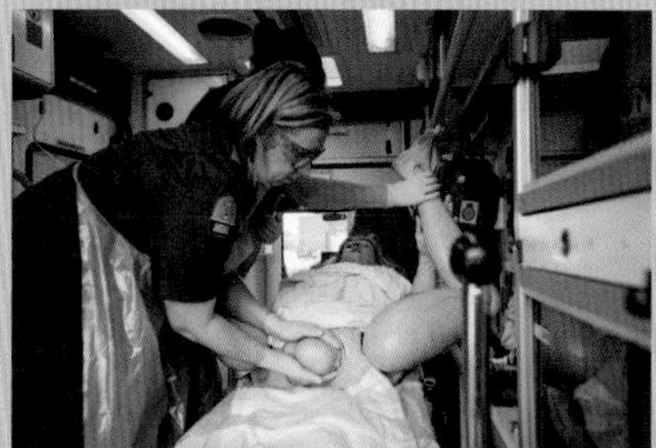

Undelivered?

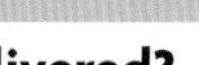

Apply suprapubic pressure with the woman in the McRoberts position
- Identify the position of the fetal back and place assistant on that maternal side
- Using a CPR grip, apply continuous pressure downwards and lateral for 30 seconds (2 fingers above symphysis pubis)
- Encourage the woman to push **OR** attempt gentle 'axial' traction to deliver baby

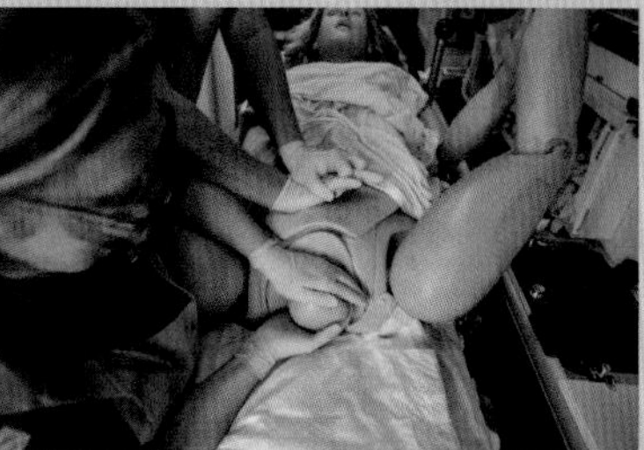

Undelivered?

- Attempt intermittent 'rocking' suprapubic pressure for 30 seconds and encourage woman to push
- Or attempt gentle 'axial' traction to deliver baby

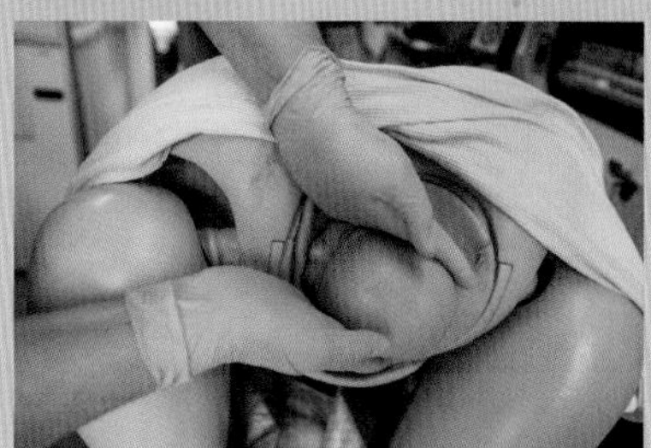

Undelivered?

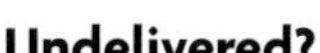

- Change the woman's position to 'all fours' and encourage her to push
- Or attempt gentle 'axial' traction to deliver baby

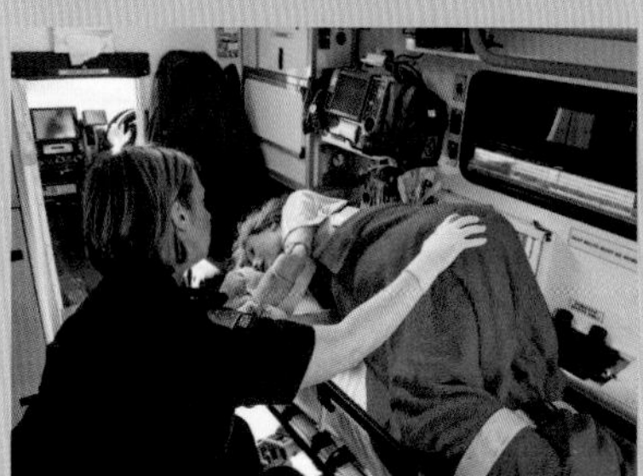

Undelivered?

- Walk the woman to the ambulance and anticipate the birth during transfer
- Convey in a lateral position with legs separated by a blanket to protect the baby's head
- Reassure the woman and provide Entonox as required.

Baby born
Refer to **Care of the Newborn**

Transfer to the nearest appropriate destination as agreed locally
Maternal safety is the prime consideration
Consider the specific clinical situation **and which interventions may be required for the woman and baby on arrival**
Refer to 'Appropriate Destination for Conveyance' in **Maternity Care**
Pre-alert stating the obstetric emergency shoulder dystocia
Keep a log of the time each intervention is attempted

Figure 5.7 – Pre-hospital maternity emergency – management of shoulder dystocia.

Bibliography

1 Woollard M, Hinshaw K, Simpson H, Wieteska S. Normal delivery. In Pre-hospital Obstetric Emergency Training. Oxford: Wiley-Blackwell, 2009: 28–37.

2 Woollard M, Hinshaw K, Simpson H, Wieteska S. Structured approach to the obstetric patient. In *Pre-hospital Obstetric Emergency Training*. Oxford: Wiley-Blackwell, 2009: 38–52.

3 Woollard M, Hinshaw K, Simpson H, Wieteska S. Emergencies in late pregnancy. In *Pre-Hospital Obstetric Emergency Training*. Oxford: Wiley-Blackwell, 2009: 62–110.

4 Woollard M, Hinshaw K, Simpson H, Wieteska S. Emergencies after delivery. In *Pre-hospital Obstetric Emergency Training*. Oxford: Wiley-Blackwell, 2009: 111–124.

5 Woollard M, Hinshaw K, Simpson H, Wieteska S. Care of the baby at birth. In *Pre-hospital Obstetric Emergency Training*. Oxford: Wiley-Blackwell, 2009: 125–135.

6 Royal College of Obstetricians and Gynaecologists. *The Management of Breech Presentation* (Green-top Guideline 20b). London: RCOG, 2006.

7 Royal College of Obstetricians and Gynaecologists. *Placenta Praevia, Placenta Praevia Accreta and Vasa Praevia: Diagnosis and Management* (Green-top Guideline 27). London: RCOG, 2011.

8 Royal College of Obstetricians and Gynaecologists. Shoulder Dystocia (Green-top Guideline 42). London RCOG, 2012.

9 Royal College of Obstetricians and Gynaecologists. *Umbilical Cord Prolapse* (Green-top Guideline 50). London: RCOG, 2008.

10 Royal College of Obstetricians and Gynaecologists. *Prevention and Management of Postpartum Haemorrhage* (Green-top guideline 52). London: RCOG, 2016.

11 Mousa HA, Alfirevic Z. Treatment for primary postpartum haemorrhage. *Cochrane Database of Systematic Reviews* 2007, 1: CD003249.

12 Starrs A, Winikoff B. Misoprostol for postpartum hemorrhage: moving from evidence to practice. *International Journal of Gynaecology and Obstetrics* 2012, 116(1): 1–3.

13 Health and Care Professions Council. *Standards of Conduct, Performance and Ethics: Your Duties as a Registrant*. London: Health Professions Council, 2003.

14 Crofts JF, Lenguerrand E, Bentham GL, Tawfik S, Claireaux HA, Odd D, Fox R, Draycott TJ. Prevention of brachial plexus injury – 12 years of shoulder dystocia training: an interrupted time-series study. *BJOG* 2016, 123(1): 111–118.

15 Griffin C. Re: Prevention of brachial plexus injury – 12 years of shoulder dystocia training: an interrupted time-series study: posterior arm delivery at the time of caesarean section. *BJOG* 2016, 123(1): 144.

16 Menticoglou S. Delivering shoulders and dealing with shoulder dystocia: should the standard of care change? *JOGC* 2016, 38(7): 655–658.

17 Gherman RB. Shoulder dystocia. *Clinical Obstetrics and Gynecology* 2016, 59(4): 789–790.

1. Introduction

- Ambulance clinicians attend births that occur at home, or on the way to hospital. Hence it is important to be aware of the differences in physiology of the newborn baby. The newborn baby has emerged from dependence on the protective uterine environment to independent life. Physiology is changing within the first few hours to weeks after birth. Hence what may apply to infants and children may not necessarily be applicable to newborn babies. Additionally, different management issues arise in premature babies.
- Most babies manage the transition to extra-uterine life by themselves, a few require assistance with that transition and even fewer require resuscitation.
- All babies should initially be kept warm. **Skin-to-skin contact is an effective measure in keeping babies warm, and early feeding is key.**

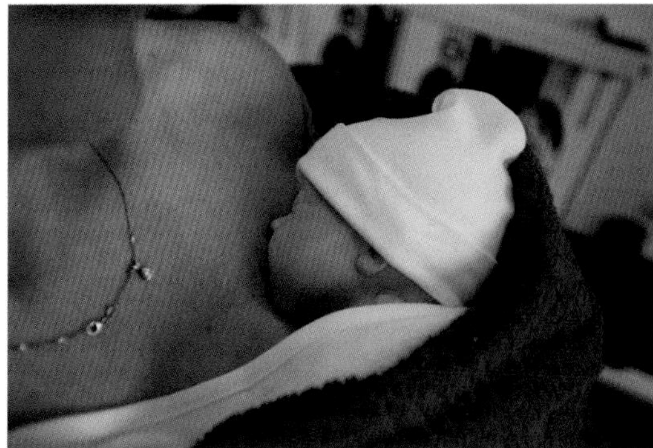

Figure 5.8 Skin-to-skin contact.

- Some babies may be born at home and a proportion of these may need to be transported to hospital because of unexpected problems.
- A newborn baby will need to be transferred to hospital for the following reasons:
  - any baby that required resuscitation
  - perinatal hypoxia (APGAR score below 5)
  - meconium staining or aspiration
  - baby of a diabetic mother
  - small for dates/growth-restricted baby
  - prematurity (gestation <37 weeks) or a term baby >37 with respiratory distress syndrome/abnormal breathing pattern
  - major congenital abnormalities, even if the baby appears well at birth
  - red flags suggesting a high risk of early onset neonatal bacterial infection
  - safeguarding concerns known to the ambulance service or communicated by the maternity unit.

2. Pathophysiology

2.1 Perinatal Hypoxia

- Perinatal hypoxia can occur for various reasons including cord prolapse, the cord being tightly wrapped around the fetal neck, significant placental or umbilical bleeding, or prolonged second stage of labour. The presence of thick meconium may indicate an episode of perinatal hypoxia.
- Severe perinatal hypoxia has a poor outlook and is often associated with neurological deficits and cerebral palsy. A low APGAR score at 10 minutes suggests a high possibility of long-term neurological complications.
- Recent studies have shown that in babies born at >36 weeks gestation with perinatal hypoxia, moderate hypothermia results in a better neurological outcome. The multicentre CoolCap, ICE and TOBY trials showed that cooling to 33.5°C within 6 hours of birth for 72 hours was associated with a decreased death rate, less neurodevelopmental disability and less cerebral palsy in survivors. This controlled cooling was done without adverse effects being seen in the babies. A meta-analysis of all the neonatal cooling trials strongly supports the use of therapeutic hypothermia in newborn infants with hypoxic ischaemic encephalopathy to reduce the risk of death and neurological impairment at 18 months.
- Researchers are currently studying the benefits of controlled therapeutic cooling using special blankets or suits during interhospital transfers when taking hypoxic babies to tertiary neonatal units. The transfer of these babies between neonatal intensive care units is, however, the only situation when babies can be transferred without ensuring the ambulance is well heated, and it will be made clear by the medical staff if this is required. Unless the specific equipment is available and requested by hospital staff, the ambulance should be as warm as possible for transfer.

2.2 Hypothermia

- Babies have a large body surface area relative to their weight, and heat loss occurs easily by convection. Premature babies are at particular risk. A wet baby will also lose heat by evaporation, especially if in a draught. Babies lose heat as a result of their proportionately large heads when compared to their bodies. Hats, towels and blankets can be used to significantly reduce these heat losses. Transfer the baby in a POD if this is available.
- The body temperature of the baby should be kept at about 36.5–37.5°C. The ambulance should therefore be kept well heated to prevent cooling during the transfer to hospital. Accidental hypothermia in all babies, but especially in the premature baby, can be harmful. For each degree below 36.5°C, the risk of mortality increases by 28%. A cold baby has increased oxygen consumption, and is at risk of hypoglycaemia and acidosis, and is associated with an increased mortality. It is therefore important that the baby is kept warm during the transfer in the ambulance, to prevent hypoglycaemia and these complications.

2.3 Hypoglycaemia

- The newborn baby has a relatively immature liver with limited glycogen stores and so low blood sugars are not an uncommon problem. It is therefore important to encourage and support early breastfeeding where possible.

- In a baby without any abnormal signs and symptoms (see list below), and no risk factors (see list below), hypoglycaemia is defined as any single blood glucose (BG) reading with a value of <1.0 mmol/l, even if a subsequent reading is normal. In a baby who is at-risk (see list below), hypoglycaemia is defined as two consecutive blood glucose readings of <2.0 mmol/l. In a baby with abnormal signs and symptoms, a single reading of <2.5 mmol/l can be used to diagnose hypoglycaemia. If the BG is <1.1 mmol/L, remains <2.6 mmol/L or if the baby is symptomatic, they must be reviewed urgently by a paediatrician and the baby requires admission to the neonatal unit.
- Glucose is the main energy source for the fetus and neonate, and the newborn brain depends almost exclusively on glucose for energy metabolism.
- Hypoglycaemia can therefore lead to convulsions and brain injury. Severe and prolonged hypoglycaemia may result in long-term neurological damage. It is therefore important to prevent and treat a low blood sugar level as soon as it is detected.
- Signs and symptoms of hypoglycaemia include:
  - jitteriness
  - irritability
  - lethargy
  - apnoeic episodes
  - convulsions
  - BG <1.5 mmol/L.

NB Many hypoglycaemic babies are asymptomatic, hence the importance of routine blood glucose checks in babies at risk. Those at risk of hypoglycaemia include babies who are:

- premature
- small for gestational age
- <2.5kg at birth
- in need of resuscitation at birth
- born to diabetic mothers, due to high circulating maternal insulin levels
- born to mothers using beta blockers (labetalol)
- suffering from perinatal hypoxia
- suffering from hypothermia
- suffering from sepsis.

After birth, encourage the mother to feed her baby as soon as possible (or at least within the first hour). Failing this, intravenous glucose may be needed, depending on (i) the baby's condition and (ii) the blood glucose level. The newborn baby's liver has very limited glycogen stores, so hypoglycaemia must not be treated using intramuscular glucagon (glucagon works by stimulating the liver to convert glycogen into glucose). A baby found to have hypoglycaemia (as previously defined) must be transported to hospital for further investigation and management.

2.4 Neonatal Jaundice

- Jaundice refers to the yellow colouration of the skin and sclera caused by a raised bilirubin level. About 60% of term and 80% of pre-term babies develop jaundice in the first week of life. Physiological jaundice occurs around day 2–7, although 10% of breast fed babies are still jaundiced at 1 month of age. Physiological jaundice is due to increased breakdown of haemoglobin in red blood cells to bilirubin, and the immature liver is unable to handle the conversion of bilirubin to a form that can be excreted in the gut. Jaundice is harmless unless the bilirubin level is very high, when this can cross the blood–brain barrier.
- Unconjugated bilirubin is potentially toxic to brain tissue causing kernicterus and brain damage. Different treatment thresholds are recommended for different gestations and ages (see graphs published by National Institute for Health and Clinical Excellence). Jaundice is treated with phototherapy or exchange transfusion, depending on the level of bilirubin and the cause. Early jaundice (occurring before day 2) or prolonged jaundice (after day 14) may be due to other pathological causes or underlying diseases and requires investigation. Babies with early jaundice occurring <2 days of age must be referred for an urgent medical review.

2.5 Preterm Delivery

- Prematurity is defined as <37 weeks gestation. Premature infants are more likely to need assistance with ventilation.
- At <32 weeks gestation spontaneous breathing will be inadequate and this group of babies are likely to be deficient in surfactant (surfactant reduces alveolar surface tension and keeps the lung alveoli open during expiration), necessitating surfactant replacement and/or ventilatory support, and immediate transfer to the nearest ED with an obstetric unit will be necessary.
- At <32 weeks gestation the risk of intracranial bleeds is increased.
- Other complications of prematurity include hypothermia, hypoglycaemia and a higher risk of infection.
- Improving neonatal intensive care has seen better outcomes for babies born pre-term (especially in babies born after 28 weeks gestation). However, the EPICure study following up babies born in the UK at the limits of viability before 26 weeks gestation showed a high mortality and morbidity. Overall survival was only 39% and survivors commonly have severe disabilities. Hypothermia was one of the factors associated with death.

Birth at Less Than 24 Weeks Gestation

Ambulance clinicians may attend births at extremes of prematurity and viability. The guidance regarding newborn resuscitation in the pre-hospital phase of care is less well defined than in a maternity unit, where access to neonatal expertise can enable a plan to be discussed with the woman based upon the clinical assessment of the pregnancy to date. The following guidance acts to enable clinicians working in the pre-hospital setting to be supported when faced with a baby born prematurely between 20 and 24 weeks gestation:

- When attending a birth at 20–24 weeks **OR** the gestation is unknown, and there are signs of life, the recommendations are:
  - Maintain ventilation using the smallest paediatric mask – size 00.
  - Provide effective ventilations with the baby lying flat, assess heart rate and do not expect the chest to move at this gestation. If ventilations are effective the heart rate will remain stable or improve.
  - Where neonatal wraps or cribs are available these should be used to minimise heat loss.
  - Ensure the head is covered with the small baby hat.
  - Place a pre-alert stating whether the mother is travelling with the baby.
  - Convey to the nearest ED with an obstetric unit, requesting the neonatal team.
- Where there are signs of life, ventilations should be continued until the neonatal team can assess the gestation and weight of the baby. The team will then consider the ongoing management in the best interests of the baby and the family.
- Neither a midwife nor an ambulance clinician should discontinue resuscitative attempts; this decision sits within the expertise of the neonatologist.

2.6 Congenital Abnormalities

- The outcome of babies born with congenital abnormalities varies but is improving with advancement in medical therapies and interventions. The abnormality may have been detected on previous antenatal scans or may have been undiagnosed until birth. Hence all babies who are known to have a congenital abnormality should be transferred to hospital where the abnormality can be assessed and treated, even when the baby appears to be normal at birth.
- Cling film the defect to reduce fluid and heat losses.

NB Do not wrap the cling film circumferentially around the newborn's body as this will inhibit breathing.

2.7 Early Onset Neonatal Sepsis

Early onset neonatal sepsis can be life-threatening and it is important that it is recognised and treated early. The following **red flags** ⚑ suggest a high risk of early onset neonatal sepsis:

- Maternal risk factors:
  - ⚑ systemic antibiotic treatment given to the mother for confirmed or suspected invasive bacteria
  - ⚑ group B streptococcus (GBS)
  - ⚑ E.coli
  - ⚑ listeria
  - ⚑ other organisms, such as anaerobes (rare)
  - ⚑ GBS colonisation, bacteriuria or infection in CURRENT pregnancy
  - ⚑ a previous baby with invasive GBS infection
  - ⚑ preterm, pre-labour rupture of membranes of any duration
  - ⚑ suspected or confirmed intrapartum rupture of membranes >18 hours.
- Neonatal risk factors
  - ⚑ convulsions in the baby
  - ⚑ signs for shock in the baby
  - ⚑ need for mechanical ventilation in a term baby
  - ⚑ suspected or confirmed infection in a co-twin.

3. Assessment and Management

The baby's condition can be assessed quickly just from their colour, heart rate and breathing effort. For the initial clinical assessment of the newborn baby the following should be undertaken (refer to Table 5.5):

- Colour – useful for assessing the initial condition of the baby at birth.
- Tone – a baby born well-flexed and with good tone is normally well.
- Breathing – usually starts spontaneously within a minute of birth.
- Heart rate – in healthy term babies the heart rate is usually greater than 100 bpm by 2 minutes of age.

Table 5.5 – ASSESSMENT and MANAGEMENT of:

The Newborn

ASSESSMENT	MANAGEMENT
● Assess **ABCD**	● If any of the following **TIME CRITICAL** features are present: – major **ABCD** problems – perinatal hypoxia – major congenital abnormalities – prematurity – hypoglycaemia. ● Start correcting **A** and **B** problems. ● Undertake a **TIME CRITICAL** transfer to the nearest appropriate destination as agreed locally. ● Expedite transferral of the baby once available resources are secured. This may require transferral separately from the mother. ● Provide a pre-alert/information call detailing the neonatal emergency.
– Assess need for resuscitation at birth (refer to **Newborn Life Support**)	● Use a quick assessment, observing: – colour – tone – breathing – heart rate. ● If time permits, perform an APGAR score at 1 and 5 minutes after birth and document within the patient record.
● Perinatal hypoxia	● If resuscitation is required at birth or there is evidence of perinatal hypoxia, transfer to the nearest appropriate destination as agreed locally.
● Suspected hypoglycaemia	● Ensure early feed. ● Check newborn temperature. If transferring to hospital, keep the baby warm during transfer. ● Where a baby is sleepy and unable to coordinate its breathing with feeding, check blood sugar from a heel prick. ● If hypoglycaemia is confirmed, treatment is **TIME CRITICAL** to prevent convulsions and brain damage. ● IM glucagon will **NOT** work due to poor glycogen stores in the newborn.
● Assess temperature	● Heat loss occurs readily because of the large body surface area. ● Ensure the newborn baby is dried after birth, as heat loss also occurs by evaporation if the baby is wet. Make sure the environment remains warm and that the baby is covered, including a hat. If well, skin-to-skin will maintain a covered baby's temperature effectively, but continuously monitor airway and breathing.
● Transfer to further care	● A baby requiring transfer for neonatal care needs to be transferred via the ED.

Table 5.6 – APGAR SCORE

Score	0	1	2
Appearance	blue or pale all over	blue at extremities body pink	body and extremities pink
Pulse rate	absent	<100	≥100
Grimace or response to stimulation	no response to stimulation	grimace/feeble cry when stimulated	cry or pull away when stimulated
Activity or muscle tone	none	some flexion	flexed arms and legs that resist extension
Respiration	absent	weak, irregular, gasping	strong, lusty cry

3.1 APGAR score

The APGAR score can also be used to assess the clinical condition of the baby at birth (refer to Table 5.6), and can be recorded retrospectively at 1 and 5 minutes after birth where a midwife is not present.

- A pink baby with a lusty cry and a heart rate >100/min will need no further treatment, and just needs to be dried and given to the mother to hold. Most babies fall into this category and only require drying, warming and some stimulation.
- A blue baby with a heart rate >60/min, who has some tone and some response to stimulation may begin to breathe spontaneously after a short wait (not >1 minute) if given a little time and some firm stimulation.
- A pale, floppy and apnoeic baby with a heart rate <60/min will need bag-and-mask ventilation, followed by cardiac compression if the heart rate does not improve or breathing does not start (refer to **Newborn Life Support**), and undertake a **TIME CRITICAL** transfer.
- Only use suctioning if the airway requires clearing. Then use gentle suctioning of the mouth and nose with a soft suction catheter (CH12–14) to remove excess secretions. Avoid deep pharyngeal suctioning as this can cause bradycardia (from vagal stimulation) or laryngospasm.
- If there has been either meconium staining of the liquor or baby, or evidence of meconium aspiration, the baby will need to be transferred to hospital quickly, as this may indicate fetal distress and possible fetal hypoxia. Meconium aspiration can lead to respiratory distress and the need for ventilatory support. The baby may additionally have associated complications from perinatal hypoxia (refer to **Newborn Life Support**).

KEY POINTS

Care of the Newborn

- **The need for resuscitation can be determined from a quick assessment of the baby's condition at birth, including its colour, tone, breathing and heart rate.**
- **Dry the baby and keep it warm.**
- **Treat hypoglycaemia as soon as it is detected to prevent convulsions or long-term neurological damage.**
- **Pre-term babies require further management in hospital.**
- **All babies with congenital abnormalities should be transferred to hospital for assessment.**
- **Be aware of red flags in mother or baby, which might suggest a high risk of early onset neonatal sepsis.**

Bibliography

1 Wyllie J, Bruinenberg J, Roehr CC, Rüdiger M, Trevisanuto D, Urlesberger B. European Resuscitation Council Guidelines for Resuscitation 2015: Section 7. Resuscitation and support of transition of babies at birth. *Resuscitation* 2015, 95: 249–263.

2 Porter A, Snooks H, Youren A, Gaze S, Whitfield R, Rapport F et al. 'Covering our backs': ambulance crews' attitudes towards clinical documentation when emergency (999) patients are not conveyed to hospital. *Emergency Medicine Journal* 2008, 25(5): 292–295.

3 Wyllie J, Perlman JM, Kattwinkel J, Atkins DL, Chameides L, Goldsmith JP, et al. Part 11: Neonatal resuscitation: 2010 International Consensus on Cardiopulmonary Resuscitation and Emergency Cardiovascular Care Science with Treatment Recommendations. *Resuscitation* 2010, 81(1): e260–287.

4 Wyllie J, Perlman JM, Kattwinkel J, et al. Part 7: Neonatal resuscitation: 2015 International Consensus on Cardiopulmonary Resuscitation and Emergency Cardiovascular Care Science with Treatment Recommendations. *Resuscitation* 2015; 95: e169–201.

5 Hawdon JM. Investigation, prevention and management of neonatal hypoglycaemia (impaired postnatal metabolic adaptation). *Paediatrics and Child Health* 2012, 22(4): 131–135.

6 Cornblath M, Hawdon JM, Williams AF, Aynsley-Green A, Ward-Platt MP, Schwartz R, et al. Controversies regarding definition of neonatal hypoglycemia: suggested operational thresholds. *Pediatrics* 2000, 105 (5): 1141–1145.

7 Woollard M, Hinshaw K, Simpson H, Wieteska S. Care of the baby at birth. In *Pre-hospital Obstetric Emergency Training*. Oxford: Wiley-Blackwell, 2009: 125–135.

8 National Collaborating Centre for Women's and Children's Health. *Diabetes in Pregnancy* (CG63). London: National Institute for Health and Clinical Excellence, 2008.

9 Beard L, Lax P, Tindall M. Physiological effects of transfer for critically ill patients. *Anaesthesia Tutorial of the Week* 2016, 330. Available from: http://anaesthesiology.gr/media/File/pdf/330-Physiological-effects-of-transfer-for-critically-ill-patients.pdf.

10 National Institute for Health and Clinical Excellence. Neonatal Jaundice: Treatment Threshold Graphs. London: NICE, 2010. Available from: https://www.nice.org.uk/guidance/cg98/evidence/full-guideline-pdf-245411821.

Haemorrhage During Pregnancy (including Miscarriage and Ectopic Pregnancy)

1. Introduction

- This guidance is for the assessment and management of women with bleeding during early and late pregnancy (including miscarriage and ectopic pregnancy). For postpartum haemorrhage refer to **Birth Imminent: Normal Birth and Birth Complications**. For complications associated with therapeutic termination ('abortion') refer to **Vaginal Bleeding: Gynaecological Causes**.
- Any bleeding from the genital tract during pregnancy is of concern and in early pregnancy may indicate miscarriage or an ectopic pregnancy. This more commonly occurs in the first three months (weeks 1–12) but can also occur in the second trimester. Haemorrhage may:
  - present with evident vaginal loss of blood (e.g. miscarriage and placenta praevia)
  - occur mainly (or completely) within the abdomen or uterus. This presents with little or no external loss, but pain and signs of hypovolaemic shock (e.g. ruptured ectopic pregnancy and placental abruption). Pregnant women may appear well even with a large amount of concealed blood loss. Tachycardia may not appear until 30% or more of the circulating volume has been depleted.
- Bleeding in pregnancy is broadly divided into two timeframes: bleeding that occurs in the early part of pregnancy, such as miscarriage or ectopic pregnancy (less than 24 weeks), and that occurring in the late second and third trimesters of pregnancy, such as placenta praevia or placental abruption (i.e. after 24 weeks).

2. Haemorrhage in Early Pregnancy (≤24 weeks)

Haemorrhage in early pregnancy may indicate miscarriage or ectopic pregnancy

2.1 Incidence

Miscarriage is most common in the first 12 weeks of gestation. The mother will often be anxious as to what is happening and can be very concerned as to the health and wellbeing of her unborn baby.

2.2 Pathophysiology

- Miscarriage is the loss of pregnancy before 24 completed weeks. It is most commonly seen at 6–14 weeks of gestation but can occur after 14 weeks.
- Miscarriage occurs when some the early fetal or placental tissue (known as 'products of conception') are partly passed through the cervix and may become trapped, leading to continuing blood loss. If shock ensues, it is often out of proportion to the amount of blood loss (i.e. there is an added vagal component from tissue trapped in the cervix).

Risk factors – miscarriage

- Previous history of miscarriage.
- Previously identified potential miscarriage at scan.
- Smoker.
- Obesity.

Symptoms:

- Bleeding – light or heavy, often with clots and or jelly-like tissue.
- Pain – central, crampy, suprapubic or backache.
- Signs of pregnancy may be subsiding, e.g. nausea or breast tenderness.
- Significant symptoms (including hypotension) without obvious external blood loss may indicate 'cervical shock' due to retained miscarriage tissue stuck in the cervix. Symptomatic bradycardia may arise due to vagal stimulation.
- Usually presents at around 6–8 weeks gestation, so usually only one period has been missed.

Symptoms characteristic of a ruptured ectopic pregnancy:

- Acute lower abdominal pain.
- Slight bleeding or brownish vaginal discharge.
- Signs of blood loss within the abdomen with tachycardia and skin coolness.

Other suspicious symptoms:

- Unexplained fainting.
- Shoulder-tip pain.
- Unusual bowel symptoms.
- Intra-uterine contraceptive device fitted.
- Previous ectopic pregnancy.
- Tubal surgery.
- Sterilisation or reversal of sterilisation.
- Endometriosis.
- Pelvic inflammatory disease.
- Subfertility (delay in conceiving).

2.3 Management of Pregnancy Loss and Fetal Tissue in Early Pregnancy (<22 weeks)

Ambulance clinicians are often called to attend women who may have miscarried before the clinicians' arrival, or during the episode of care. This can be a very distressing time for the woman, her family and the ambulance clinicians involved.

Fetal tissue, including the baby, may be passed by the mother during the miscarriage. It may resemble blood-stained tissue, or demonstrate a discernible baby with placenta still attached. The management of fetal tissue must follow the principles below to ensure that all staff comply with the Human Tissue Act (March 2015).

- Where a woman has passed a pregnancy, whether miscarriage or following a medical induction, she may choose to handle the pregnancy remains herself; she should, however, have been given advice by the service provider (this is likely to be an early pregnancy unit or termination service). In **ALL** cases, offer the woman the opportunity to transfer the early pregnancy tissue/baby with her into the hospital.

Practical guidance:

- In **ALL** cases, inform the woman, and discuss her preferences about management of the fetal tissue or 'her baby'.
- Where it is difficult to identify fetal tissue, transport this tissue, using a soft item from the maternity pack.
- Where the baby is noticeably developed and small, the mother may wish to have the baby wrapped within a towel and placed with her during conveyance to hospital, this may be an important part of her grieving process.
- If the mother declines to see or hold the pregnancy tissue or baby, wrap it accordingly in a sensitive way using a towel or soft item from the maternity pack and convey to hospital.
- Where the pregnancy remains have been passed into a toilet and are no longer accessible, document the inspection undertaken.
- Where the mother is unable to make a decision, or is not able to articulate her wishes at that time, in order to act in the best interests of the mother, it is appropriate to remove the pregnancy remains from the toilet, wrapping them sensitively as detailed above.
- In **ALL** cases, document how the fetal tissue/baby was conveyed, and hand the fetal tissue/baby to the nurse or midwife at transfer of care.

3. Haemorrhage in Late Pregnancy

Antepartum or prepartum haemorrhage (>24 weeks) may indicate placenta praevia or placental abruption.

3.1 Incidence

Placenta praevia occurs in 1 in 200 pregnancies and usually presents at 24–32 weeks with small episodes of painless bleeding.

3.2 Pathophysiology

- **Placenta Praevia:** the placenta develops low down in the uterus and partially or completely covers the internal opening of the cervical canal, the internal cervical os. With the development and growth of the uterus, bleeding is inevitable. This can lead to severe haemorrhage during the pregnancy (i.e. painless bleeding) or when labour begins.
- **Placental Abruption:** Any vaginal bleeding in late pregnancy or during labour which is accompanied by severe/sudden continuous abdominal/back pain, or with signs of shock, may be due to placental abruption. Bleeding occurs between the placenta and the wall of the uterus, detaching an area of the placenta from the uterine wall. It can be associated with severe pregnancy-induced hypertension (PIH) and trauma. Placental abruption causes continuous severe/sudden abdominal/back pain, tightening of the uterus and/or signs of hypovolaemic shock, and puts the baby at immediate risk. There may be some external blood loss, but more commonly the haemorrhage is **concealed** behind the placenta. Where there is a combination of **revealed** (external) blood loss and concealed haemorrhage, this can be particularly dangerous, as it can lead to an underestimation of the amount of total blood lost. The woman's abdomen will be tender when felt and the uterus will feel rigid or 'woody' with no signs of relaxation.

NOTE:

Because the true amount of bleeding is concealed, placental abruption is also associated with disseminated intravascular coagulation (DIC), which can worsen the tendency to bleed.

Table 5.7 – ASSESSMENT and MANAGEMENT of:

Haemorrhage During Pregnancy

ASSESSMENT	MANAGEMENT
• Quickly assess the woman and scene as you approach • Undertake a primary survey **<C>ABCDEF** • Assess for **TIME CRITICAL** features	• If any time critical features are present correct **<C>ABC** and transport to nearest suitable receiving hospital (refer to **Medical Emergencies in Adults – Overview** and **Medical Emergencies in Children – Overview**). • Provide an alert/information call.
• Monitor SpO_2	• If **oxygen** (O_2) <94% administer O_2 to aim for a target saturation within the range of 94–98%.

Haemorrhage During Pregnancy *continued*	
• Assess volume of blood loss	• Obtain IV access – insert **LARGE BORE** (16G) cannula. • Visually inspect sanitary towels if worn. • A large sanitary towel can absorb 50 ml of blood. Blood loss will appear greater if mixed with amniotic fluid. 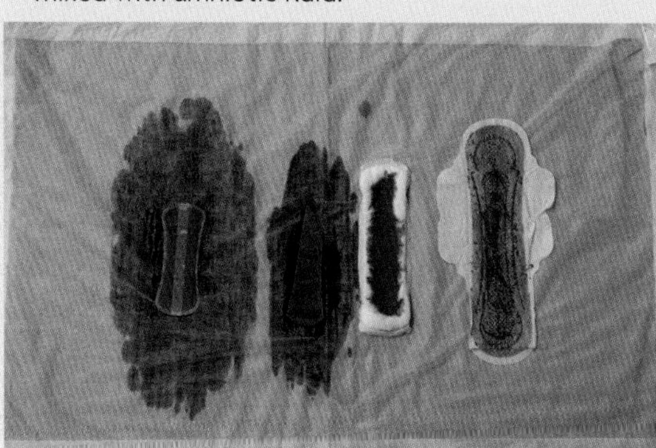 Four sanitary towels each soaked with 50 ml blood.
• In the event of **LIFE-THREATENING HAEMORRHAGE AND** a **confirmed diagnosis of miscarriage** (e.g. where a patient has gone home with medical management and starts to bleed)	• Administer Syntometrine intramuscularly if available (refer to **Syntometrine**). • If Syntometrine is **NOT** available or the woman is hypertensive (≥140/90), administer misoprostol 800 micrograms sublingually (4 tablets) (refer to **Misoprostol**). **CAUTION: DO NOT** administer Syntometrine or misoprostol with a fetus in situ.
• Assess for signs of shock (e.g. tachycardia >100 bpm, systolic <90 mmHg with cool sweaty skin) • Undertake a capillary refill test **NOTE:** hypovolaemia is manifested late in pregnant women; the woman may be very unwell and the fetus may be compromised; therefore **ADMINISTER** fluid replacement early (refer to **Intravascular Fluid Therapy (Adults)** and **Intravascular Fluid Therapy (Children)**)	• If >20 weeks, the gravid uterus may compress the inferior vena cava in a patient who is supine. Therefore, it is important to ensure adequate venous return before determining the need for fluid resuscitation; this can be achieved by using manual uterine displacement (see **Maternal Resuscitation**) or alternatively by placing the woman in a full lateral ('recovery') position or by lying her supine with lateral tilt (towards her left side where possible). • Administer 250 ml of sodium chloride 0.9% IV to maintain SBP of 90 mmHg (refer to **Intravascular Fluid Therapy (Adults)** and **Intravascular Fluid Therapy (Children)**). • Re-assess vital signs prior to further fluid therapy. • Take any blood-soaked pads to hospital. **NB:** Symptoms of hypovolaemic shock occur very late in otherwise fit young women; tachycardia may not appear until 30% of circulating volume has been lost, by which stage the patient is very unwell.
Ask 'When did you last feel the baby move?'	• Record when the mother last felt her baby move.
• If no **TIME CRITICAL** features, perform a more thorough assessment with secondary survey including fetal assessment (refer to **Maternity Care**) • Check the handheld maternity records for scan results confirming a 'low-lying' placenta	
• Assess woman's level of pain	• Titrate pain relief against pain (refer to **Pain Management in Adults** and **Pain Management in Children**): – **Paracetamol**. – **Entonox**. – **Morphine**: **NOTE** administer cautiously if the woman is hypotensive.

Haemorrhage During Pregnancy *continued*	
	• Nil by mouth.
	• Symptomatic bradycardia due to vagal stimulation can be treated with atropine (refer to **Atropine** and **Cardiac Rhythm Disturbance**).
	• Adjust woman's position as required.
	• If **TIME CRITICAL** features present, transfer to the nearest appropriate destination with a pre-alert stating the emergency. • Dependent upon locally agreed pathways and the gestational age of the pregnancy, it may be necessary to take the woman directly to the nearest maternity unit.

KEY POINTS

Haemorrhage During Pregnancy (including Miscarriage and Ectopic Pregnancy)

- **Haemorrhage during pregnancy is broadly divided into two categories, occurring in early and late pregnancy.**
- **Haemorrhage may be revealed (evident vaginal blood loss) or concealed (little or no obvious loss).**
- **Pregnant women may appear well even when a large amount of blood has been lost (tachycardia may not appear until 30% of circulating volume as symptoms of hypovolaemic shock occur very late, by which stage the woman is critically ill).**
- **Obtain venous access with large bore cannulae (16G).**
- **In the presence of a confirmed miscarriage, intramuscular Syntometrine administration should be considered.**

Bibliography

1. Soar J, Perkins GD, Abbas G, Alfonzo A, Barelli A, Bierens JJLM, et al. European Resuscitation Council Guidelines for Resuscitation 2010 Section 8: Cardiac arrest in special circumstances: electrolyte abnormalities, poisoning, drowning, accidental hypothermia, hyperthermia, asthma, anaphylaxis, cardiac surgery, trauma, pregnancy, electrocution. *Resuscitation* 2010, 81(10): 1400–1433.
2. Woollard M, Simpson H, Hinshaw K, Wieteska S. Obstetric services. In *Pre-hospital Obstetric Emergency Training*. Oxford: Wiley-Blackwell, 2009: 1–6.
3. Woollard M, Hinshaw K, Simpson H, Wieteska S. Anatomical and physiological changes in pregnancy. In *Pre-hospital Obstetric Emergency Training*. Oxford: Wiley-Blackwell, 2009: 18–27.
4. Woollard M, Hinshaw K, Simpson H, Wieteska S. Structured approach to the obstetric patient. In *Pre-hospital Obstetric Emergency Training*. Oxford: Wiley-Blackwell, 2009: 38–52.
5. Woollard M, Hinshaw K, Simpson H, Wieteska S. Emergencies in early pregnancy and complications following gynaecological surgery. In *Pre-hospital Obstetric Emergency Training*. Oxford: Wiley-Blackwell, 2009: 53–61.
6. Woollard M, Hinshaw K, Simpson H, Wieteska S. Emergencies in late pregnancy. In *Pre-Hospital Obstetric Emergency Training*. Oxford: Wiley-Blackwell, 2009: 62–110.
7. Human Tissue Authority (2015) *Guidance on the Disposal of Pregnancy Remains Following Pregnancy Loss or Termination*. Available from: https://www.hta.gov.uk/sites/default/files/Guidance_on_the_disposal_of_pregnancy_remains.pdf, 2015.
8. Royal College of Nursing. *Managing the Disposal of Pregnancy Remains. RCN Guidance for Nursing and Midwifery Practice*. Available from: https://www2.rcn.org.uk/__data/assets/pdf_file/0008/645884/RCNguide_disposal_pregnancy_remains_WEB.pdf, 2015.

Haemorrhage During Pregnancy (including Miscarriage and Ectopic Pregnancy)

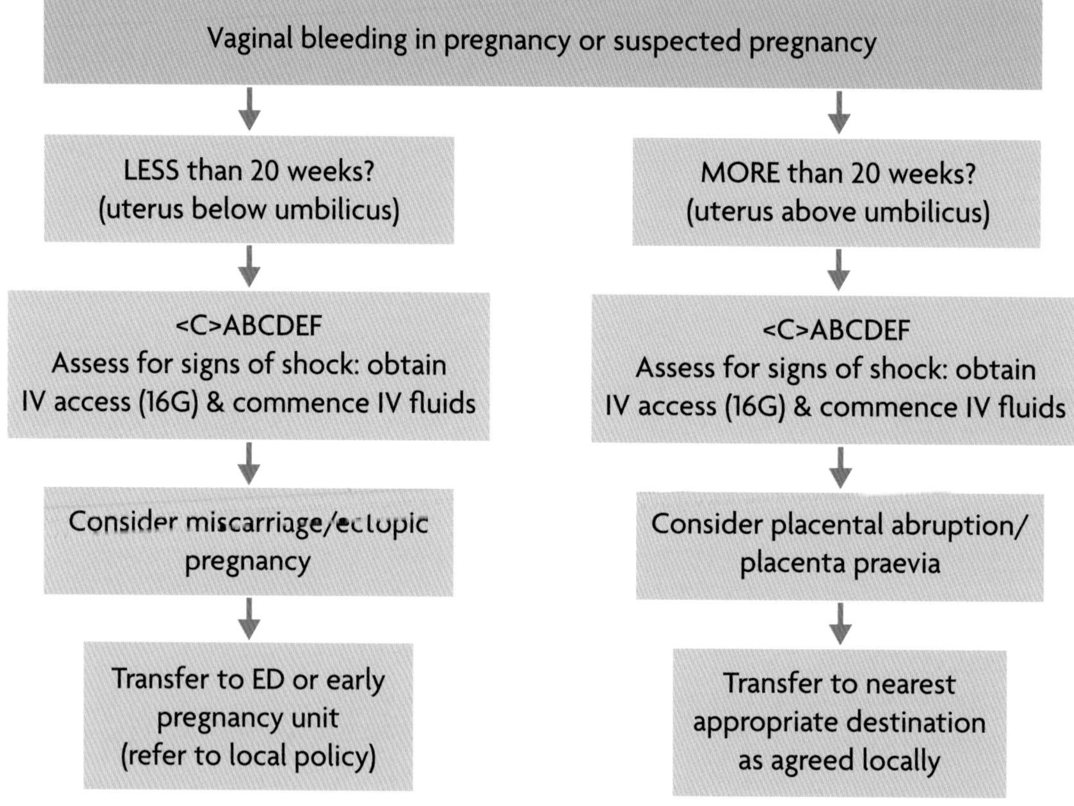

Maternal safety is the prime consideration

Consider the specific clinical situation **and which interventions may be required for the woman and baby on arrival**

Refer to 'Appropriate Destination for Conveyance' in **Maternity Care**

- If significant shock or compromise, consider ED in the first instance
- Take maternity notes if available

Figure 5.9 – Pre-hospital maternity emergency management – haemorrhage during pregnancy.

SECTION 1 – Pregnancy-induced Hypertension and Severe Pre-eclampsia

1. Introduction

- Pregnancy-induced hypertension (PIH) or gestational hypertension are generic terms used to define a significant rise in blood pressure after 20 weeks gestation, in the absence of proteinuria or other features of pre-eclampsia.
- Collapse related to hypertension is rare and usually related to eclampsia. Treatment and resuscitation of the mother will also resuscitate the fetus.

2. Incidence

- Hypertension from all causes is a common medical problem affecting 10–15% of all pregnancies.
- Approximately 15% of women who present with pregnancy-induced hypertension will develop pre-eclampsia.

3. Severity and Outcome

- PIH is usually mild (i.e. blood pressure (BP) 140/90 mmHg) and there is only a 10% risk of developing pre-eclampsia with mild rises in BP beyond 37 weeks.
- Fetal outcomes are good; however, pre-eclampsia accounted for 13.6% of maternal deaths related to pregnancy causes.

4. Pathophysiology

4.1 Pre-eclampsia

- Pre-eclampsia is PIH associated with proteinuria. It commonly occurs beyond 24–28 weeks gestation, but rarely can occur as early as 22 weeks.
- Although the underlying pathophysiology is not fully understood, pre-eclampsia is primarily a placental disorder associated with poor placental perfusion, which often results in a fetus that is growth-restricted (i.e. smaller than expected because of the poor placental blood flow).
- In the UK, the diagnosis of pre-eclampsia includes an increase in BP above 140/90 mmHg, oedema and detection of protein in the woman's urine.
- Pre-eclampsia is usually diagnosed at routine antenatal visits and may require admission to hospital and early delivery.
- The disease may be of mild, moderate or severe degree.

4.2 Severe Pre-eclampsia

- May present in a patient with known mild pre-eclampsia or may present with little or no prior warning.

4.3 Signs and Symptoms of Severe Pre-eclampsia

- Blood pressure is significantly raised and the diagnosis should be considered with any systolic >160 mmHg and diastolic >110 mmHg. There is proteinuria. Severe pre-eclampsia is usually associated with one or more of the following symptoms:
  - headache – severe and frontal
  - visual disturbances
  - epigastric pain – often mistaken for heartburn
  - right-sided upper abdominal pain – due to stretching of the liver capsule
  - muscle twitching or tremor
  - nausea
  - vomiting
  - confusion
  - rapidly progressive oedema.
- **Note** – the absence of these symptoms does not exclude severe pre-eclampsia and still requires critical assessment and management of the blood pressure alone.
- Agitation and restlessness may be signs of an underlying problem or impending deterioration in women with hypertension.

Pre-existing risk factors for development of pre-eclampsia

- Primiparity or first child with a new partner.
- Previous severe pre-eclampsia.
- Essential hypertension.
- Diabetes.
- Obesity.
- Twins or higher multiples.
- Renal disease.
- Advanced maternal age (over 35 years).
- Young maternal age (less than 16 years).
- Pre-existing cardiovascular disease.

Severe pre-eclampsia is:

- a 'multi-organ' disease; although hypertension is a cardinal feature, other complications include:
  - intracranial haemorrhage
  - stroke
  - renal failure
  - liver failure
  - abnormal blood clotting, e.g. disseminated intravascular coagulation (DIC).

5. Assessment and Management

- For the assessment and management of mild/moderate pre-eclampsia, refer to Table 5.8.
- For the assessment and management of severe pre-eclampsia, refer to Table 5.9.

Pregnancy-induced Hypertension (including Eclampsia)

Table 5.8 – ASSESSMENT and MANAGEMENT of:

Mild/Moderate Pre-eclampsia

Definition – raised blood pressure >140/90 mmHg, detection of proteinuria and sometimes oedema.

- Any woman with a blood pressure >140 mmHg systolic or >90 mmHg diastolic on **TWO** occasions in labour or immediately after birth should be transferred to a consultant obstetric unit.
- Blood pressure of 150/100 in pregnancy, labour or immediately after birth **requires urgent treatment**, and therefore rapid transfer to a consultant-led obstetric unit should be arranged.

ASSESSMENT	MANAGEMENT
• Undertake a quick assessment • Undertake a primary survey **ABCDEF** • Assess for **TIME CRITICAL** features (see definition and symptoms of severe pre-eclampsia below)	• If any time critical features are present correct **A** and **B** and transport to nearest suitable receiving hospital (refer to **Medical Emergencies in Adults – Overview** and **Medical Emergencies in Children – Overview**). • Provide an alert/information call.
• If **NON-TIME CRITICAL**, perform a more thorough assessment of the woman with secondary survey, including fetal assessment (refer to **Maternity Care** for guidance)	
• Measure blood pressure	Transfer to further care: • If pregnant >20 weeks and systolic blood pressure is >140/90 mmHg, discuss management directly with the BOOKED OBSTETRIC UNIT or MIDWIFE.

Table 5.9 – ASSESSMENT and MANAGEMENT of:

Severe Pre-eclampsia

Definition and symptoms – raised blood pressure >160 mmHg systolic and diastolic >110 mmHg, detection of proteinuria, particularly with one or more of the following: headache (severe and frontal), visual disturbances, epigastric pain, right-sided upper abdominal pain, muscle twitching or tremor, nausea, vomiting, confusion, rapidly progressive oedema.

ASSESSMENT	MANAGEMENT
• Undertake a quick assessment • Undertake a primary survey ABCDEF • Assess for signs of severe pre-eclampsia (see definition and symptoms above). Signs of severe pre-eclampsia are **TIME CRITICAL FEATURES**	• If any time critical features are present correct **A** and **B** problems (refer to **Medical Emergencies in Adults – Overview** and **Medical Emergencies in Children – Overview**) and transfer to a consultant-led obstetric unit. **NB** Caution with 'lights and sirens', as strobe lights and noise may precipitate convulsions. • If the patient is convulsing refer to **Convulsions (Adults)** and **Convulsions (Children)**. • Provide an alert/information call. • If the convulsion is NOT self-limiting, transfer to consultant-led obstetric unit.
• Monitor SpO_2 (94–98%)	• Attach pulse oximeter; if SpO_2 <94%, administer O_2 to aim for a target saturation within the range of 94–98%.
	• Obtain IV access – insert a LARGE BORE (16G) cannula en-route. • DO NOT administer intravenous fluid boluses because of the risk of provoking pulmonary oedema.
• Measure blood glucose level	• Refer to **Glycaemic Emergencies (Adults)** and **Glycaemic Emergencies (Children)**.

SECTION 2 – Eclampsia

1. Introduction

- Eclampsia is generalised tonic/clonic convulsion and identical to an epileptic convulsion.
- Many patients will have had pre-existing pre-eclampsia (of a mild, moderate or severe degree), but cases of eclampsia can present acutely with no prior warning – ONE THIRD of cases present for the FIRST TIME post-delivery (usually in the first 48 hours). **THE BP MAY ONLY BE MILDLY ELEVATED AT PRESENTATION** (i.e. 140/80–90 mmHg).
- Refer to **Convulsions (Adults)** and **Convulsions (Children)**.

2. Incidence

- Eclampsia occurs in approximately 2.7:10,000 deliveries, usually beyond 24 weeks.

3. Severity and Outcome

- Eclampsia is one of the most dangerous complications of pregnancy, and is a significant cause of maternal mortality, with a mortality rate of 2% in the UK.
- Convulsions are usually self-limiting, but may be severe and repeated.
- Other complications associated with eclampsia include renal failure, hepatic failure and DIC.

4. Pathophysiology

- The hypoxia caused during a tonic/clonic convulsion may lead to significant fetal compromise and death.

Risk factors – eclampsia

- Known pre-eclampsia.
- Primiparity or first child with a new partner.
- Previous severe pre-eclampsia.
- Essential hypertension.
- Diabetes.
- Obesity.
- Twins or higher multiples.
- Renal disease.
- Advanced maternal age (over 35 years).
- Young maternal age (less than 16 years).

5. Assessment and Management

- For the assessment and management of eclampsia and eclamptic convulsion, refer to Table 5.10.

Table 5.10 – ASSESSMENT and MANAGEMENT of:

Eclampsia

Definition – generalised tonic/clonic convulsion and identical to an epileptic convulsion.

ASSESSMENT	MANAGEMENT
• Undertake a primary survey **ABCDEF** • Assess for **TIME CRITICAL** features such as recurrent convulsions	• Correct **A** and **B** and transport to a consultant-led obstetric unit (refer to **Medical Emergencies in Adults – Overview** and **Medical Emergencies in Children – Overview**). • Obtain IV (LARGE BORE cannulae) or IO access. DO NOT administer fluid boluses because of the risk of provoking pulmonary oedema. • Provide a pre-alert stating the obstetric emergency of eclampsia.
• If **NON-TIME CRITICAL**, perform a more thorough assessment of the woman with secondary survey, including fetal assessment (refer to **Maternity Care** for guidance)	**NOTE:** epileptic patients may suffer tonic/clonic convulsions. • If >20 weeks gestation with a history of hypertension or pre-eclampsia, treat as for eclampsia – refer to Table 5.8 and Table 5.9. • If there is no history of hypertension or pre-eclampsia and blood pressure is normal, treat as for epilepsy (refer to **Convulsions (Adults)** and **Convulsions (Children)**). • Protect the airway. Place the woman in a full lateral ('recovery') position – do not use the supine position with left lateral tilt. If formal resuscitation is required, use the supine position with manual uterine displacement (refer to **Maternal Resuscitation**).
• Monitor SpO_2 (94–98%)	• Attach pulse oximeter; if SpO_2 <94%, administer O_2 to aim for a target saturation within the range of 94–98%.
• Continuous or recurrent convulsion	• If the patient convulses for longer than 2–3 minutes or has a second or subsequent convulsion, administer diazepam IV/PR titrated against effect (refer to **Diazepam** for dosages and information). **NOTE:** IV magnesium sulphate (4 g slow IV over 10 minutes) can be given if available and avoids the use of multiple drugs.

Pregnancy-induced Hypertension (including Eclampsia)

KEY POINTS

Pregnancy-induced Hypertension (including Eclampsia)

- **Pregnancy-induced hypertension and pre-eclampsia commonly occur beyond 24–28 weeks gestation but can occur as early as 22 weeks.**
- **Pre-eclampsia can present up to 6 weeks post-delivery.**
- **Diagnosis of pre-eclampsia includes an increase in blood pressure above 140/90 mmHg, oedema and detection of protein in the woman's urine.**
- **Eclampsia is one of the most dangerous complications of pregnancy.**
- **Only administer diazepam or magnesium sulphate if the convulsions are prolonged or recurrent.**
- **Severe pre-eclampsia and eclampsia are TIME CRITICAL EMERGENCIES for both mother and fetus.**

Bibliography

1 Soar J, Perkins GD, Abbas G, Alfonzo A, Barelli A, Bierens JJLM, et al. European Resuscitation Council Guidelines for Resuscitation 2010 Section 8: Cardiac arrest in special circumstances: electrolyte abnormalities, poisoning, drowning, accidental hypothermia, hyperthermia, asthma, anaphylaxis, cardiac surgery, trauma, pregnancy, electrocution. *Resuscitation* 2010, 81(10): 1400–1433.

2 Centre for Maternal and Child Enquiries. Saving mothers' lives: reviewing maternal deaths to make motherhood safer: 2006–2008. *BJOG: An International Journal of Obstetrics & Gynaecology* 2011, 118 (suppl. 1).

3 Woollard M, Simpson H, Hinshaw K, Wieteska S. Obstetric services. In *Pre-hospital Obstetric Emergency Training*. Oxford: Wiley-Blackwell, 2009: 1–6.

4 Woollard M, Hinshaw K, Simpson H, Wieteska S. Anatomical and physiological changes in pregnancy. In *Pre-hospital Obstetric Emergency Training*. Oxford: Wiley-Blackwell, 2009: 18–27.

5 Woollard M, Hinshaw K, Simpson H, Wieteska S. Structured approach to the obstetric patient. In *Pre-hospital Obstetric Emergency Training*. Oxford: Wiley-Blackwell, 2009: 38–52.

6 Woollard M, Hinshaw K, Simpson H, Wieteska S. Emergencies in late pregnancy. In *Pre-Hospital Obstetric Emergency Training*. Oxford: Wiley-Blackwell, 2009: 62–110.

Vaginal Bleeding: Gynaecological Causes

1. Introduction

- A number of conditions can cause vaginal bleeding that is different from normal menstruation. Such conditions may result in a call to the ambulance service, including:
  - excessive menstrual period
  - normal or excessive menstrual period associated with severe abdominal pain
  - following surgical or medical therapeutic termination ('abortion') (**NB** – bleeding often continues for up to 10 days after treatment)
  - following gynaecological surgery (e.g. hysterectomy) (**NB** – heavy, ongoing bleeding commencing 7-14 days after surgery can indicate pelvic infection requiring antibiotics and may require hospital assessment)
  - colposcopy (**NB** – slight bleeding may occur up to 10 days after a colposcopy). A colposcopy is an outpatient test where the cervix is inspected following an abnormal cervical smear. Treatment such as cone biopsy for the abnormal smear may have been undertaken. Heavy bleeding post-colposcopy affects very few women in this situation. Heavy, ongoing bleeding at 7–14 days post-procedure can indicate infection requiring antibiotics and may require hospital assessment
  - gynaecological cancers, either before diagnosis or after treatment (i.e. cervix, uterus or vagina) may present with heavy vaginal bleeding
  - trauma; this can include post-coital tears and may be caused by sexual assault/rape.
- This guideline provides guidance for the assessment and management of gynaecological vaginal bleeding. For causes of bleeding in early or late pregnancy, refer to **Haemorrhage During Pregnancy**.

2. Incidence

- Women over 50 years are more at risk of cancers of the uterus and cervix.

3. Severity and Outcome

- The majority of causes of vaginal bleeding do not compromise the circulation, but blood loss can be alarming.

Sexual assault

- In sexual assault cases, there may be other injuries.
- When sexual assault is suspected (especially in a child or vulnerable adult), there are clear safeguarding issues (refer to **Safeguarding Children** and **Safeguarding Adults at Risk**).
- It is not the role of the ambulance service to investigate. This is a police matter.
- Remember that the victim of sexual assault has physical forensic evidence on their body and clothing, and represents a 'crime scene' (refer to **Sexual Assault – Table 1.8**).

4. Assessment and Management

For the assessment and management of vaginal bleeding, refer to Table 5.11.

Table 5.11 – ASSESSMENT and MANAGEMENT of:

Vaginal Bleeding

ASSESSMENT	MANAGEMENT
• Quickly assess the woman and scene as you approach	• If any **TIME CRITICAL** features are present, correct **A** and **B** and transport to nearest suitable receiving hospital (refer to **Medical Emergencies in Adults – Overview** and **Medical Emergencies in Children – Overview**).
• Undertake a primary survey **<C>ABCDEF**	• Provide an alert/information call.
• Evaluate whether the woman has any **TIME CRITICAL** features or any signs of hypovolaemic shock	

Vaginal Bleeding *continued*

• Assess blood loss – ask about clots, blood-soaked clothes, bed sheets, number of soaked tampons/towels/pads, and where necessary, visibly inspect **NB** Blood under the feet or between toes indicates significant bleeding	• Obtain IV access – insert a **LARGE BORE (16G)** cannula. • If there is visible external blood loss >500 ml, refer to **Intravascular Fluid Therapy (Adults)** and **Intravascular Fluid Therapy (Children)**. 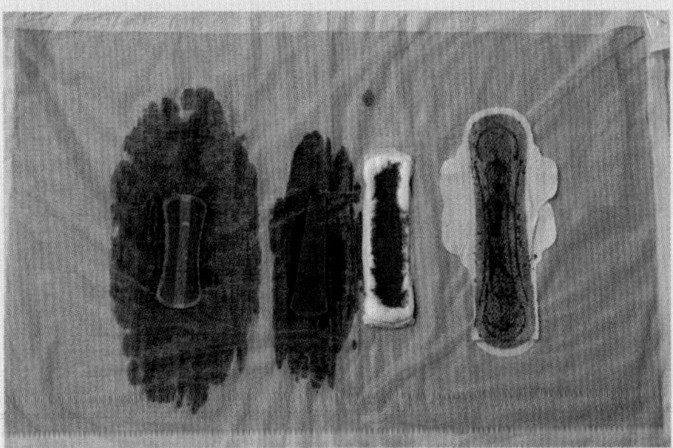 50 ml blood loss on various sanitary towels. 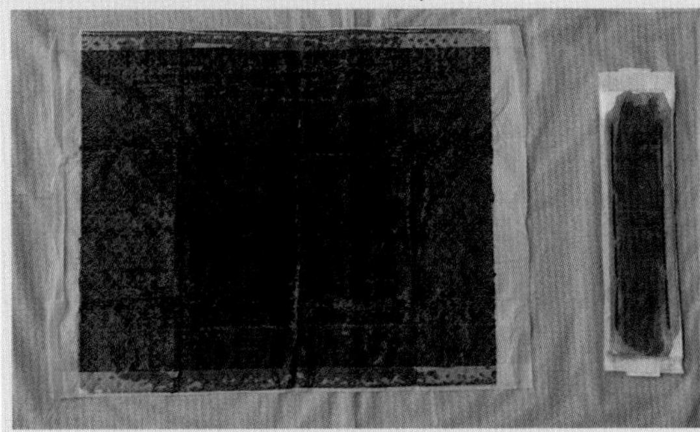 500 ml blood loss on maternity pad and 50 ml on maternity towel.
• If **NON-TIME CRITICAL**, perform a more thorough assessment of the woman with brief secondary survey for lower abdominal tenderness or guarding	
• Measure temperature and consider sepsis (refer to **Sepsis**)	
• Check the woman's age: – >50 years – more at risk of cancers of the uterus/cervix – <50 years – may be pregnant	
• Monitor SpO_2 (94–98%)	• If oxygen (SpO_2) <94%, administer O_2 to aim for a target saturation within the range of 94–98%.
• Assess the woman's level of pain	• Titrate analgesia against pain (refer to **Pain Management in Adults** and **Pain Management in Children**): – Paracetamol – Entonox – Morphine – **NB** administer cautiously if the patient is hypotensive.
• Assess the woman's comfort	• Nil by mouth. • Adjust the woman's position as required. • Transfer to further care.

KEY POINTS

Vaginal Bleeding: Gynaecological Causes

- **The majority of vaginal bleeding episodes do not compromise circulation, but blood loss can be alarming.**
- **Following gynaecological surgical interventions, heavy, ongoing vaginal bleeding commencing 7–14 days post-procedure may indicate underlying infection.**
- **Assess blood loss; ask about number of soaked tampons/towels/pads and visually inspect.**
- **Provide analgesia where indicated.**
- **If you suspect a miscarriage or ectopic pregnancy refer to Haemorrhage During Pregnancy.**

Bibliography

1 Centre for Maternal and Child Enquiries. Saving mothers' lives: reviewing maternal deaths to make motherhood safer: 2006–2008. *BJOG: An International Journal of Obstetrics & Gynaecology* 2011, 118 (suppl. 1).

2 Woollard M, Hinshaw K, Simpson H, Wieteska S. Emergencies in early pregnancy and complications following gynaecological surgery. In *Pre-hospital Obstetric Emergency Training*. Oxford: Wiley-Blackwell, 2009: 53–61.

3 Woollard M, Hinshaw K, Simpson H, Wieteska S. Management of non-obstetric emergencies. In *Pre-hospital Obstetric Emergency Training*. Oxford: Wiley-Blackwell, 2009: 136–165.

Maternal Resuscitation

1. Introduction

- As outlined by the Mother and Babies: Reducing Risk through Audits and Confidential Enquiries Across the UK (MBRRACE) report, 'for women in the United Kingdom, giving birth remains safer than ever – less than 9 in every 100,000 women die in pregnancy and around childbirth. Overall the maternal mortality rate in the UK continues to fall.'
- Between 2012–2014, deaths from 'indirect' causes remain the largest group of deaths; these are deaths from conditions not directly due to pregnancy but existing conditions which are exacerbated by pregnancy, for example women with heart problems. Given the very gradual rate of decline and the complexity of medical conditions now experienced by women during pregnancy, achieving the Government's ambition to reduce maternal deaths by 20% by 2020 and 50% by 2030 presents a major challenge for the health service that will require co-ordination of care across multiple specialities.[1]
- A maternal death is defined internationally as the death of a woman during or up to six weeks (42 days) after the end of pregnancy (whether the pregnancy ended by termination, miscarriage or a birth, or was an ectopic pregnancy) through causes associated with, or exacerbated by, pregnancy.[2]
- A late maternal death is one that occurs between six weeks and one year after the end of pregnancy.
- Deaths are further subdivided on the basis of cause into:
  - direct deaths, from pregnancy-specific causes, such as pre-eclampsia
  - indirect deaths, from other medical conditions made worse by pregnancy, such as cardiac disease
  - coincidental deaths, where the cause is considered to be unrelated to pregnancy, such as road traffic accidents.

These definitions are summarised in Table 5.12.

Table 5.12 – DEFINITIONS OF MATERNAL DEATHS[2]

Maternal Death is the death of a women while pregnant or within 42 days of the end of the pregnancy, including giving birth, ectopic pregnancy, miscarriage or termination of pregnancy, from any cause related to or aggravated by the pregnancy or its management, but not from accidental or incidental causes.	
• ***Direct Death***	• Resulting from obstetric complications of the pregnant state (pregnancy, labour and puerperium), from interventions, omissions, incorrect treatment or from a chain of events resulting from any of the above.
• ***Indirect Death***	• Resulting from previous existing disease, or disease that developed during pregnancy and which was not the result of direct obstetric causes, but which was aggravated by the physiological effects of pregnancy.
• ***Late Death***	• Occurring between 42 days and 1 year after the end of pregnancy, including giving birth, ectopic pregnancy, miscarriage or termination of pregnancy, as the result of Direct or Indirect maternal causes.
• ***Coincidental Death***	• From unrelated causes that happen to occur in pregnancy or the puerperium. Termed 'Fortuitous' in the International Classification of Diseases (ICD).

- It is important to recognise that there are two patients.
- Effective resuscitation of the mother may provide effective resuscitation of the fetus.
- Resuscitation of the mother is the primary concern.
- If there is no response to CPR after 5 minutes, undertake a **TIME CRITICAL** transfer to the nearest ED with an obstetric unit attached. Place a pre-alert as soon as possible to enable the ED team to organise a maternity team, as an immediate peri-mortem caesarean section (resuscitative hysterotomy) may be performed.

2. Cardiac Arrest

Undertake a TIME CRITICAL transfer as soon as ventilation is achieved and CPR commenced.

2.1 Introduction

- The approach to resuscitating a pregnant woman is the same as that of any adult in cardiac arrest. However, from 20 weeks gestation onwards, the weight of the gravid uterus can cause 30% of cardiac output to be sequestered into the lower limbs with a woman lying supine.
- Immediately manually displace the uterus to the maternal left side (relieving pressure on the inferior vena cava (refer to Figure 5.10)).
- CPR should not be terminated in the pre-hospital setting on a pregnant woman.

2.2 Pathophysiology

Cardiac arrest in pregnancy is very rare. Common causes of sudden maternal death include haemorrhage, embolism (thromboembolic and amniotic fluid) and hypertensive disorders. Figure 5.11 and Table 5.13 detail the common reversible causes of maternal collapse in the pregnant woman.

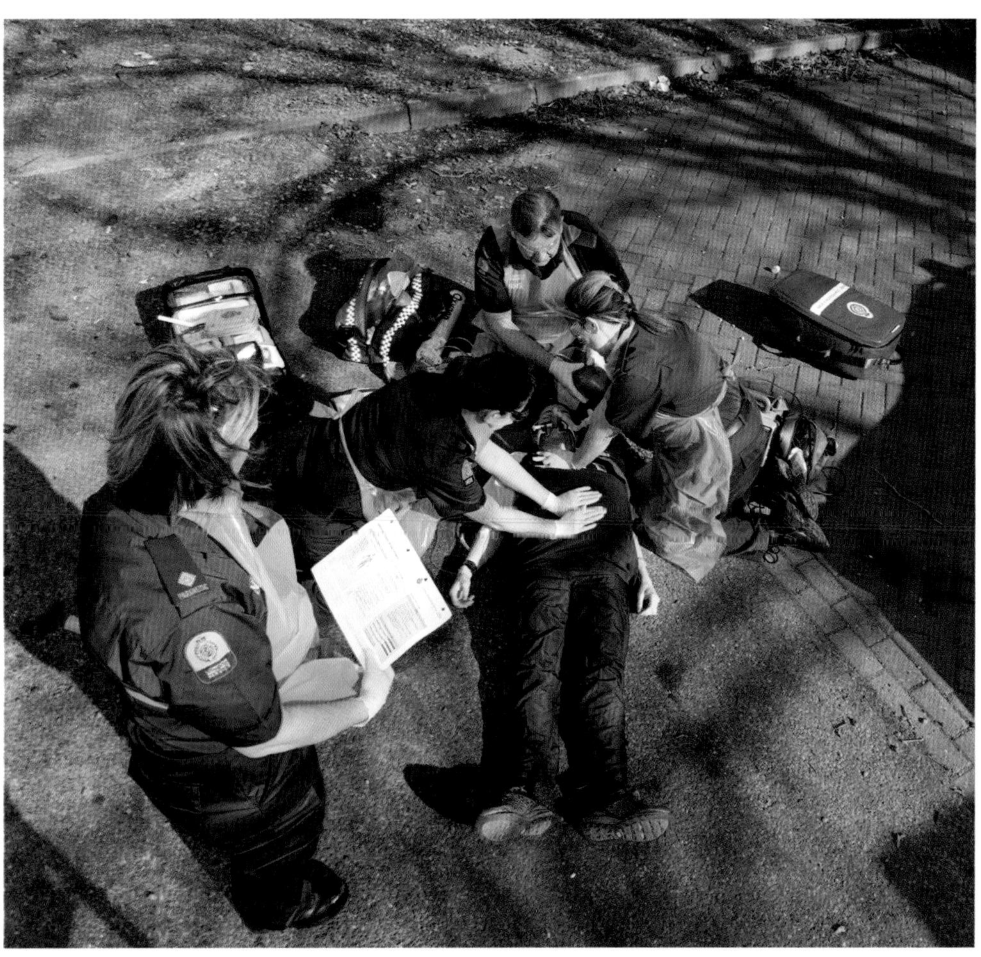

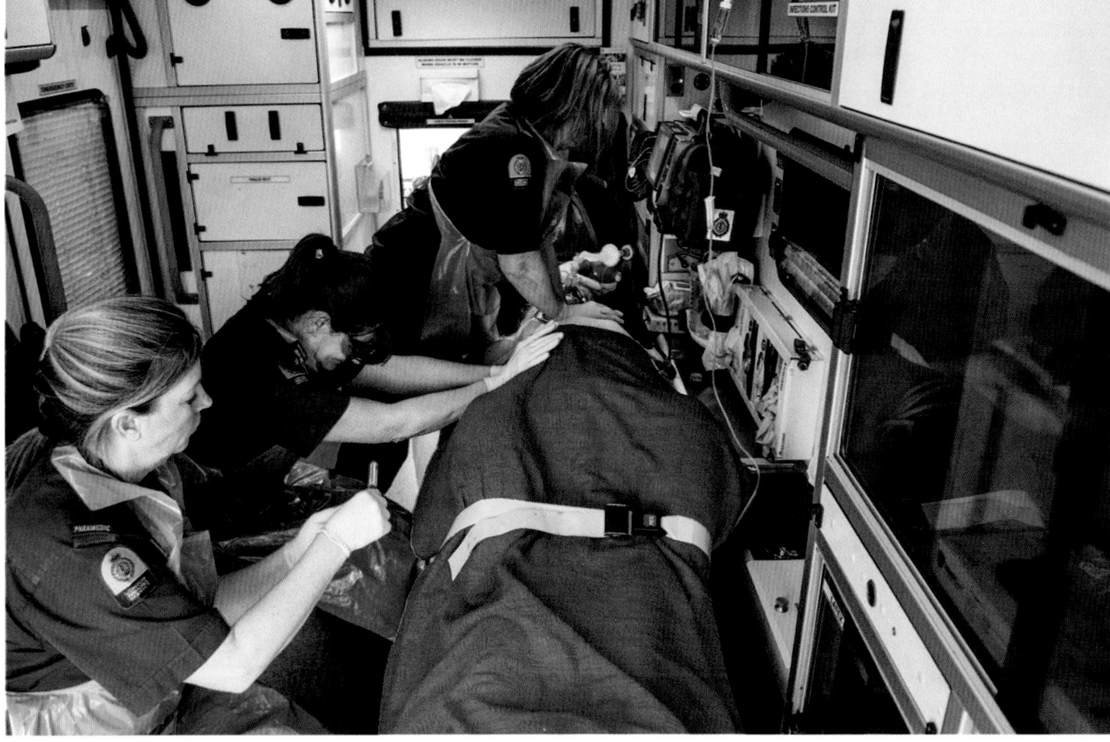

Figure 5.10 – Manual uterine displacement during resuscitation.

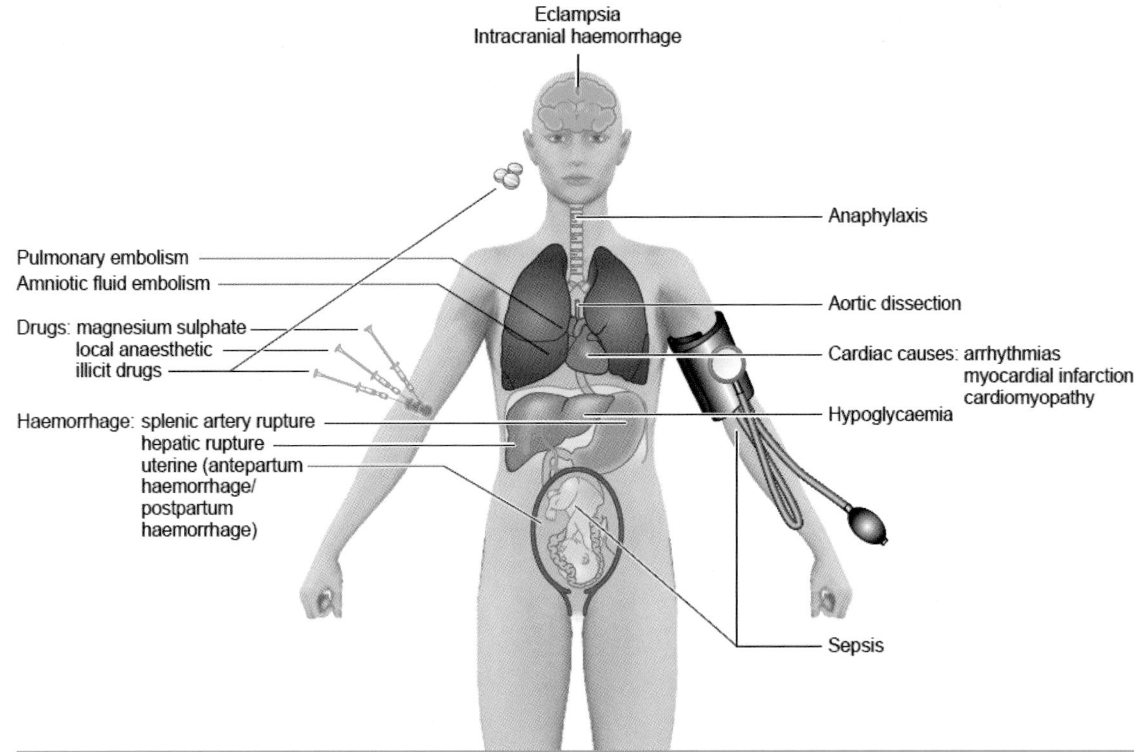

Figure 5.11 – Causes of maternal collapse.[3]
Republished with kind permission of the Royal College of Obstetricians and Gynaecologists.

Table 5.13 – REVERSIBLE CAUSES OF MATERNAL COLLAPSE[3]

REVERSIBLE CAUSE		CAUSE IN PREGNANCY
4Hs	• Hypovolaemia • Hypoxia • Hypo/hyperkalaemia and other electrolyte disturbances • Hypothermia	• Bleeding (may be concealed) (obstetric/other) or relative hypovolaemia of dense spinal block; septic or neurogenic shock. • Pregnant women become hypoxic rapidly. • Cardiac events: peripartum cardiomyopathy, myocardial infarction, aortic dissection, large-vessel aneurysms. • No more likely.
4Ts	• Thromboembolism • Toxicity • Tension pneumothorax • Tamponade (cardiac)	• Amniotic fluid embolus, pulmonary embolus, air embolus, myocardial infarction. • Local anaesthetic, magnesium, other. • Following trauma/suicide attempt
	• Eclampsia and pre-eclampsia	• Includes intracranial haemorrhage.

2.3 Modifications for Cardiac Arrest in Pregnancy

For the assessment and management of cardiac arrest during pregnancy refer to Table 5.14.

Key points are listed below:

- Start resuscitation according to standard ALS guidelines with manual displacement of the uterus to the maternal left to minimise inferior vena caval compression (spinal board will not achieve the required left lateral tilt).
- The hand position for chest compressions may need to be slightly higher (2–3 cm) on the sternum for patients with advanced pregnancy (e.g. >28 weeks).
- Consider using a tracheal tube 0.5–1.0 mm smaller than usual as the trachea can be narrowed by oedema and swelling. Supraglottic airway devices are a suitable alternative in the pre-hospital setting and may provide a more rapid means of oxygenation than potentially prolonged intubation attempts.[4]
- Defibrillation energy levels are as recommended for

standard defibrillation. If large breasts make it difficult to place an apical defibrillator electrode, use an antero-posterior or bi-axillary electrode position.

- Establish IV or IO access as soon as possible, preferably at a level above the diaphragm.
- Identify and correct the cause of the arrest using 4Hs and 4Ts as appropriate.
- Administer 100% supplemental oxygen (refer to Oxygen).
- Undertake a **TIME CRITICAL** transfer to the nearest ED with an obstetric unit attached. Place a pre-alert as soon as possible to enable the ED team to organise a maternity team, as an immediate peri-mortem caesarean section (resuscitative hysterotomy) may be performed.

2.4 The Team Approach to Pre-hospital Resuscitation (Resuscitation Council 2015)

- Resuscitation requires a system to be in place to achieve the best possible chance of survival. The system requires technical and non-technical skills (teamwork, situational awareness, leadership, decision making) in the pregnant woman, this will also involve consideration for manual uterine displacement.

Allocation of Roles

- Appoint a team leader as early as possible; ideally they should be a paramedic or clinician experienced in pre-hospital resuscitation.
- The team leader should assign team members specific roles, which they clearly understand and are capable of undertaking. This will promote teamwork, reduce confusion and ensure organised and effective management of resuscitation.
- Minimum of four trained staff is required to deliver high quality resuscitation. This will necessitate dispatch of more than one ambulance resource.
- Ensure there is 360° access to the patient ('Circle of Life'):
  - Position 1: Airway (at head of patient) – the person must be trained and equipped to provide the full range of airway skills.
  - Position 2: High quality chest compressions and defibrillation if needed – at patient's left side. Be prepared to alternate with the operator at position 3 to avoid fatigue.
  - Position 3: High quality chest compressions and access to the circulation (intravenous, intraosseous) – at patient's right side.
  - Position 4: Team leader – stand back and oversee the resuscitation attempt, only becoming involved if required. The team leader should have an awareness of the whole incident and ensure high quality resuscitation is maintained and appropriate decisions made.

The team leader will need to allocate the role of manual uterine displacement and may necessitate the involvement of additional resources where available.

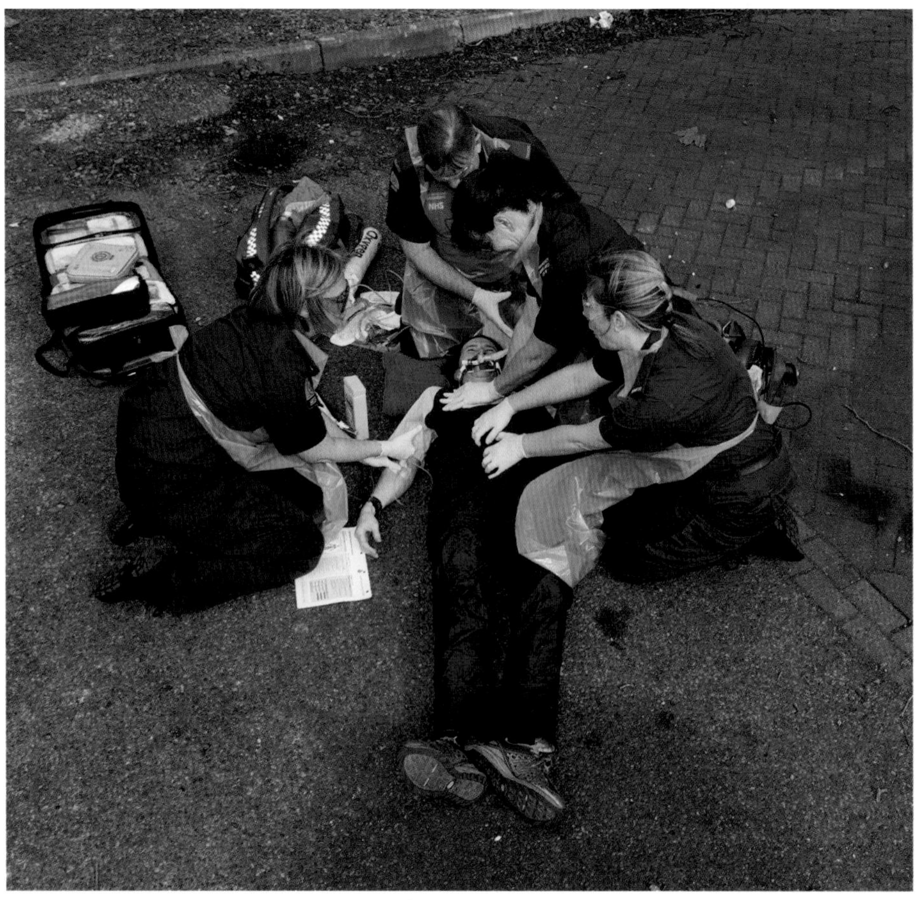

Figure 5.12 – Working as a team.

Maternal Resuscitation

Table 5.14 – ASSESSMENT and MANAGEMENT of:

Cardiac Arrest During Pregnancy

ASSESSMENT	MANAGEMENT
• Undertake a primary survey **ABCDE** • At 20 weeks, the uterine fundus will be below the umbilicus	• Manage as per standard advanced life support (refer to Advanced Life Support (Adult)). • Assess and exclude reversible causes (see Table 5.13).
	• Caution – ventilation with a bag-valve-mask may lead to regurgitation and aspiration. A supraglottic airway device may reduce the risk of gastric aspiration and make ventilation of the lungs easier (refer to Airway and Breathing Management). • If there is no response to CPR after 5 minutes, undertake a **TIME CRITICAL** transfer to the nearest ED with an obstetric unit attached. Place a pre-alert as soon as possible to enable the ED team to organise a maternity team, as an immediate peri-mortem caesarean section (resuscitative hysterotomy) may be performed.
	• For pregnant women at 20 weeks gestation or more, use manual uterine displacement (to the maternal left side) to avoid compression of the inferior vena cava. • Manual displacement can be applied from either the maternal left or right side with the assistant ensuring the uterus is displaced toward the maternal left. (Resuscitation Council, 2015) • Within the ambulance saloon, manual uterine displacement must be maintained.
	• Establish IV or IO access as soon as possible, preferably at a level above the diaphragm.

KEY POINTS

Maternal Resuscitation

- **DO NOT withhold or terminate maternal resuscitation.**
- **ALWAYS manage pregnant women in cardiac arrest at greater than 20 weeks' gestation with manual displacement of the uterus to the maternal left.**
- **If resuscitation attempts fail to achieve ROSC within 5 minutes of the cardiac arrest, undertake a TIME CRITICAL transfer to the nearest ED with an obstetric unit attached.**
- **Provide an early pre-alert to enable the ED team to summon the maternity team, as an immediate peri-mortem caesarean section (resuscitative hysterotomy) may be performed.**

Further Reading

Further important information and evidence in support of this guideline can be found in the Bibliography.[5, 6, 7, 8]

Bibliography

1 Knight M, Tuffnell D, Kenyon S, Shakespeare J, Gray R, Kurinczuk JJ (eds) on behalf of MBRRACE-UK. *Saving Lives, Improving Mothers' Care – Surveillance of maternal deaths in the UK 2011–13 and lessons learned to inform maternity care from the UK and Ireland Confidential Enquiries into Maternal Deaths and Morbidity 2009–13*. Oxford: National Perinatal Epidemiology Unit, University of Oxford, 2015.

2 World Health Organization. International Classification of Diseases (ICD) 10. Available from: http://apps.who.int/classifications/icd10/browse/2016/en#/XV, 2010.

3 Royal College of Obstetricians and Gynaecologists. *Maternal Collapse in Pregnancy and the Puerperium* (Green-top Guideline 56). London: RCOG, 2010, updated 2014. Available from: https://www.rcog.org.uk/globalassets/documents/guidelines/gtg_56.pdf.

4 Resuscitation Council. Prehospital resuscitation. Available from: https://www.resus.org.uk/resuscitation-guidelines/prehospital-resuscitation, 2015.

5 Deakin CD, Nolan JP, Soar J, Sunde K, Koster RW, Smith GB, et al. European Resuscitation Council Guidelines for Resuscitation 2010 Section 4: Adult advanced life support. *Resuscitation* 2010, 81(10): 1305–1352.

6 Koster RW, Baubin MA, Bossaert LL, Caballero A, Cassan P, Castren M, et al. European Resuscitation Council Guidelines for Resuscitation 2010 Section 2: Adult basic life support and use

of automated external defibrillators. *Resuscitation* 2010, 81(10): 1277–1292.

7 Soar J, Perkins GD, Abbas G, Alfonzo A, Barelli A, Bierens JJLM, et al. European Resuscitation Council Guidelines for Resuscitation 2010 Section 8: Cardiac arrest in special circumstances: electrolyte abnormalities, poisoning, drowning, accidental hypothermia, hyperthermia, asthma, anaphylaxis, cardiac surgery, trauma, pregnancy, electrocution. *Resuscitation* 2010, 81(10): 1400–1433.

8 Deakin CD, Nolan JP, Sunde K, Koster RW. European Resuscitation Council Guidelines for Resuscitation 2010 Section 3: Electrical therapies: automated external defibrillators, defibrillation, cardioversion and pacing. *Resuscitation* 2010, 81(10): 1293–1304.

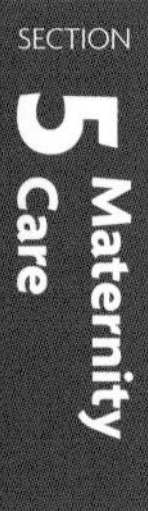

1. Introduction

- Passage through the birth canal is a hypoxic event for the fetus, since placental respiratory exchange is prevented for the 50–75 seconds duration of the average contraction. Most babies tolerate this well, and are able to make the transition to normal breathing within a minute of birth, but for those few that do not, help will be required to establish normal breathing.
- The newborn life support guideline outlines this help and comprises the following elements:
  a. drying and covering the baby to conserve heat
  b. assessing the need for any intervention
  c. opening the airway
  d. lung aeration
  e. ventilation breaths
  f. chest compressions.
- The use of a radiant heat source, such as a heated mattress, may offer the possibility to provide a controlled heat source within which it becomes appropriate to consider the use of plastic bags and polythene wraps. This should be undertaken in a research capacity where the uncontrolled environment of the pre-hospital setting and the changing temperature within the ambulance chamber during conveyance are accounted for.
- Where a tested, proven radiant heat source is available, significantly preterm infants (<32 weeks gestation) and all those requiring resuscitation are best placed, after drying, into polyethylene wrapping, up to their armpits, to maintain their temperature. Food-grade or purpose-made plastic bags or wraps can be used for this. The ambulance heaters should be at maximum.

2. Physiology

- In the face of in utero hypoxia, the breathing centre in the fetal brain becomes depressed and spontaneous breathing ceases. The fetus can maintain an effective circulation during periods of hypoxia, so the most urgent requirement for a hypoxic baby at birth is aeration of the lungs. Provided the circulation has remained intact, oxygenated blood will be conveyed from the lungs to the heart and onwards to the brain. The breathing centre should then recover and the baby will breathe spontaneously.

3. Sequence of Actions

Refer to Figure 5.13.

Keep the baby warm.

- Babies are born wet and can become cold very easily, particularly if they remain wet and exposed.
- Dry the baby paying particular attention to the head; apply a newborn hat and cover with a dry towel.
- A newborn that does not require resuscitation can be placed with the mother and skin-to-skin contact provided. Use a blanket covering the baby to protect from drafts. Make continuous observations of the baby's airway position and breathing. This will afford the opportunity for early feeding and reduce the risk of hypoglycaemia.
- Do not place the baby in a plastic bag or polythene wrap as there is a lack of pre-hospital evidence demonstrating the role of these in the prevention of newborn hypothermia in either significantly preterm (<32 weeks) or term infants, contrary to the evidence within both hospital settings and low income settings, where access to radiant heat sources and controlled ambient temperatures are feasible and have been shown to reduce the number of newborns with a temperature <36.5°C at one hour of age.[1, 2]
- Preterm babies (<37 weeks gestation) who are breathing and do not require resuscitation, may be wrapped in a towel and placed next to the mother. However, the use of foil cribs or heating mattresses may afford benefits to minimise heat loss in this group of babies, where the airway and breathing can be continuously monitored.
- After birth a temperature must be recorded as soon as practicable and repeated during conveyance.

4. Assessment and Management

- A healthy baby will be born blue but will have a good tone and will breathe spontaneously within a minute of birth. In a healthy term baby, the heart rate is greater than 100 beats per minute by two minutes of age and will become pink within the first minute or two.
- A less healthy baby will be born blue, will have reduced tone, may have a slow heart rate (60 to 100 beats per minute) and may not establish adequate breathing by two minutes.
- An ill (very hypoxic) baby will be born pale and floppy, not breathing and with a very slow heart rate (less than 60 beats per minute).

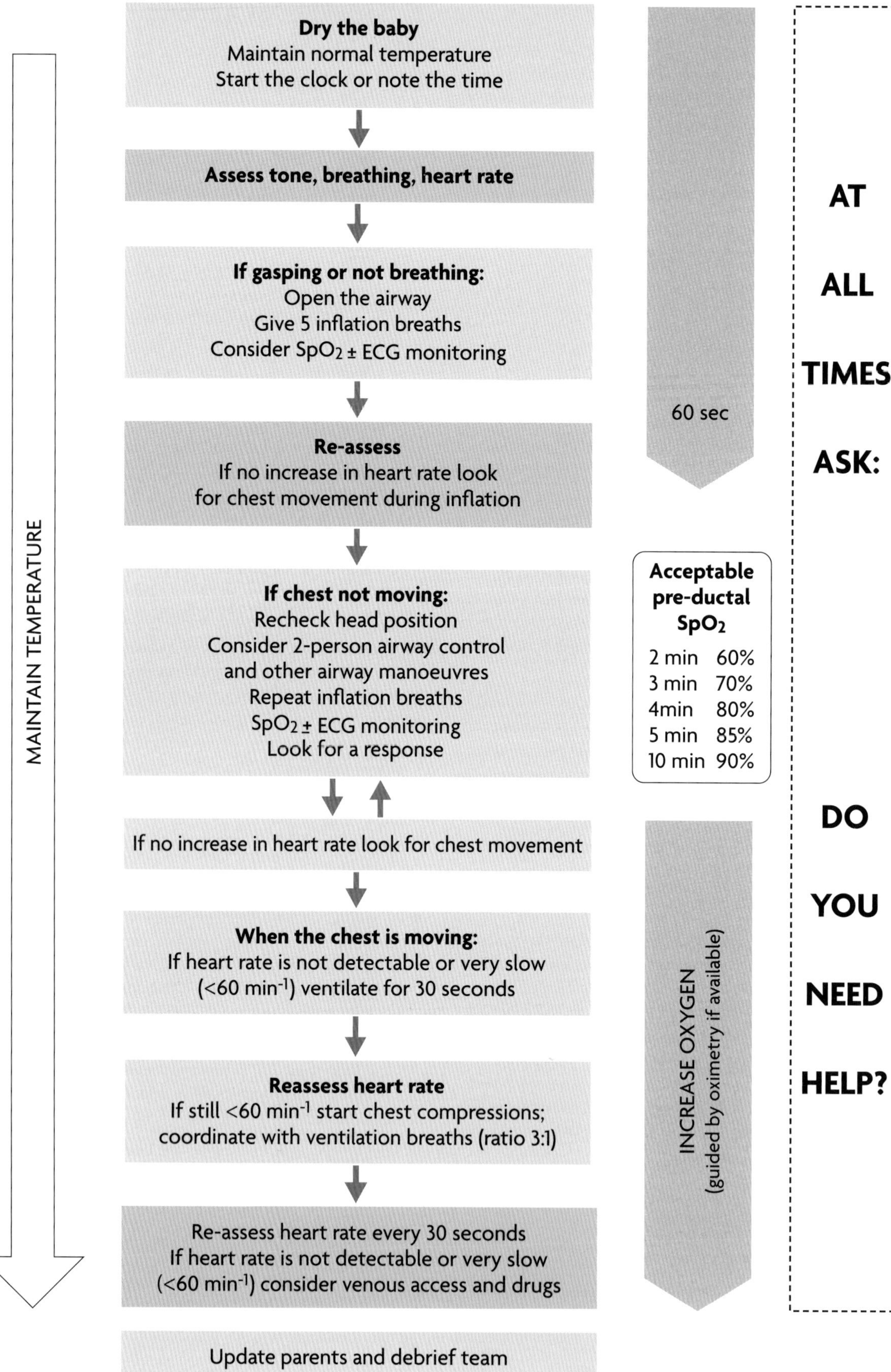

Figure 5.13 – Newborn life support algorithm – modified from the Resuscitation Council (UK) Guidelines 2015 algorithm (www.resus.org.uk).

Table 5.15 – ASSESSMENT and MANAGEMENT of:

Newborn Life Support

ASSESSMENT	MANAGEMENT
• In all cases	• Ensure the ambient temperature is as high as possible. • Close windows and doors to reduce cold draughts. • Position the baby where there is 360-degree access to enable management of the airway and chest in case further intervention is required. • Dry the baby from head to toe while completing **ABC** assessment. • Apply appropriately sized newborn hat and wrap in a warm dry towel. • Delay clamping and cutting of the umbilical cord unless resuscitation is required.
• Assess	• Colour. • Tone. • Breathing rate. • Heart rate: – Assess heart rate by listening with a stethoscope (feeling for a peripheral pulse is not reliable). – In noisy or very cold environments, palpating the pulse at the umbilical cord may be an alternative and may save unwrapping the baby (this is only reliable when the pulse is >100 bpm). – Attach a pulse oximeter. **NB** Attaching to the right wrist using an infant probe can give an accurate heart rate in approximately 90 seconds, and provides an accurate oxygen saturation.
• Re-assess breathing and heart rate, every 30 seconds	• An increase in heart rate is usually the first clinical sign of improvement.
• Decide whether help is required (and likely to be available) and whether rapid evacuation to hospital is indicated. If transferring to hospital, follow pre-alert procedure	• Ensure the heater in the ambulance is set to maximum. • Once the baby is in the ambulance, continue to monitor its condition and repeat the temperature en-route.
Airway	• Place the baby on its back with the head in a neutral position, neither flexed nor extended. • If the baby is very floppy, a chin lift or jaw thrust may be required. • A small pad (2 cm) can be placed under the shoulders to assist in maintaining the neutral position. 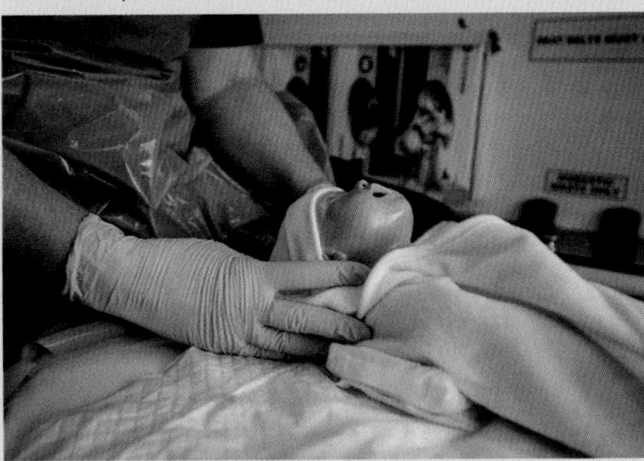

Newborn Life Support *continued*	
Breathing ● If the baby is not breathing adequately by approximately 60 seconds	● Give 5 inflation breaths, sustaining the inflation pressure at about 30cm of water for two to three seconds with each breath – use a 500 ml bag-valve-mask device. 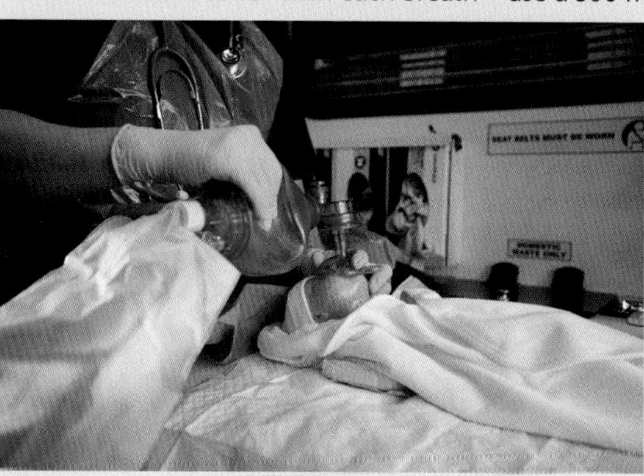 **NB** The first two or three breaths replace the fluid in the lungs with air without changing the volume in the chest. Therefore, you may not observe the chest wall rise until the fourth or fifth breath.
Heart rate ● If the heart rate increases	● Assume that lung aeration has been successful.
● If the heart rate increases but the baby does not start breathing	● Continue to provide regular breaths (ventilation breaths) at a rate of about 30–40 per minute until the baby starts to breathe on their own. **NB** Ventilation breaths are given at a rate of one every two seconds; the aim is to establish 30–40 per minute. Continue to monitor the heart rate. If the rate should drop to <100 bpm it suggests insufficient ventilation. In this situation, increase the rate of inflation or use a longer inspiratory time.
● If the heart rate does not increase following inflation breaths	● Either lung aeration has not been adequate or the baby requires more than lung aeration alone. It is most likely that you have not aerated the lungs effectively. **Repeat the procedure of inflation breaths.** **NB** If the heart rate does not increase and the chest does not move with each inflation, you have not aerated the lungs; in this situation consider: 1. Is the head in the neutral position? 2. Do you need to do a jaw thrust? 3. Do you need a longer inflation time? 4. Do you need help with the airway from a second person? 5. Is there obstruction in the oropharynx (where an appropriately sized laryngoscope is available, it may be used to inspect the airway and remove any obvious obstructions, where the clinician has the expertise)? 6. Do you need an oropharyngeal airway?
● **If after a further set of 5 inflation breaths and 30 seconds of ventilation breaths**, the heart rate remains less than 60 bpm, or the heart beat is absent despite chest wall rise	● Commence chest compressions ensuring the baby is on a flat, hard surface (not a mattress or sofa).
● If the baby does not respond very rapidly to bag-valve-mask ventilation and cardiac compressions are commenced	● Undertake a **TIME CRITICAL** transfer. ● Provide a pre-alert and convey to the nearest ED with an obstetric unit.

Newborn Life Support *continued*	
Circulation • If chest compressions are necessary	• Ensure that the lungs have been successfully aerated. • Encircle the lower chest with both hands in such a way that the two thumbs can compress the lower third of the sternum, at a point just below an imaginary line joining the nipples, with the fingers over the spine at the back. • Compress the chest quickly and firmly in such a way as to reduce the antero-posterior diameter of the chest by a third. • The ratio of compressions to inflations in newborn resuscitation is 3:1. • ECG complexes do not indicate the presence of a cardiac output and should not be the sole means of monitoring the infant. However, improving heart rate on ECG is likely to indicate successful ventilation and some cardiac output.
Meconium	• Attempting to aspirate meconium from a baby's mouth and nose while their head is still on the perineum does not prevent meconium aspiration and is not recommended. • Attempts to aspirate meconium from a vigorous baby's airway after birth will not prevent meconium aspiration and are not recommended. • If a baby is born through thick meconium and is unresponsive at birth, the oropharynx must be inspected and cleared of meconium first. The focus should be on inflating the lungs and the trachea should only be suctioned if a suitable laryngoscope and the expertise is available and the trachea is thought to be blocked. Attempts at lung inflation and ventilation must not be unduly delayed.
	Additional information • Commence resuscitation with air. Introduce supplemental oxygen if there is not a rapid improvement in the baby's condition and compressions are required. • For uncompromised term and pre-term infants, delay cord clamping at least two minutes from the complete delivery of the infant and until the cord stops pulsating.

KEY POINTS

Newborn Life Support

- **Passage through the birth canal is a hypoxic event and some babies may require help to establish normal breathing after birth.**
- **Babies become cold very easily; dry the baby, remove any wet towels and wrap with dry ones. Once in the ambulance keep the compartment as warm as possible.**
- **Ensure the airway is open by placing the baby on its back with the head in a neutral position.**
- **If the baby is very floppy, it may be necessary to apply a chin lift or jaw thrust.**
- **If the baby is not breathing adequately within 60 seconds, give 5 inflation breaths.**
- **If chest compressions are necessary, compress the chest quickly and firmly at a ratio of 3:1 compressions to inflations using a two-thumbs encircling technique.**

Further Reading

Further important information and evidence in support of this guideline can be found in the Bibliography.[3, 4]

Bibliography

1 Belsches TC, Tilly AE, Miller TR, Kambeyanda RH, Leadford A, Manasyan A, Chomba E et al. Randomised trial of plastic bags to prevent term neonatal hypothermia in a resource-poor setting. Pediatrics 2013, 132(3). Available from: http://pediatrics.aappublications.org/content/132/3/e656.

2 Leadford AE, Warren JB, Manasyan A, Chomba E, Salas AA, Schelonka R, Carlo WA. Plastic bags for prevention of hypothermia in preterm and low birth weight infants. Pediatrics 2013, 132(1). Available from: http://pediatrics.aappublications.org/content/132/1/e128.

3 Wyllie J, Bruinenberg J, Roehr CC, Rüdiger M, Trevisanuto D, Urlesberger B. European Resuscitation Council Guidelines for Resuscitation 2015: Section 7. Resuscitation and support of transition of babies at birth. *Resuscitation* 2015, 95: 249–263.

4 Wyllie J, Perlman JM, Kattwinkel J, et al. Part 7: Neonatal resuscitation: 2015 International Consensus on Cardiopulmonary Resuscitation and Emergency Cardiovascular Care Science with Treatment Recommendations. *Resuscitation* 2015, 95:e169–201.

Trauma in Pregnancy

1. Introduction

- The management of pregnant women with traumatic injuries requires a special approach.
- Mechanism of injury may indicate possible trauma to enlarged internal organs and structures, especially trauma occurring in the third trimester. For example, trauma to the gravid uterus during domestic violence can be linked to placental abruption (refer to **Birth Imminent**).
- It is important to remember that resuscitation of the mother may facilitate resuscitation of the fetus.

2. Incidence

- In the UK, 5% of maternal deaths are as a result of trauma, with a high proportion related to domestic violence and road traffic collisions.

Mechanism of injury

- Domestic violence.
- High energy transfer (especially road traffic accidents).
- Fall from height.

3. Severity and Outcome

- Managing a pregnant woman with major trauma is rare; however, both blunt and penetrating trauma can cause catastrophic haemorrhage.
- Trauma can lead to major placental abruption (separation) with significant hidden blood loss within the uterus and no visible vaginal bleeding abruption (refer to **Birth Imminent**).

4. Pathophysiology

- There are a number of physiological and anatomical changes during pregnancy that may influence the management of the pregnant woman with trauma (refer to **Maternity Care**).

Table 5.16 – ASSESSMENT and MANAGEMENT of:

Trauma in Pregnancy

ASSESSMENT	MANAGEMENT
• Quickly assess the scene and the woman as you approach • Undertake a primary survey **<C>ABCDEF** – specifically assess for: – abdominal pain – should be presumed to be significant and may be associated with internal concealed blood loss – vaginal blood loss – abruption may occur 3–4 days after the initial incident – stage of the pregnancy and impact on resuscitation if >20 weeks gestation – any medical problems with the pregnancy or relevant previous medical history – twins or multiple pregnancy – fetal movements (refer to **Maternity Care**) • Review the maternity handheld record if available • If domestic violence is suspected, consider any other children/adults present who may be at risk (refer to **Safeguarding Adults at Risk** and **Safeguarding Children**)	• Control external catastrophic haemorrhage using direct and indirect pressure or tourniquets where indicated (refer to **Trauma Emergencies Overview**). • Refer to **Maternal Resuscitation** where cardiac/respiratory arrest is identified. • Open, maintain and protect the airway in accordance with the woman's clinical need. • Administer high levels of supplemental oxygen and aim for a target saturation within the range of 94–98% (refer to **Oxygen**). Provide assisted ventilation as indicated (refer to **Airway and Breathing Management**). • If the woman is unable to position herself (e.g. if she is unconscious), she should be positioned on the left (right side up) by using a spinal board and monitor the airway. Where resources allow, the uterus can be manually displaced to the maternal left side (and this must be recorded on the patient record form) as illustrated in Figure 5.1. • Provide cervical spine protection as necessary (refer to **Spinal Injury and Spinal Cord Injury**). • Manage thoracic injuries (refer to **Thoracic Trauma**). **NB** The management of thoracic injuries is the same as for the non-pregnant woman. • Insert a minimum of one large bore IV cannula (16G) – do not delay transfer. • Administer intravascular fluids as indicated to maintain a systolic blood pressure above 90 mmHg (refer to **Intravascular Fluid Therapy**).

Trauma in Pregnancy *continued*	
● Undertake a secondary survey **<C>ABCDEF**	
● Assess the woman's level of pain	● Pain management (refer to **Pain Management in Adults**). **NB** Administer morphine cautiously if the patient is hypotensive. ● Apply splints as appropriate, for example to pelvis (refer to **Pelvic Trauma**) or long bone fractures (refer to **Limb Trauma**).
● Assess blood glucose	● Measure blood glucose en-route to the appropriate facility.
	● Nil by mouth.
● Assess for burns and scalds	● For the management of burns, treat as non-pregnant woman (refer to **Burns and Scalds** and **Intravascular Fluid Therapy**).

KEY POINTS

Trauma in Pregnancy

- **All trauma is significant.**
- **If the pregnant woman is found in cardiac arrest or develops cardiac/respiratory arrest en-route, commence advanced life support and pre-alert the nearest ED with an obstetric unit.**
- **Resuscitation of the woman may facilitate resuscitation of the fetus.**
- **Compression of the inferior vena cava by the gravid uterus (>20 weeks) is a serious potential complication; manually displace the uterus to the maternal left. Maintain during transfer.**
- **Due to the physiological changes in pregnancy, signs of shock may be slow to appear following trauma, hypotension being an extremely late indication of volume loss. Signs of hypovolaemia during pregnancy are likely to indicate a 35% (class III) blood loss and must be treated aggressively.**
- **Abruption may occur 3–4 days after the initial incident.**
- **If sexual assault or domestic violence is suspected, consideration must be given to potential safeguarding issues and provision made to ensure safety is maintained (refer to Safeguarding Adults at Risk).**

Bibliography

1 Centre for Maternal and Child Enquiries. Saving mothers' lives: reviewing maternal deaths to make motherhood safer: 2006–2008. *BJOG: An International Journal of Obstetrics & Gynaecology* 2011, 118 (suppl. 1).

2 Woollard M, Simpson H, Hinshaw K, Wieteska S. Obstetric services. In *Pre-hospital Obstetric Emergency Training*. Oxford: Wiley-Blackwell, 2009: 1–6.

3 Woollard M, Hinshaw K, Simpson H, Wieteska S. Anatomical and physiological changes in pregnancy. In *Pre-hospital Obstetric Emergency Training*. Oxford: Wiley-Blackwell, 2009: 18–27.

4 Woollard M, Hinshaw K, Simpson H, Wieteska S. Structured approach to the obstetric patient. In *Pre-hospital Obstetric Emergency Training*. Oxford: Wiley-Blackwell, 2009: 38–52.

5 Woollard M, Hinshaw K, Simpson H, Wieteska S. Emergencies in late pregnancy. In *Pre-Hospital Obstetric Emergency Training*. Oxford: Wiley-Blackwell, 2009: 62–110.

6 Woollard M, Hinshaw K, Simpson H, Wieteska S. Emergencies after delivery. In *Pre-hospital Obstetric Emergency Training*. Oxford: Wiley-Blackwell, 2009: 111–124.

7 Woollard M, Hinshaw K, Simpson H, Wieteska S. Management of non-obstetric emergencies. In *Pre-hospital Obstetric Emergency Training*. Oxford: Wiley-Blackwell, 2009: 136–165.

6

Drugs

Drugs Overview

1. Introduction

- The guidelines contained in this section are the current medicines that can be administered by registered paramedics.[a]
- The Medicines Act 1968 governs what paramedics can administer and this is regulated by The Medicines and Healthcare Products Regulatory Agency (MHRA).
- Where a Prescription-Only Medicines (POMs) exemption exists, the MHRA has agreed a Patient Group Direction (PGD) is no longer required for paramedics to administer drugs where a JRCALC drug protocol is issued. Currently POMs exemptions have not been issued for tranexamic acid, therefore a PGD is required. A POMs exemption is not required for dexamethasone as the intravenous preparation is administered orally.
- The drugs administered by ambulance clinicians fall into two categories:

1. **Non-prescription drugs** (e.g. aspirin).
2. **Prescription-only medicines (POMs)** (e.g. morphine).

POMs can only be prescribed by a qualified doctor (or dentist) and non-medical prescribers but exemptions exist under Part III of Schedule 5 to the Prescription Only Medicines (Human Use) Order 1997, which allows suitably trained paramedics to administer these drugs in specified circumstances.

1.1 Safety aspects

- Always check the following:
  - the drug type
  - the drug strength
  - whether the packaging is intact
  - the clarity of fluid
  - the expiry date.

1.2 Prescribing terms

In the case of prescription medicines, a variety of abbreviations are used, some of which are described – refer to Table 6.2.

NB Internationally recognised units and symbols should be used where possible.

Table 6.1 – DOCUMENTATION

Note the following:	✓	✗
• Avoid unnecessary use of decimal points	3 mg	3.0 mg
• Quantities of 1 gram or more should be written as	1 g	
• Quantities less than 1 gram should be written in milligrams	500 mg	0.5 g
• Quantities less than 1 mg should be written in micrograms	100 micrograms	0.1 mg
• When decimals are unavoidable a zero should be written in front of the decimal point where there is no other figure	0.5 ml	not .5 ml
• Use of the decimal point is acceptable to express a range	0.5 to 1 g	
• 'Micrograms' and 'nanograms' should not be abbreviated nor should 'units'		
• The term 'millilitre' is used	ml or mL	cubic centimetre, c.c., or cm^3

1.3 Drug routes

- Drug routes are classified as **parenteral** and **non-parenteral**:
  - **Parenteral routes** are those where a physical breach of the skin or mucous membrane is made, for example, by injection.
  - **Non-parenteral routes** are those where the drug is absorbed passively, for example, via the gastrointestinal tract, mucous membranes or skin.
- Drugs can be administered via a number of routes – refer to Table 6.3. It is important that the most appropriate route is selected – refer to Table 6.4 – taking into account the patient's condition and the urgency of the situation.
- Drugs and their possible routes of administration are listed in Table 6.4. In cases of parenteral administration, where at all possible, intravenous (IV) cannulation should be attempted, except for children in cardiac arrest where intraosseous cannulation is the preferred method. NB If a vein cannot be found it is not necessary to attempt IV cannulation. With intramuscular and subcutaneous routes, absorption may be erratic or incomplete if the patient is hypovolaemic or clinically unstable.

SECTION 6 Drugs

a Paramedic is defined as being on the register of paramedics maintained by the Health and Care Professions Council pursuant to paragraph 11 of Schedule 2 to the Health Professions Order 2001.

Table 6.2 – COMMON ABBREVIATIONS

Abbreviation	Translation
ac	ante cibum (before food)
approx	approximately
bd	twice daily
CD	controlled drug preparation subject to prescription requirements control – The Misuse of Drugs Act
ec	enteric-coated (termed gastro-resistant in British Pharmacopoeia)
f/c	film-coated
IM	intramuscular
IV	intravenous
m/r	modified-release
MAOI	monoamine-oxidase inhibitors
max	maximum
NSAID	non-steroidal anti-inflammatory drug
o.d	omni die (every day)
o.m	omni mane (every morning)
o.n	omni nocte (every night)
p.c	post cibum (after food)
PGD	patient group direction
POM	prescription only medicine
pr	per rectum (rectally)
prn	when required
q.d.s	quater die sumendus (to be taken four times daily)
q.q.h	quarta quaque hora (every four hours)
s/c	sugar-coated
SSRI	selective serotonin re-uptake inhibitor
SOS	when required
SR	slow release
stat	immediately
t.d.s	ter die sumendus (to be taken three times daily)
t.i.d	ter in die (three times daily)
top	topical

1.4 Paediatric doses

- Paediatric drug doses are based on a child's **weight**, on a milligram per kilogram basis.
- When a child's weight **is** known, it is better to administer according to their **weight** rather than their **age**.
- Often the child's weight is **not** known; in these situations **Page for Age** can provide an estimated drug dose, calculated according to 'average' growth chart weights for child of a given age.
- When a child is clearly larger or smaller than would be expected for their age (their parents/carers will often be aware of this), an 'older' or 'younger' **Page for Age** chart should be selected for that child, dependent on the chart that most closely reflects their actual weight.

1.5 Drug codes

The drug codes listed in Table 6.5 are provided for **INFORMATION ONLY** and represent drugs that may be commonly encountered in the emergency/urgent care environment. **ONLY** the drugs listed in the guidelines are for use by registered paramedics; the remaining drugs are for use by physicians or under patient group directions by paramedics who have undertaken extended training.

Table 6.3 – DRUG ROUTES

Parenteral routes

Intramuscular – Injection of the drug into muscle, which is then absorbed into the blood. Absorption may be decreased in poor perfusion states.

Intraosseous – A rigid needle inserted directly into the bone marrow. Resuscitation drugs and fluid replacement may be administered by this route. Absorption is as quick as by the intravenous route.

Intravenous – Direct introduction of the drug into the cardiovascular system that normally delivers the drug to the target organs very quickly.

Subcutaneous – Injection of the drug into subcutaneous tissue. This usually has a slower rate of absorption than from intramuscular injection and may be decreased in poor perfusion states.

Non-parenteral routes

Inhaled – Gaseous drugs that are absorbed via the lungs.

Nebulisation – Liquid drugs agitated in a stream of gas such as oxygen to create fine droplets that are absorbed rapidly from the lungs.

Oral – The drug is swallowed and is absorbed into the blood from the gut. In serious trauma or illness, absorption may be delayed.

Rectal – The drug is absorbed from the wall of the rectum. This route is used for patients who are having seizures and who cannot be cannulated without risk to themselves or ambulance personnel. Effects usually occur 5–15 minutes after administration.

Sub-lingual – Tablet or aerosol spray is absorbed from the mucous membrane beneath the tongue. Effects usually occur within 2–3 minutes.

Transdermal – Absorption of a drug through the skin.

Buccal – Absorption via the mucous membrane.

Intranasal – Aerosol spray absorbed from the mucous membrane

KEY POINTS

Drugs Overview

- **Check the drug type, strength, whether the packaging is intact, the clarity of fluid and the expiry date.**
- **Select the most appropriate route taking into account the patient's condition and the urgency of the situation.**
- **Only administer drugs via the routes you have been trained for.**
- **The drug codes are provided for INFORMATION ONLY.**
- **Complete documentation.**

Table 6.4 – SUGGESTED DRUG ROUTES

Drug/ Route	IV	IO	IM	SC	Oral	Sub-lingual	Buccal	Intranasal	Rectal	Inhaled	Nebulised	Transdermal	Flush
Adrenaline	✓	✓	✓	✓	N/A	N/A	N/A	N/A	N/A	N/A	N/A	N/A	N/A
Amiodarone	✓	✓	N/A	N/A	N/A	N/A	N/A	N/A	N/A	N/A	N/A	N/A	N/A
Aspirin	N/A	N/A	N/A	N/A	✓	N/A	N/A	N/A	N/A	N/A	N/A	N/A	N/A
Atropine	✓	✓	N/A	N/A	N/A	N/A	N/A	N/A	N/A	N/A	N/A	N/A	N/A
Atropine (CBRNE)	N/A	N/A	✓	N/A	N/A	N/A	N/A	N/A	N/A	N/A	N/A	N/A	N/A
Benzylpenicillin	✓	✓	✓	N/A	N/A	N/A	N/A	N/A	N/A	N/A	N/A	N/A	N/A
Chlorphenamine	✓	✓	✓	N/A	✓	N/A	N/A	N/A	N/A	N/A	N/A	N/A	N/A
Ciprofloxacin (CBRNE)	N/A	N/A	N/A	N/A	✓	N/A	N/A	N/A	N/A	N/A	N/A	N/A	N/A
Clopidogrel	N/A	N/A	N/A	N/A	✓	N/A	N/A	N/A	N/A	N/A	N/A	N/A	N/A
Dexamethasone	✓	✓	✓	N/A	✓	N/A	N/A	N/A	N/A	N/A	N/A	N/A	N/A
Diazepam	✓	✓	N/A	N/A	N/A	N/A	N/A	N/A	✓	N/A	N/A	N/A	N/A
Dicobalt (CBRNE)	✓	✓	N/A	N/A	N/A	N/A	N/A	N/A	N/A	N/A	N/A	N/A	N/A
Doxycycline (CBRNE)	N/A	N/A	N/A	N/A	✓	N/A	N/A	N/A	N/A	N/A	N/A	N/A	N/A
Entonox	N/A	N/A	N/A	N/A	N/A	N/A	N/A	N/A	N/A	✓	N/A	N/A	N/A
Furosemide	✓	✓	N/A	N/A	N/A	N/A	N/A	N/A	N/A	N/A	N/A	N/A	N/A
Glucagon	N/A	N/A	✓	N/A	N/A	N/A	N/A	N/A	N/A	N/A	N/A	N/A	N/A
Glucose 10%	✓	✓	N/A	N/A	N/A	N/A	N/A	N/A	N/A	N/A	N/A	N/A	N/A
Glucose 40% gel	N/A	N/A	N/A	N/A	N/A	N/A	✓	N/A	N/A	N/A	N/A	N/A	N/A
Glyceryl trinitrate	N/A	N/A	N/A	N/A	N/A	✓	✓	N/A	N/A	N/A	N/A	N/A	N/A
Heparin	✓	✓	N/A	N/A	N/A	N/A	N/A	N/A	N/A	N/A	N/A	N/A	N/A
Hydrocortisone	✓	✓	✓	N/A	N/A	N/A	N/A	N/A	N/A	N/A	N/A	N/A	N/A
Ibuprofen	N/A	N/A	N/A	N/A	✓	N/A	N/A	N/A	N/A	N/A	N/A	N/A	N/A
Ipratropium bromide	N/A	N/A	N/A	N/A	N/A	N/A	N/A	N/A	N/A	N/A	✓	N/A	N/A
Ketamine	✓	✓	✓	N/A	N/A	N/A	N/A	N/A	N/A	N/A	N/A	N/A	N/A
Metoclopramide	✓	✓	✓	N/A	N/A	N/A	N/A	N/A	N/A	N/A	N/A	N/A	N/A
Patient's own midazolam	N/A	N/A	N/A	N/A	N/A	N/A	✓	✓	N/A	N/A	N/A	N/A	N/A
Misoprostol	N/A	N/A	N/A	N/A	✓	✓	N/A	N/A	✓	N/A	N/A	N/A	N/A
Morphine sulphate	✓	✓	✓	✓	✓	N/A	N/A	N/A	N/A	N/A	N/A	N/A	N/A
Naloxone hydrochloride	✓	✓	✓	✓	N/A	N/A	N/A	✓	N/A	N/A	N/A	N/A	N/A
Obidoxime (CBRNE)	✓	✓	N/A	N/A	N/A	N/A	N/A	N/A	N/A	N/A	N/A	N/A	N/A

Table 6.4 – SUGGESTED DRUG ROUTES *continued*

Drug/ Route	IV	IO	IM	SC	Oral	Sub-lingual	Buccal	Intranasal	Rectal	Inhaled	Nebulised	Transdermal	Flush
Ondansetron	✓	✓	✓	N/A	N/A	N/A	N/A	N/A	N/A	N/A	N/A	N/A	N/A
Oxygen	N/A	N/A	N/A	N/A	N/A	N/A	N/A	N/A	N/A	✓	N/A	N/A	N/A
Paracetamol	✓	✓	N/A	N/A	✓	N/A	N/A	N/A	N/A	N/A	N/A	N/A	N/A
Potassium iodate (CBRNE)	N/A	N/A	N/A	N/A	✓	N/A	N/A	N/A	N/A	N/A	N/A	N/A	N/A
Pralidoxime mesylate (CBRNE)	✓	✓	N/A	N/A	N/A	N/A	N/A	N/A	N/A	N/A	N/A	N/A	N/A
Reteplase	✓	N/A	N/A	N/A	N/A	N/A	N/A	N/A	N/A	N/A	N/A	N/A	N/A
Salbutamol	N/A	N/A	N/A	N/A	N/A	N/A	N/A	N/A	N/A	✓	✓	N/A	N/A
0.9% Sodium chloride	✓	✓	N/A	N/A	N/A	N/A	N/A	N/A	N/A	N/A	N/A	N/A	✓
Sodium lactate	✓	✓	N/A	N/A	N/A	N/A	N/A	N/A	N/A	N/A	N/A	N/A	N/A
Syntometrine	N/A	N/A	✓	N/A	N/A	N/A	N/A	N/A	N/A	N/A	N/A	N/A	N/A
Tenecteplase	✓	N/A	N/A	N/A	N/A	N/A	N/A	N/A	N/A	N/A	N/A	N/A	N/A
Tetracaine	N/A	N/A	N/A	N/A	N/A	N/A	N/A	N/A	N/A	N/A	N/A	✓	N/A
Tranexamic acid	✓	N/A	N/A	N/A	N/A	N/A	N/A	N/A	N/A	N/A	N/A	N/A	N/A

Table 6.5 – JRCALC DRUG CODES

Drug	Code	Drug	Code
Adenosine	**ADE**	Cetirizine	**CTZ**
Adrenaline (Epinephrine) 1:1,000	**ADM**	Ciprofloxacin	**CXN**
Adrenaline (Epinephrine) 1:10,000	**ADX**	Co-amoxiclav	**CXV**
Aminophylline	**AMN**	Cyclimorph	**CYM**
Amiodarone	**AMO**	Cyclizine	**CYZ**
Amoxicillin	**AMX**	Clotrimazole	**CZL**
Alteplase	**APL**	Diclofenac	**DCF**
Aspirin	**ASP**	Dicobalt Edetate	**DCO**
Atracurium	**ATC**	Dexamethasone	**DEX**
Atropine	**ATR**	Dihydrocodeine	**DHC**
Benzylpenicillin	**BPN**	Diamorphine	**DMO**
Co-dydramol	**CDY**	Domperidone	**DMP**
Cefalexin	**CEF**	Doxycycline	**DXN**
Cefotaxime	**CFT**	Diazepam	**DZP**
Ceftriaxone	**CFX**	Enoxaparin (Low Molecular Weight Heparin)	**ENP**
Chlorpromazine	**CHZ**	Ergometrine Maleate	**ERG**
Clopidogrel	**CLO**	Erythromycin	**ERY**
Clarithromycin	**CMY**	Etomidate	**ETO**
Codeine	**COD**	Flucloxacillin	**FCX**
Colloid Gel Solution	**COL**	Fluorescein Sodium	**FLR**
Codeine-Paracetamol Combination	**CPC**	Flumazenil	**FLZ**
Chlorphenamine	**CPH**	Furosemide	**FRM**
Chloramphenicol Eye Preparation	**CPL**	Fusidic Acid Eye Preparation	**FUA**

Table 6.5 – JRCALC DRUG CODES *continued*

Drug	Code
Glucose 40% Gel	**GLG**
Glucose 50%	**GLL**
Glycerol Suppositories	**GLS**
Glucagon	**GLU**
Dextrose 5%	**GLV**
Glucose 5%	**GLX**
Glucose 10%	**GLX**
Glyceryl Trinitrate (GTN)	**GTN**
Heparin (Standard Unfractionated)	**HEP**
Haloperidol	**HPD**
Hydrocortisone	**HYC**
Ibuprofen	**IBP**
Ipratropium Bromide	**IPR**
Ketamine	**KET**
Lidocaine	**LID**
Lidocaine Gel (Mucocutaneous Anaesthesia)	**LDU**
Lorazepam	**LRZ**
Levonorgestrel	**LVG**
Midazolam (Patient's Own Midazolam)	**MDZ**
Midazolam	**MDZ**
Misoprostol	**MIS**
Morphine Sulphate	**MOR**
Metoclopramide	**MTC**
Methylprednisolone	**MTP**
Metronidazole	**MTZ**
Nitrofurantoin	**NFT**
Naloxone Hydrochloride	**NLX**
Entonox	**NOO**
Naproxen	**NPN**
Nystatin	**NST**
Oxybuprocaine Benoxinate	**OBP**
Obidoxime Chloride	**ODC**
Ondansetron	**ODT**
Oral Rehydration Salts	**ORS**
Oseltamivir	**OSV**
Otosporin Ear Drops	**OTS**
Oxygen	**OXG**
Oxytetracycline	**OXL**
Oxytocin	**OXT**
Paracetamol	**PAR**
Procyclidine	**PCY**
Prochlorperazine	**PCZ**
Pralidoxime Mesylate	**PDM**
Potassium Iodate	**PIO**
Penicillin V	**PNV**
Propofol	**PPL**
Prednisolone	**PRD**
Pethidine	**PTH**
Rocuronium	**RCR**
Reteplase	**RPA**
0.9% Sodium Chloride	**SCP**
Salbutamol	**SLB**
Sodium Lactate Compound	**SLC**
Sodium Thiopentone	**STP**
Suxamethonium	**SUX**
Syntometrine	**SYN**
Tenecteplase	**TNK**
Terbutaline	**TER**
Tetanus Immunoglobulin	**TIG**
Trimethoprim	**TMP**
Tramadol	**TRM**
Tetracaine (Amethocaine)	**TTC**
Tetanus/Low Dose Diphtheria Vaccine	**TTD**
Tranexamic Acid	**TXA**
Vecuronium	**VEC**
Water for Injection	**WFI**

Bibliography

1 The British National Formulary, British National Formulary for Children. Available from: http://www.bnf.org/bnf/index.htm, 2012.

2 NHS Evidence. *List of Drug Interactions.* Available from: http://www.evidence.nhs.uk/formulary/bnf/current/a1-interactions/list-of-drug-interactions, 2012.

3 The Medicines and Healthcare Products Regulatory Agency. Available from: http://www.mhra.gov.uk, 2012.

4 The Medicines and Healthcare products Regulatory Agency. *Patient Group Directions in the NHS.* Available from: http://www.medicinesresources.nhs.uk/en/Communities/NHS/PGDs/, 2012.

Atropine

Presentation

Pre-filled syringe containing 1 milligram atropine in 10 ml.

Pre-filled syringe containing 1 milligram atropine in 5 ml.

Pre-filled syringe containing 3 milligrams atropine in 10 ml.

An ampoule containing 600 micrograms in 1 ml.

Indications

Symptomatic bradycardia in the presence of **ANY** of these adverse signs:

- Absolute bradycardia (pulse <40 beats per minute).
- Systolic blood pressure below expected for age (refer to **Page-for-Age** for age related blood pressure readings in children).
- Paroxysmal ventricular arrhythmias requiring suppression.
- Inadequate perfusion causing confusion, etc.
- Bradycardia following return of spontaneous circulation (ROSC)

NB Hypoxia is the most common cause of bradycardia in children, therefore interventions to support ABC and oxygen therapy should be the first-line therapy.

Contra-indications

Should **NOT** be given to treat bradycardia in suspected hypothermia.

Actions

May reverse effects of vagal overdrive.

May increase heart rate by blocking vagal activity in sinus bradycardia, second or third degree heart block.

Enhances A-V conduction.

Side Effects

Dry mouth, visual blurring and pupil dilation.

Confusion and occasional hallucinations.

Tachycardia.

In older people retention of urine may occur.

Do not use small (<100 micrograms) doses as they may cause paradoxical bradycardia.

Additional Information

May induce tachycardia when used after myocardial infarction, which will increase myocardial oxygen demand and worsen ischaemia. Hence, bradycardia in a patient with an MI should **ONLY** be treated if the low heart rate is causing problems with perfusion.

Dosage and Administration

SYMPTOMATIC BRADYCARDIA

NB BRADYCARDIA in children is most commonly caused by **HYPOXIA,** requiring immediate ABC care, **NOT** drug therapy; therefore **ONLY** administer atropine in cases of bradycardia caused by vagal stimulation (e.g. suction).

Route: Intravenous/intra-osseous administer as a rapid bolus.

AGE	INITIAL DOSE	REPEAT DOSE	DOSE INTERVAL	CONCENTRATION	VOLUME	MAXIMUM DOSE
≥12 years	600 micrograms[a]	600 micrograms[a]	3–5 minutes	600 micrograms per ml	1 ml	3 milligrams
11 years	500 micrograms	NONE	N/A	600 micrograms per ml	0.8 ml	500 micrograms
10 years	500 micrograms	NONE	N/A	600 micrograms per ml	0.8 ml	500 micrograms
9 years	500 micrograms	NONE	N/A	600 micrograms per ml	0.8 ml	500 micrograms
8 years	500 micrograms	NONE	N/A	600 micrograms per ml	0.8 ml	500 micrograms
7 years	400 micrograms	NONE	N/A	600 micrograms per ml	0.7 ml	400 micrograms
6 years	400 micrograms	NONE	N/A	600 micrograms per ml	0.7 ml	400 micrograms
5 years	300 micrograms	NONE	N/A	600 micrograms per ml	0.5 ml	300 micrograms
4 years	300 micrograms	NONE	N/A	600 micrograms per ml	0.5 ml	300 micrograms
3 years	240 micrograms	NONE	N/A	600 micrograms per ml	0.4 ml	240 micrograms
2 years	240 micrograms	NONE	N/A	600 micrograms per ml	0.4 ml	240 micrograms
18 months	200 micrograms	NONE	N/A	600 micrograms per ml	0.3 ml	200 micrograms
12 months	200 micrograms	NONE	N/A	600 micrograms per ml	0.3 ml	200 micrograms
9 months	120 micrograms	NONE	N/A	600 micrograms per ml	0.2 ml	120 micrograms
6 months	120 micrograms	NONE	N/A	600 micrograms per ml	0.2 ml	120 micrograms
3 months	120 micrograms	NONE	N/A	600 micrograms per ml	0.2 ml	120 micrograms
1 month	90 micrograms	NONE	N/A	600 micrograms per ml	0.15 ml	90 micrograms
Birth	60 micrograms	NONE	N/A	600 micrograms per ml	0.1 ml	60 micrograms

a The adult dosage can be given as 500 or 600 micrograms to a maximum of 3 milligrams depending on presentation available.

Atropine

Route: Intravenous/intraosseous **administer as a rapid bolus.**

AGE	INITIAL DOSE	REPEAT DOSE	DOSE INTERVAL	CONCENTRATION	VOLUME	MAXIMUM DOSE
≥12 years	600 micrograms[a]	600 micrograms[a]	3–5 minutes	300 micrograms per ml	2 ml	3 milligrams
11 years	500 micrograms	NONE	N/A	300 micrograms per ml	1.7 ml	500 micrograms
10 years	500 micrograms	NONE	N/A	300 micrograms per ml	1.7 ml	500 micrograms
9 years	500 micrograms	NONE	N/A	300 micrograms per ml	1.7 ml	500 micrograms
8 years	500 micrograms	NONE	N/A	300 micrograms per ml	1.7 ml	500 micrograms
7 years	400 micrograms	NONE	N/A	300 micrograms per ml	1.3 ml	400 micrograms
6 years	400 micrograms	NONE	N/A	300 micrograms per ml	1.3 ml	400 micrograms
5 years	300 micrograms	NONE	N/A	300 micrograms per ml	1 ml	300 micrograms
4 years	300 micrograms	NONE	N/A	300 micrograms per ml	1 ml	300 micrograms
2 years	240 micrograms	NONE	N/A	300 micrograms per ml	0.8 ml	240 micrograms
18 months	200 micrograms	NONE	N/A	300 micrograms per ml	0.7 ml	200 micrograms
12 months	200 micrograms	NONE	N/A	300 micrograms per ml	0.7 ml	200 micrograms
9 months	120 micrograms	NONE	N/A	300 micrograms per ml	0.4 ml	120 micrograms
6 months	120 micrograms	NONE	N/A	300 micrograms per ml	0.4 ml	120 micrograms
3 months	120 micrograms	NONE	N/A	300 micrograms per ml	0.4 ml	120 micrograms
1 month	90 micrograms	NONE	N/A	300 micrograms per ml	0.3 ml	90 micrograms
Birth	60 micrograms	NONE	N/A	300 micrograms per ml	0.2 ml	60 micrograms

Route: Intravenous/intraosseous **administer as a rapid bolus**.

AGE	INITIAL DOSE	REPEAT DOSE	DOSE INTERVAL	CONCENTRATION	VOLUME	MAXIMUM DOSE
≥12 years	600 micrograms[a]	600 micrograms[a]	3–5 minutes	200 micrograms per ml	3 ml	3 milligrams
11 years	500 micrograms	NONE	N/A	200 micrograms per ml	2.5 ml	500 micrograms
10 years	500 micrograms	NONE	N/A	200 micrograms per ml	2.5 ml	500 micrograms
9 years	500 micrograms	NONE	N/A	200 micrograms per ml	2.5 ml	500 micrograms
8 years	500 micrograms	NONE	N/A	200 micrograms per ml	2.5 ml	500 micrograms
7 years	400 micrograms	NONE	N/A	200 micrograms per ml	2 ml	400 micrograms
6 years	400 micrograms	NONE	N/A	200 micrograms per ml	2 ml	400 micrograms
5 years	300 micrograms	NONE	N/A	200 micrograms per ml	1.5 ml	300 micrograms
4 years	300 micrograms	NONE	N/A	200 micrograms per ml	1.5 ml	300 micrograms
3 years	240 micrograms	NONE	N/A	200 micrograms per ml	1.2 ml	240 micrograms
2 years	240 micrograms	NONE	N/A	200 micrograms per ml	1.2 ml	240 micrograms
18 months	200 micrograms	NONE	N/A	200 micrograms per ml	1 ml	200 micrograms
12 months	200 micrograms	NONE	N/A	200 micrograms per ml	1 ml	200 micrograms
9 months	120 micrograms	NONE	N/A	200 micrograms per ml	0.6 ml	120 micrograms
6 months	120 micrograms	NONE	N/A	200 micrograms per ml	0.6 ml	120 micrograms
3 months	120 micrograms	NONE	N/A	200 micrograms per ml	0.6 ml	120 micrograms
1 month	100 micrograms	NONE	N/A	200 micrograms per ml	0.5 ml	100 micrograms
Birth[b]	80 micrograms	NONE	N/A	200 micrograms per ml	0.4 ml	80 micrograms

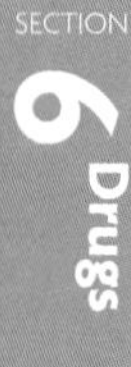

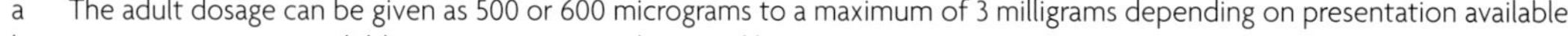

a The adult dosage can be given as 500 or 600 micrograms to a maximum of 3 milligrams depending on presentation available.

b **NB** BRADYCARDIA in children is most commonly caused by **HYPOXIA,** requiring immediate ABC care, **NOT** drug therapy; therefore **ONLY** administer atropine in cases of bradycardia caused by vagal stimulation (e.g. suction).

Atropine

Route: Intravenous/Intra-osseous **administer as a rapid bolus**.

AGE	INITIAL DOSE	REPEAT DOSE	DOSE INTERVAL	CONCENTRATION	VOLUME	MAXIMUM DOSE
≥12 years	600 micrograms[a]	600 micrograms[a]	3–5 minutes	100 micrograms per ml	6 ml	3 milligrams
11 years	500 micrograms	NONE	N/A	100 micrograms per ml	5 ml	500 micrograms
10 years	500 micrograms	NONE	N/A	100 micrograms per ml	5 ml	500 micrograms
9 years	500 micrograms	NONE	N/A	100 micrograms per ml	5 ml	500 micrograms
8 years	500 micrograms	NONE	N/A	100 micrograms per ml	5 ml	500 micrograms
7 years	400 micrograms	NONE	N/A	100 micrograms per ml	4 ml	400 micrograms
6 years	400 micrograms	NONE	N/A	100 micrograms per ml	4 ml	400 micrograms
5 years	300 micrograms	NONE	N/A	100 micrograms per ml	3 ml	300 micrograms
4 years	300 micrograms	NONE	N/A	100 micrograms per ml	3 ml	300 micrograms
3 years	240 micrograms	NONE	N/A	100 micrograms per ml	2.4 ml	240 micrograms
2 years	240 micrograms	NONE	N/A	100 micrograms per ml	2.4 ml	240 micrograms
18 months	200 micrograms	NONE	N/A	100 micrograms per ml	2 ml	200 micrograms
12 months	200 micrograms	NONE	N/A	100 micrograms per ml	2 ml	200 micrograms
9 months	120 micrograms	NONE	N/A	100 micrograms per ml	1.2 ml	120 micrograms
6 months	120 micrograms	NONE	N/A	100 micrograms per ml	1.2 ml	120 micrograms
3 months	120 micrograms	NONE	N/A	100 micrograms per ml	1.2 ml	120 micrograms
1 month	90 micrograms	NONE	N/A	100 micrograms per ml	0.9 ml	90 micrograms
Birth	70 micrograms	NONE	N/A	100 micrograms per ml	0.7 ml	70 micrograms

Bibliography

1 NHS Evidence. *Atropine.* Available from: https://www.evidence.nhs.uk/formulary/bnf/current/15-anaesthesia/151-general-anaesthesia/1513-antimuscarinic-drugs/atropine-sulfate, 2011.

a The adult dosage can be given as 500 or 600 micrograms to a maximum of 3 milligrams depending on presentation available.

Diazepam

Presentation

Ampoule containing 10 milligrams diazepam in an oil-in-water emulsion making up 2 ml.

Rectal tube containing 2.5 milligrams, 5 milligrams or 10 milligrams diazepam.

Indications

Patients who have prolonged (lasting 5 minutes or more) **OR** repeated (three or more in an hour) convulsions who are **CURRENTLY CONVULSING** – not secondary to an uncorrected hypoxic or hypoglycaemic episode (see 'Additional Information' below).

Eclamptic convulsions (initiate treatment if seizure lasts over 2–3 minutes or if it is recurrent).

Symptomatic cocaine toxicity (severe hypertension, chest pain or convulsions).

Actions

Central nervous system depressant, acts as an anticonvulsant and sedative.

Cautions

Should be used with caution if alcohol, antidepressants or other CNS depressants have been taken as side effects are more likely.

Recent doses by carers/relatives of any benzodiazepine (e.g. midazolam or diazepam) should be taken into account when calculating the maximum cumulative dose.

Contra-indications

Patients with known hypersensitivity.

Side Effects

Respiratory depression may occur, especially in the presence of alcohol (which enhances the depressive side effect of diazepam). Opioid drugs similarly enhance diazepam's cardiac and respiratory depressive effects.

Hypotension may occur. This may be significant if the patient has to be moved from a horizontal position to allow for extrication from an address. Caution should therefore be exercised and consideration given to either removing the patient flat or, if the convulsion has stopped and it is considered safe, allowing a 10-minute recovery period prior to removal.

Other side effects include light-headedness, unsteadiness, drowsiness, confusion and amnesia.

Additional Information

If the patient has their own supply of buccal midazolam this should be used in preference to PR diazepam.

Diazepam should only be used if the patient has been convulsing for 5 minutes or more (and is still convulsing), or if convulsions recur in rapid succession without time for full recovery in between. There is no value in giving 'preventative' diazepam if the convulsion has ceased. In any clearly sick or ill child, there must be no delay at the scene while administering the drug – it can be administered en-route to hospital.

Where IV diazepam can be given rapidly, this should be used in preference to rectal diazepam.

Early consideration should be given to using the PR route when IV access cannot be rapidly and safely obtained, **commonly the case in children.** In small children the PR route should be considered the first treatment option (with IV access being sought subsequently). When giving rectal medication, offer parental explanation and maintain patient dignity.

All patients who continue to convulse should receive **TWO** doses of benzodiazepine (midazolam or diazepam) 10 minutes apart, the second dose should be IV/IO if possible. Only give a second rectal dose if IV/IO access cannot be obtained in the 10 minutes between the first and second doses.

Care must be taken when inserting rectal tubes. They should be inserted no more than 2.5 cm in children or 4–5 cm in adults. (All tubes have an insertion marker on the nozzle.)

The **full** dose should be given at the appropriate times. It is **not** appropriate to either i) gradually 'titrate the dose upwards' or ii) to only give a partial dose if the convulsion stops (once started, even if the convulsion stops, that dose must be given). If this approach is followed, convulsion recurrence is much less likely.

Dosage and Administration

Route: Rectal

For convulsions give the full dose.

***NB** In recurrent or ongoing convulsions, a second rectal dose should ONLY be given if it is not possible to gain IV/IO access in the 10 minutes between the first and second dose.

AGE	INITIAL DOSE	REPEAT DOSE*	DOSE INTERVAL	CONCENTRATION	RECTAL TUBE VOLUME	MAXIMUM DOSE
Adult 70 yrs and over	10 milligrams	10 milligrams	10 minutes	10 milligrams in 2.5 ml	1 x 10 milligram tube	20 milligrams
Adult under 70 yrs	20 milligrams	10 milligrams	10 minutes	10 milligrams in 2.5 ml	1 or 2 x 10 milligram tube	30 milligrams
11 years	10 milligrams	10 milligrams	10 minutes	10 milligrams in 2.5 ml	1 x 10 milligram tube	20 milligrams
10 years	10 milligrams	10 milligrams	10 minutes	10 milligrams in 2.5 ml	1 x 10 milligram tube	20 milligrams
9 years	10 milligrams	10 milligrams	10 minutes	10 milligrams in 2.5 ml	1 x 10 milligram tube	20 milligrams
8 years	10 milligrams	10 milligrams	10 minutes	10 milligrams in 2.5 ml	1 x 10 milligram tube	20 milligrams
7 years	10 milligrams	10 milligrams	10 minutes	10 milligrams in 2.5 ml	1 x 10 milligram tube	20 milligrams
6 years	10 milligrams	10 milligrams	10 minutes	10 milligrams in 2.5 ml	1 x 10 milligram tube	20 milligrams
5 years	10 milligrams	10 milligrams	10 minutes	10 milligrams in 2.5 ml	1 x 10 milligram tube	20 milligrams
4 years	5 milligrams	5 milligrams	10 minutes	5 milligrams in 2.5 ml	1 x 5 milligram tube	10 milligrams
3 years	5 milligrams	5 milligrams	10 minutes	5 milligrams in 2.5 ml	1 x 5 milligram tube	10 milligrams
2 years	5 milligrams	5 milligrams	10 minutes	5 milligrams in 2.5 ml	1 x 5 milligram tube	10 milligrams
18 months	5 milligrams	5 milligrams	10 minutes	5 milligrams in 2.5 ml	1 x 5 milligram tube	10 milligrams
12 months	5 milligrams	5 milligrams	10 minutes	5 milligrams in 2.5 ml	1 x 5 milligram tube	10 milligrams
9 months	5 milligrams	5 milligrams	10 minutes	5 milligrams in 2.5 ml	1 x 5 milligram tube	10 milligrams
6 months	5 milligrams	5 milligrams	10 minutes	5 milligrams in 2.5 ml	1 x 5 milligram tube	10 milligrams
3 months	2.5 milligrams	2.5 milligrams	10 minutes	2.5 milligrams in 1.25 ml	1 x 2.5 milligram tube	5 milligrams
1 month	2.5 milligrams	2.5 milligrams	10 minutes	2.5 milligrams in 1.25 ml	1 x 2.5 milligram tube	5 milligrams
Birth[a]	1.25 milligrams	1.25 milligrams	10 minutes	2.5 milligrams in 1.25 ml	0.5 x 2.5 milligram tube	2.5 milligram

a Birth and neonatal dose, up to 1 month.

Diazepam

Route: Intravenous/intraosseous – administer **SLOWLY** over 2 minutes for adults (3–5 minutes for children).

For convulsions give the full dose. In symptomatic cocaine toxicity titrate slowly to response.

NB The second benzodiazepine dose should be IV/IO wherever possible (i.e. IV/IO diazepam).

Be ready to support ventilations.

AGE	INITIAL DOSE	REPEAT DOSE	DOSE INTERVAL	CONCENTRATION	DRUG VOLUME	MAXIMUM DOSE
Adult	10 milligrams	10 milligrams	10 minutes	10 milligrams in 2 ml	2 ml	20 milligrams
11 years	10 milligrams	10 milligrams	10 minutes	10 milligrams in 2 ml	2ml	20 milligrams
10 years	10 milligrams	10 milligrams	10 minutes	10 milligrams in 2 ml	2 ml	20 milligrams
9 years	9 milligrams	9 milligrams	10 minutes	10 milligrams in 2 ml	1.8 ml	18 milligrams
8 years	8 milligrams	8 milligrams	10 minutes	10 milligrams in 2 ml	1.6 ml	16 milligrams
7 years	7 milligrams	7 milligrams	10 minutes	10 milligrams in 2 ml	1.4 ml	14 milligrams
6 years	6.5 milligrams	6.5 milligrams	10 minutes	10 milligrams in 2 ml	1.3 ml	13 milligrams
5 years	6 milligrams	6 milligrams	10 minutes	10 milligrams in 2 ml	1.2 ml	12 milligrams
4 years	5 milligrams	5 milligrams	10 minutes	10 milligrams in 2 ml	1 ml	10 milligrams
3 years	4.5 milligrams	4.5 milligrams	10 minutes	10 milligrams in 2 ml	0.9 ml	9 milligrams
2 years	4 milligrams	4 milligrams	10 minutes	10 milligrams in 2 ml	0.8ml	8 milligrams
18 months	3.5 milligrams	3.5 milligrams	10 minutes	10 milligrams in 2 ml	0.7 ml	7 milligrams
12 months	3 milligrams	3 milligrams	10 minutes	10 milligrams in 2 ml	0.6 ml	6 milligrams
9 months	3 milligrams	3 milligrams	10 minutes	10 milligrams in 2 ml	0.6 ml	6 milligrams
6 months	2.5 milligrams	2.5 milligrams	10 minutes	10 milligrams in 2 ml	0.5 ml	5 milligrams
3 months	2 milligrams	2 milligrams	10 minutes	10 milligrams in 2 ml	0.4 ml	4 milligrams
1 month	1.5 milligrams	1.5 milligrams	10 minutes	10 milligrams in 2 ml	0.3 ml	3 milligrams
Birth	1 milligram	1 milligram	10 minutes	10 milligrams in 2 ml	0.2 ml	2 milligrams

Bibliography

1 American Epilepsy Society. Available from: https://www.aesnet.org/clinical_resources/guidelines.

2 NHS Evidence. *Diazepam*. Available from: https://bnf.nice.org.uk/.

3 National Institute for Health and Care Excellence. *Epilepsies: Diagnosis and Management* (CG137), 2012. Available from: https://www.nice.org.uk/guidance/cg137.

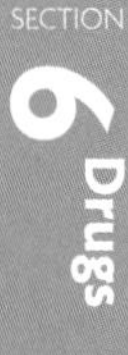

Entonox

Presentation

Entonox is a combination of nitrous oxide 50% and oxygen 50%. It is stored in medical cylinders that have a blue body with white shoulders.

Indications

Moderate to severe pain.

Labour pains.

Actions

Inhaled analgesic agent.

Contra-indications

Nitrous oxide may have a deleterious effect if used with patients in an air-containing closed space since nitrous oxide diffuses into such a space with a resulting increase in pressure.

Do not give entonox to patients with:

- Severe head injuries with impaired consciousness.
- Decompression sickness (the bends) where entonox can cause nitrogen bubbles within the blood stream to expand, aggravating the problem further. Consider anyone that has been diving within the previous 24 hours to be at risk.
- Violently disturbed psychiatric patients.
- Intraocular injection of gas within the last four weeks.
- Abdominal pain where intestinal obstruction is suspected.

Cautions

Any patient at risk of having a pneumothorax, pneumomediastinum and/or a pneumoperitoneum (e.g. polytrauma, penetrating torso injury).

Side Effects

Minimal side effects.

Additional Information

Prolonged use for more than 24 hours, or more frequently than every four days, can lead to vitamin B12 deficiency.

Administration of entonox should be in conjunction with pain score monitoring.

Entonox's advantages include:

- Rapid analgesic effect with minimal side effects.
- No cardiorespiratory depression.
- Self-administered.
- Analgesic effect rapidly wears off.
- The 50% oxygen concentration is valuable in many medical and trauma conditions.
- Entonox can be administered whilst preparing to deliver other analgesics.

The usual precautions must be followed with regard to caring for the entonox equipment and the cylinder MUST be inverted several times to mix the gases when temperatures are low.

Dosage and Administration

Adults:

- Entonox should be self-administered via a facemask or mouthpiece, after suitable instruction. It takes about **3–5 minutes** to be effective, but it may be **5–10 minutes** before maximum effect is achieved.

Children:

- Entonox is effective in children provided they are capable of following the administration instructions and can activate the demand valve.

Hydrocortisone

Presentation

An ampoule containing 100 milligrams hydrocortisone as either sodium succinate or sodium phosphate in 1 ml.

An ampoule containing 100 milligrams hydrocortisone sodium succinate for reconstitution with up to 2 ml of water.

Indications

Severe or life-threatening asthma.

Anaphylaxis.

Adrenal crisis (including Addisonian crisis) which is a time-critical medical emergency with an associated mortality.

Adrenal crisis may occur in patients on long-term steroid therapy, either:

- as replacement therapy for adrenal insufficiency from any cause
- in long-term therapy at doses of 5+mg prednisolone, eg for immune-suppression.

Administer hydrocortisone to:

1 Patients in an established adrenal crisis (IV administration preferable). Ensure parenteral hydrocortisone is given prior to transportation.

2 Patients with suspected adrenal insufficiency or on long-term steroid therapy who have become unwell, to prevent them having an adrenal crisis. (IM administration is usually sufficient).

3 If in doubt, it is better to administer hydrocortisone.

Actions

Glucocorticoid drug that restores blood pressure, blood sugar, cardiac synchronicity and volume. High levels are important to survive shock. Therapeutic actions include suppression of inflammation and immune response.

Contra-indications

Known allergy to the product/excipients.

Where a patient has adrenal crisis it is preferable to give whatever preparation is available.

Cautions

None relevant to a single dose.

Avoid intramuscular administration if patient likely to require thrombolysis.

Side Effects

Both sodium phosphate and sodium succinate solutions contain significant amounts of phosphate preservative and may cause stinging or burning sensations.

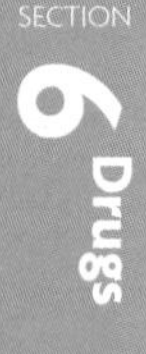

Dosage and Administration

1. **Severe or life-threatening asthma and adrenal crisis.** NB If there is any doubt about previous steroid administration, it is better to administer further hydrocortisone. There is no toxic dose for hydrocortisone, where advanced hypocortisolaemia may rapidly prove fatal.

Route: Preferably, intravenous (**SLOW** injection over a minimum of 2 minutes to avoid side effects).

Otherwise: intramuscular (upper arm or thigh) where IV access is not possible.

Note that patients with a larger BMI will need a longer IM needle.

AGE	INITIAL DOSE	REPEAT DOSE	DOSE INTERVAL	CONCENTRATION	VOLUME	MAXIMUM DOSE
Adult	100 milligrams	NONE	N/A	100 milligrams in 1 ml	1 ml	100 milligrams
11 years	100 milligrams	NONE	N/A	100 milligrams in 1 ml	1 ml	100 milligrams
10 years	100 milligrams	NONE	N/A	100 milligrams in 1 ml	1 ml	100 milligrams
9 years	100 milligrams	NONE	N/A	100 milligrams in 1 ml	1 ml	100 milligrams
8 years	100 milligrams	NONE	N/A	100 milligrams in 1 ml	1 ml	100 milligrams
7 years	100 milligrams	NONE	N/A	100 milligrams in 1 ml	1 ml	100 milligrams
6 years	100 milligrams	NONE	N/A	100 milligrams in 1 ml	1 ml	100 milligrams
5 years	50 milligrams	NONE	N/A	100 milligrams in 1 ml	0.5 ml	50 milligrams
4 years	50 milligrams	NONE	N/A	100 milligrams in 1 ml	0.5 ml	50 milligrams
3 years	50 milligrams	NONE	N/A	100 milligrams in 1 ml	0.5 ml	50 milligrams
2 years	50 milligrams	NONE	N/A	100 milligrams in 1 ml	0.5 ml	50 milligrams
18 months	50 milligrams	NONE	N/A	100 milligrams in 1 ml	0.5 ml	50 milligrams
12 months	50 milligrams	NONE	N/A	100 milligrams in 1 ml	0.5 ml	50 milligrams
9 months	50 milligrams	NONE	N/A	100 milligrams in 1 ml	0.5 ml	50 milligrams
6 months	50 milligrams	NONE	N/A	100 milligrams in 1 ml	0.5 ml	50 milligrams
3 months	25 milligrams	NONE	N/A	100 milligrams in 1 ml	0.25 ml	25 milligrams
1 month	25 milligrams	NONE	N/A	100 milligrams in 1 ml	0.25 ml	25 milligrams
Birth	10 milligrams	NONE	N/A	100 milligrams in 1 ml	0.1 ml	10 milligrams

Route: Intravenous (**SLOW** injection over a minimum of 2 minutes to avoid side effects)/intraosseous OR intramuscular (when IV access is impossible).

AGE	INITIAL DOSE	REPEAT DOSE	DOSE INTERVAL	CONCENTRATION	VOLUME	MAXIMUM DOSE
Adult	100 milligrams	NONE	N/A	100 milligrams in 2 ml	2 ml	100 milligrams
11 years	100 milligrams	NONE	N/A	100 milligrams in 2 ml	2 ml	100 milligrams
10 years	100 milligrams	NONE	N/A	100 milligrams in 2 ml	2 ml	100 milligrams
9 years	100 milligrams	NONE	N/A	100 milligrams in 2 ml	2 ml	100 milligrams
8 years	100 milligrams	NONE	N/A	100 milligrams in 2 ml	2 ml	100 milligrams
7 years	100 milligrams	NONE	N/A	100 milligrams in 2 ml	2 ml	100 milligrams
6 years	100 milligrams	NONE	N/A	100 milligrams in 2 ml	2 ml	100 milligrams
5 years	50 milligrams	NONE	N/A	100 milligrams in 2 ml	1 ml	50 milligrams
4 years	50 milligrams	NONE	N/A	100 milligrams in 2 ml	1 ml	50 milligrams
3 years	50 milligrams	NONE	N/A	100 milligrams in 2 ml	1 ml	50 milligrams
2 years	50 milligrams	NONE	N/A	100 milligrams in 2 ml	1 ml	50 milligrams
18 months	50 milligrams	NONE	N/A	100 milligrams in 2 ml	1 ml	50 milligrams
12 months	50 milligrams	NONE	N/A	100 milligrams in 2 ml	1 ml	50 milligrams
9 months	50 milligrams	NONE	N/A	100 milligrams in 2 ml	1 ml	50 milligrams
6 months	50 milligrams	NONE	N/A	100 milligrams in 2 ml	1 ml	50 milligrams
3 months	25 milligrams	NONE	N/A	100 milligrams in 2 ml	0.5 ml	25 milligrams
1 month	25 milligrams	NONE	N/A	100 milligrams in 2 ml	0.5 ml	25 milligrams
Birth	10 milligrams	NONE	N/A	100 milligrams in 2 ml	0.2 ml	10 milligrams

2. **Anaphylaxis**

Route: Intravenous (**SLOW** injection over a minimum of 2 minutes to avoid side effects)/intraosseous OR intramuscular (when IV access is impossible).

AGE	INITIAL DOSE	REPEAT DOSE	DOSE INTERVAL	CONCENTRATION	VOLUME	MAXIMUM DOSE
Adult	200 milligrams	NONE	N/A	100 milligrams in 1 ml	2 ml	200 milligrams
11 years	100 milligrams	NONE	N/A	100 milligrams in 1 ml	1 ml	100 milligrams
10 years	100 milligrams	NONE	N/A	100 milligrams in 1 ml	1 ml	100 milligrams
9 years	100 milligrams	NONE	N/A	100 milligrams in 1 ml	1 ml	100 milligrams
8 years	100 milligrams	NONE	N/A	100 milligrams in 1 ml	1 ml	100 milligrams
7 years	100 milligrams	NONE	N/A	100 milligrams in 1 ml	1 ml	100 milligrams
6 years	100 milligrams	NONE	N/A	100 milligrams in 1 ml	1 ml	100 milligrams
5 years	50 milligrams	NONE	N/A	100 milligrams in 1 ml	0.5 ml	50 milligrams
4 years	50 milligrams	NONE	N/A	100 milligrams in 1 ml	0.5 ml	50 milligrams
3 years	50 milligrams	NONE	N/A	100 milligrams in 1 ml	0.5 ml	50 milligrams
2 years	50 milligrams	NONE	N/A	100 milligrams in 1 ml	0.5 ml	50 milligrams
18 months	50 milligrams	NONE	N/A	100 milligrams in 1 ml	0.5 ml	50 milligrams
12 months	50 milligrams	NONE	N/A	100 milligrams in 1 ml	0.5 ml	50 milligrams
9 months	50 milligrams	NONE	N/A	100 milligrams in 1 ml	0.5 ml	50 milligrams
6 months	50 milligrams	NONE	N/A	100 milligrams in 1 ml	0.5 ml	50 milligrams
3 months	25 milligrams	NONE	N/A	100 milligrams in 1 ml	0.25 ml	25 milligrams
1 month	25 milligrams	NONE	N/A	100 milligrams in 1 ml	0.25 ml	25 milligrams
Birth	10 milligrams	NONE	N/A	100 milligrams in 1 ml	0.1 ml	10 milligrams

Hydrocortisone

Route: Intravenous (**SLOW** injection over a minimum of 2 minutes to avoid side effects)/intraosseous OR intramuscular (when IV access is impossible).

AGE	INITIAL DOSE	REPEAT DOSE	DOSE INTERVAL	CONCENTRATION	VOLUME	MAXIMUM DOSE
Adult	200 milligrams	NONE	N/A	100 milligrams in 2 ml	4 ml	200 milligrams
11 years	100 milligrams	NONE	N/A	100 milligrams in 2 ml	2 ml	100 milligrams
10 years	100 milligrams	NONE	N/A	100 milligrams in 2 ml	2 ml	100 milligrams
9 years	100 milligrams	NONE	N/A	100 milligrams in 2 ml	2 ml	100 milligrams
8 years	100 milligrams	NONE	N/A	100 milligrams in 2 ml	2 ml	100 milligrams
7 years	100 milligrams	NONE	N/A	100 milligrams in 2 ml	2 ml	100 milligrams
6 years	100 milligrams	NONE	N/A	100 milligrams in 2 ml	2 ml	100 milligrams
5 years	50 milligrams	NONE	N/A	100 milligrams in 2 ml	1 ml	50 milligrams
4 years	50 milligrams	NONE	N/A	100 milligrams in 2 ml	1 ml	50 milligrams
3 years	50 milligrams	NONE	N/A	100 milligrams in 2 ml	1 ml	50 milligrams
2 years	50 milligrams	NONE	N/A	100 milligrams in 2 ml	1 ml	50 milligrams
18 months	50 milligrams	NONE	N/A	100 milligrams in 2 ml	1 ml	50 milligrams
12 months	50 milligrams	NONE	N/A	100 milligrams in 2 ml	1 ml	50 milligrams
9 months	50 milligrams	NONE	N/A	100 milligrams in 2 ml	1 ml	50 milligrams
6 months	50 milligrams	NONE	N/A	100 milligrams in 2 ml	1 ml	50 milligrams
3 months	25 milligrams	NONE	N/A	100 milligrams in 2 ml	0.5 ml	25 milligrams
1 month	25 milligrams	NONE	N/A	100 milligrams in 2 ml	0.5 ml	25 milligrams
Birth	10 milligrams	NONE	N/A	100 milligrams in 2 ml	0.2 ml	10 milligrams

Bibliography

1 NHS Evidence. *Hydrocortisone.* Available from: https://bnf.nice.org.uk/drug/hydrocortisone.html.

Misoprostol

Presentation

Tablet containing misoprostol:

- 200 micrograms.

Indications

Post-partum haemorrhage within 24 hours of delivery of the newborn baby where bleeding from the uterus is uncontrollable by uterine massage.

Miscarriage with life-threatening bleeding and a confirmed diagnosis (e.g. where a patient has gone home with medical management and starts to bleed).

Both syntometrine and ergometrine are contra-indicated in hypertension (BP >140/90); in this case misoprostol (or preferably syntocinon if available) should be administered instead.

In all other circumstances misoprostol should only be used if syntometrine or other oxytocics are unavailable or if they have been ineffective at reducing haemorrhage after 15 mins.

Actions

Stimulates contraction of the uterus.

Onset of action 7–10 minutes.

Contra-indications

- Known hypersensitivity to misoprostol.
- Active labour.
- Possible multiple pregnancy/known or suspected fetus in utero.

Side Effects

- Abdominal pain.
- Nausea and vomiting.
- Diarrhoea.
- Pyrexia.
- Shivering.

Additional Information

Syntometrine and misoprostol reduce bleeding from a pregnant uterus through different pathways; therefore if one drug has not been effective after 15 mins, the other may be administered in addition.

Dosage and Administration

- Administer sublingually unless the patient is unable to maintain their airway.
- The vaginal route is not appropriate in post-partum haemorrhage or for miscarriage, but the rectal route may be considered when appropriate (e.g. impaired consciousness).

Route: Sublingual.

AGE	INITIAL DOSE	REPEAT DOSE	DOSE INTERVAL	CONCENTRATION	TABLETS	MAXIMUM DOSE
Adult	800 micrograms	**None**	N/A	200 micrograms per tablet	4 tablets	800 micrograms

Route: Rectal.

NB At the time of publication there is no rectal preparation of misoprostol – therefore the same tablets can be administered orally or rectally.

AGE	INITIAL DOSE	REPEAT DOSE	DOSE INTERVAL	CONCENTRATION	TABLETS	MAXIMUM DOSE
Adult	800 micrograms	**None**	N/A	200 micrograms per tablet	4 tablets	800 micrograms

Bibliography

1. Woollard M, Hinshaw K, Simpson H, Wieteska S. Emergencies in early pregnancy and complications following gynaecological surgery. In *Pre-hospital Obstetric Emergency Training*. Oxford: Wiley-Blackwell, 2009: 53–61.
2. Woollard M, Hinshaw K, Simpson H, Wieteska S. Emergencies after delivery. In *Pre-hospital Obstetric Emergency Training*. Oxford: Wiley-Blackwell, 2009: 111–124.
3. Royal College of Obstetricians and Gynaecologists. *Prevention and Management of Postpartum Haemorrhage* (Green-top guideline 52). London: RCOG, 2016.
4. Mousa HA, Alfirevic Z. Treatment for primary postpartum haemorrhage. *Cochrane Database of Systematic Reviews* 2007, 1: CD003249.
5. Starrs A, Winikoff B. Misoprostol for postpartum hemorrhage: moving from evidence to practice. *International Journal of Gynaecology and Obstetrics* 2012, 116(1): 1–3.

Naloxone Hydrochloride (Narcan)

Presentation

Naloxone hydrochloride 400 micrograms per 1 ml ampoule.

Indications

Opioid overdose producing respiratory, cardiovascular and central nervous system depression.

Overdose of either an opioid analgesic (e.g. dextropropoxyphene, codeine), or a compound analgesic (refer to Table 6.6 e.g. co-codamol, combination of codeine and paracetamol).

Unconsciousness, associated with respiratory depression of unknown cause, where opioid overdose is a possibility, refer to **Altered Level of Consciousness**.

Actions

Antagonism of the effects (including respiratory depression) of opioid drugs.

Contra-indications

Neonates born to opioid addicted mothers – produces serious withdrawal effects. Emphasis should be on bag-valve-mask ventilation and oxygenation – as with all patients.

Side Effects

In patients who are physically dependent on opiates, naloxone may precipitate violent withdrawal symptoms, including cardiac dysrrhythmias. It is better, in these cases, to titrate the dose of naloxone as described (see dosing charts below), to effectively reverse the cardiac and respiratory depression, but still leave the patient in a 'groggy' state with regular re-assessment of ventilation and circulation.

Additional information

When indicated, naloxone should be administered via the intravenous route.

If IV access is impossible, naloxone may be administered intramuscularly, **undiluted** (into the outer aspect of the thigh or upper arm), but absorption may be unpredictable.

Opioid induced respiratory and cardiovascular depression can be fatal.

When used, naloxone's effects are **short lived** and once its effects have worn off respiratory and cardiovascular depression can recur with fatal consequences. **All** cases of opioid overdose should be transported to hospital, even if the initial response to naloxone has been good. If the patient refuses hospitalisation, consider, if the patient consents, a loading dose of **800 micrograms IM** to minimise the risk described above.

Table 6.6 – EXAMPLES OF PRESCRIPTION OPIOID DRUGS

Buprenorphine	Temgesic
Codeine	Used in combination in Codis, Diarrest, Migraleve, Paracodol, Phensedyl, Solpadeine, Solpadol, Syndol, Terpoin, Tylex, Veganin
Dextromoramide	Palfium
Dipipanone	Dicanol
Dextropropoxyphene	Used in combination in Distalgesic/co-proxamol
Diamorphine	'Heroin'
Dihydrocodeine	Co-dydramol, DF 118
Meptazinol	Meptid
Methadone	Physeptone, Methadose
Morphine	Oramorph, Sevredol, MST Continus, SRM Rhotard
Oxycodone	Oxycontin
Pentazocine	Fortral
Pethidine	Pamergan
Phenazocine	Narphen

NB This list is not comprehensive; other opioid drugs are available.

Naloxone Hydrochloride (Narcan)

Dosage and Administration

Respiratory arrest/extreme respiratory depression.

- If there is no response after the initial dose, repeat every 3 minutes, up to the maximum dose, until an effect is noted. NB The half-life of naloxone is short.
- Known or potentially aggressive adults suffering respiratory depression: dilute up to 800 micrograms (2 ml) of naloxone into 8 ml of water for injections or sodium chloride 0.9% to a total volume of 10 ml and administer **SLOWLY,** titrating to response, 1 ml at a time.

Route: Intravenous/intraosseous – administer **SLOWLY** 1 ml at a time. Titrated to response relieving respiratory depression but maintain patient in 'groggy' state.

AGE	INITIAL DOSE	REPEAT DOSE	DOSE INTERVAL	CONCENTRATION	VOLUME	MAXIMUM DOSE
12 years–adult	400 micrograms	400 micrograms	3 minutes	400 micrograms in 1 ml	1 ml	4,400 micrograms
11 years	350 micrograms	350 micrograms	3 minutes	400 micrograms in 1 ml	0.9 ml	3,850 micrograms
10 years	320 micrograms	320 micrograms	3 minutes	400 micrograms in 1 ml	0.8 ml	3,520 micrograms
9 years	280 micrograms	280 micrograms	3 minutes	400 micrograms in 1 ml	0.7 ml	3,080 micrograms
8 years	280 micrograms	280 micrograms	3 minutes	400 micrograms in 1 ml	0.7 ml	3,080 micrograms
7 years	240 micrograms	240 micrograms	3 minutes	400 micrograms in 1 ml	0.6 ml	2,640 micrograms
6 years	200 micrograms	200 micrograms	3 minutes	400 micrograms in 1 ml	0.5 ml	2,200 micrograms
5 years	200 micrograms	200 micrograms	3 minutes	400 micrograms in 1 ml	0.5 ml	2,200 micrograms
4 years	160 micrograms	160 micrograms	3 minutes	400 micrograms in 1 ml	0.4 ml	1,760 micrograms
3 years	160 micrograms	160 micrograms	3 minutes	400 micrograms in 1 ml	0.4 ml	1,760 micrograms
2 years	120 micrograms	120 micrograms	3 minutes	400 micrograms in 1 ml	0.3 ml	1,320 micrograms
18 months	120 micrograms	120 micrograms	3 minutes	400 micrograms in 1 ml	0.3 ml	1,320 micrograms
12 months	100 micrograms	100 micrograms	3 minutes	400 micrograms in 1 ml	0.25 ml	1,100 micrograms
9 months	80 micrograms	80 micrograms	3 minutes	400 micrograms in 1 ml	0.2 ml	880 micrograms
6 months	80 micrograms	80 micrograms	3 minutes	400 micrograms in 1 ml	0.2 ml	880 micrograms
3 months	60 micrograms	60 micrograms	3 minutes	400 micrograms in 1 ml	0.15 ml	660 micrograms
1 month	40 micrograms	40 micrograms	3 minutes	400 micrograms in 1 ml	0.1 ml	440 micrograms
Birth	N/A	N/A	N/A	N/A	N/A	N/A

Naloxone Hydrochloride (Narcan)

Respiratory arrest/extreme respiratory depression where the IV/IO route is unavailable or the ambulance clinician is not trained to administer drugs via the IV/IO route.

- If there is no response after the initial dose, repeat every 3 minutes, up to the maximum dose, until an effect is noted. NB The half-life of naloxone is short.
- **For adults when administering naloxone via the intramuscular route:** administering large volumes intramuscularly could lead to poor absorption and/or tissue damage; therefore divide the dose where necessary and practicable. Vary the site of injection for repeated doses; appropriate sites include: buttock (gluteus maximus), thigh (vastus lateralis), lateral hip (gluteus medius) and upper arm (deltoid).

Route: Intramuscular – initial dose.

AGE	INITIAL DOSE	REPEAT DOSE	DOSE INTERVAL	CONCENTRATION	VOLUME	MAXIMUM DOSE
12 years–adult	400 micrograms	See repeat dose	3 minutes	400 micrograms in 1 ml	1 ml	See repeat dose
11 years	350 micrograms	See repeat dose	3 minutes	400 micrograms in 1 ml	0.9 ml	See repeat dose
10 years	320 micrograms	See repeat dose	3 minutes	400 micrograms in 1 ml	0.8 ml	See repeat dose
9 years	280 micrograms	See repeat dose	3 minutes	400 micrograms in 1 ml	0.7 ml	See repeat dose
8 years	280 micrograms	See repeat dose	3 minutes	400 micrograms in 1 ml	0.7 ml	See repeat dose
7 years	240 micrograms	See repeat dose	3 minutes	400 micrograms in 1 ml	0.6 ml	See repeat dose
6 years	200 micrograms	See repeat dose	3 minutes	400 micrograms in 1 ml	0.5 ml	See repeat dose
5 years	200 micrograms	See repeat dose	3 minutes	400 micrograms in 1 ml	0.5 ml	See repeat dose
4 years	160 micrograms	See repeat dose	3 minutes	400 micrograms in 1 ml	0.4 ml	See repeat dose
3 years	160 micrograms	See repeat dose	3 minutes	400 micrograms in 1 ml	0.4 ml	See repeat dose
2 years	120 micrograms	See repeat dose	3 minutes	400 micrograms in 1 ml	0.3 ml	See repeat dose
18 months	120 micrograms	See repeat dose	3 minutes	400 micrograms in 1 ml	0.3 ml	See repeat dose
12 months	100 micrograms	See repeat dose	3 minutes	400 micrograms in 1 ml	0.25 ml	See repeat dose
9 months	80 micrograms	See repeat dose	3 minutes	400 micrograms in 1 ml	0.2 ml	See repeat dose
6 months	80 micrograms	See repeat dose	3 minutes	400 micrograms in 1 ml	0.2 ml	See repeat dose
3 months	60 micrograms	See repeat dose	3 minutes	400 micrograms in 1 ml	0.15 ml	See repeat dose
1 month	40 micrograms	See repeat dose	3 minutes	400 micrograms in 1 ml	0.1 ml	See repeat dose
Birth	N/A	N/A	N/A	N/A	N/A	N/A

Naloxone Hydrochloride (Narcan)

Route: Intramuscular – repeat dose.

NB In the event of IV access being unavailable for the administration of naloxone in children it is advised that the initial IM dose be given dependent on age and, if required, a single subsequent IM dose of 400 micrograms to be given once only. If IV access becomes available and further doses of naloxone are clinically indicated then revert to the IV dosage table.

AGE	INITIAL DOSE	REPEAT DOSE	DOSE INTERVAL	CONCENTRATION	VOLUME	MAXIMUM DOSE
12 years–adult	See initial dose	400 micrograms	3 minutes	400 micrograms in 1 ml	1 ml	4,400 micrograms
11 years	See initial dose	400 micrograms	3 minutes	400 micrograms in 1 ml	1 ml	750 micrograms
10 years	See initial dose	400 micrograms	3 minutes	400 micrograms in 1 ml	1 ml	720 micrograms
9 years	See initial dose	400 micrograms	3 minutes	400 micrograms in 1 ml	1 ml	680 micrograms
8 years	See initial dose	400 micrograms	3 minutes	400 micrograms in 1 ml	1 ml	680 micrograms
7 years	See initial dose	400 micrograms	3 minutes	400 micrograms in 1 ml	1 ml	640 micrograms
6 years	See initial dose	400 micrograms	3 minutes	400 micrograms in 1 ml	1 ml	600 micrograms
5 years	See initial dose	400 micrograms	3 minutes	400 micrograms in 1 ml	1 ml	600 micrograms
4 years	See initial dose	400 micrograms	3 minutes	400 micrograms in 1 ml	1 ml	560 micrograms
3 years	See initial dose	400 micrograms	3 minutes	400 micrograms in 1 ml	1 ml	560 micrograms
2 years	See initial dose	400 micrograms	3 minutes	400 micrograms in 1 ml	1 ml	520 micrograms
18 months	See initial dose	400 micrograms	3 minutes	400 micrograms in 1 ml	1 ml	520 micrograms
12 months	See initial dose	400 micrograms	3 minutes	400 micrograms in 1 ml	1 ml	500 micrograms
9 months	See initial dose	400 micrograms	3 minutes	400 micrograms in 1 ml	1 ml	480 micrograms
6 months	See initial dose	400 micrograms	3 minutes	400 micrograms in 1 ml	1 ml	480 micrograms
3 months	See initial dose	400 micrograms	3 minutes	400 micrograms in 1 ml	1 ml	460 micrograms
1 month	See initial dose	400 micrograms	3 minutes	400 micrograms in 1 ml	1 ml	440 micrograms
Birth	N/A	N/A	N/A	N/A	N/A	N/A

Bibliography

1 NHS Evidence. *Naloxone*. Available from: https://www.evidence.nhs.uk/formulary/bnf/current/15-anaesthesia/151-general-anaesthesia/1517-antagonists-for-central-and-respiratory-depression/naloxone-hydrochloride, 2011–12.

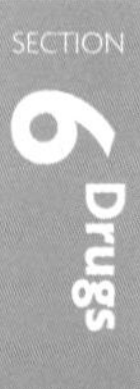

Oxygen

Presentation

Oxygen (O_2) is a gas provided in compressed form in a cylinder. It is also available in liquid form, in a system adapted for ambulance use. It is fed via a regulator and flow meter to the patient by means of plastic tubing and an oxygen mask/nasal cannulae.

Indications

Children

- Significant illness and/or injury.

Adults

- Critical illnesses requiring high levels of supplemental oxygen (refer to Table 6.11).
- Serious illnesses requiring moderate levels of supplemental oxygen if the patient is hypoxaemic (refer to Table 6.12).
- COPD and other conditions requiring controlled or low-dose oxygen therapy (refer to Table 6.13).
- Conditions for which patients should be monitored closely but oxygen therapy is not required unless the patient is hypoxaemic (refer to Table 6.14).

Actions

Essential for cell metabolism. Adequate tissue oxygenation is essential for normal physiological function.

Oxygen assists in reversing hypoxia, by raising the concentration of inspired oxygen. Hypoxia will, however, only improve if respiratory effort or ventilation and tissue perfusion are adequate.

If ventilation is inadequate or absent, assisting or completely taking over the patient's ventilation is essential to reverse hypoxia.

Contra-indications

Explosive environments.

Cautions

Oxygen increases the fire hazard at the scene of an incident.

Defibrillation – ensure pads firmly applied to reduce spark hazard.

Side Effects

Non-humidified O_2 is drying and irritating to mucous membranes over a period of time.

In patients with COPD there is a risk that even moderately high doses of inspired oxygen can produce increased carbon dioxide levels which may cause respiratory depression and this may lead to respiratory arrest. Refer to Table 6.9 for guidance.

Dosage and Administration

- Measure oxygen saturation (SpO_2) in all patients using pulse oximetry.
- For the administration of **moderate** levels of supplemented oxygen nasal cannulae are recommended in preference to simple face mask as they offer a more flexible dose range.
- Patients with tracheostomy or previous laryngectomy may require alternative appliances (e.g. tracheostomy masks).
- Entonox may be administered when required.
- Document oxygen administration.

Children

- **ALL** children with significant illness and/or injury should receive **HIGH** levels of supplementary oxygen.

Adults

- Administer the initial oxygen dose until a reliable oxygen saturation reading is obtained.
- If the desired oxygen saturation cannot be maintained with a simple face mask, change to a reservoir mask (non-rebreathe mask).
- For dosage and administration of supplemental oxygen refer to Tables 6.7–6.10.
- For conditions where **NO** supplemental oxygen is required unless the patient is hypoxaemic refer to Table 6.10.

Table 6.7 – High levels of supplemental oxygen for adults with critical illnesses

Target saturation 94–98%

Administer the initial oxygen dose until the vital signs are normal, then reduce oxygen dose and aim for target saturation within the range of **94–98%** as per table below.

Condition	Initial dose	Method of administration
• Cardiac arrest or resuscitation: – basic life support – advanced life support – foreign body airway obstruction – traumatic cardiac arrest – maternal resuscitation. • Carbon monoxide poisoning **NOTE– Some oxygen saturation monitors cannot differentiate between carboxyhaemoglobin and oxyhaemoglobin owing to carbon monoxide poisoning.**	Maximum dose until the vital signs are normal	Bag-valve-mask
• Major trauma: – abdominal trauma – burns and scalds – electrocution – head trauma – limb trauma – spinal injury and spinal cord injury – pelvic trauma – the immersion incident – thoracic trauma – trauma in pregnancy. • Anaphylaxis • Decompression illness • Major pulmonary haemorrhage • Sepsis (e.g. meningococcal septicemia) • Shock • Drowning	15 litres per minute	Reservoir mask (non-rebreathe mask)
• Active convulsion • Hypothermia	Administer 15 litres per minute until a reliable SpO_2 measurement can be obtained and the adjust oxygen flow to aim for target saturation within the range of **94–98%**	Reservoir mask (non-rebreathe mask)

<table>
<tr><th colspan="3">Table 6.8 – Moderate levels of supplemental oxygen for adults with serious illnesses if the patient is hypoxaemic</th></tr>
<tr><td colspan="3">Target saturation 94–98%
Administer the initial oxygen dose until a reliable SpO_2 measurement is available, then adjust oxygen flow to aim for target saturation within the range of 94–98% as per the table below.</td></tr>
<tr><th>Condition</th><th>INITIAL DOSE</th><th>Method of administration</th></tr>
<tr><td rowspan="3">• Acute hypoxaemia (cause not yet diagnosed)
• Deterioration of lung fibrosis or other interstitial lung disease
• Acute asthma
• Acute heart failure
• Pneumonia
• Lung cancer
• Postoperative breathlessness
• Pulmonary embolism
• Pleural effusions
• Pneumothorax
• Severe anaemia
• Sickle cell crisis</td><td>SpO_2 <85%
10–15 litres per minute</td><td>Reservoir mask (non-rebreathe mask)</td></tr>
<tr><td>SpO_2 ≥85–93%
2–6 litres per minute</td><td>Nasal cannulae</td></tr>
<tr><td>SpO_2 ≥85–93%
5–10 litres per minute</td><td>Simple face mask</td></tr>
</table>

<table>
<tr><th colspan="3">Table 6.9 – Controlled or low-dose supplemental oxygen for adults with COPD and other conditions requiring controlled or low-dose oxygen therapy</th></tr>
<tr><td colspan="3">Target saturation 88–92%
Administer the initial oxygen dose until a reliable SpO_2 measurement is available, then adjust oxygen flow to aim for target saturation within the range of 88–92% or pre-specified range detailed on the patient's alert card, as per the table below.</td></tr>
<tr><th>Condition</th><th>Initial dose</th><th>Method of administration</th></tr>
<tr><td rowspan="2">• Chronic obstructive pulmonary disease (COPD)
• Exacerbation of cystic fibrosis</td><td>4 litres per minute</td><td>28% Venturi mask or patient's own mask</td></tr>
<tr><td colspan="2">NB If respiratory rate is >30 breaths/min using Venturi mask set flow rate to 50% above the minimum specified for the mask.</td></tr>
<tr><td>• Chronic neuromuscular disorders
• Chest wall disorders
• Morbid obesity (body mass index >40 kg/m^2)</td><td>4 litres per minute</td><td>28% Venturi mask or patient's own mask</td></tr>
<tr><td>NB If the oxygen saturation remains below 88% change to simple face mask.</td><td>5–10 litres per minute</td><td>Simple face mask</td></tr>
<tr><td>NB Critical illness AND COPD/or other risk factors for hypercapnia.</td><td colspan="2">If a patient with COPD or other risk factors for hypercapnia sustains or develops critical illness/injury ensure the same target saturations as indicated in Table 6.7.</td></tr>
</table>

Oxygen

Table 6.10 – No supplemental oxygen required for adults with these conditions unless the patient is hypoxaemic but patients should be monitored closely

Target saturation 94–98%

If hypoxaemic (SpO_2 <94%) administer the initial oxygen dose, then adjust oxygen flow to aim for target saturation within the range of **94–98%**, as per table below.

Condition	Initial dose	Method of administration
• Myocardial infarction and acute coronary syndromes • Stroke	**SpO_2 <85%** 10–15 litres per minute	Reservoir mask (non-rebreathe mask)
• Cardiac rhythm disturbance	**SpO_2 ≥85–93%** 2–6 litres per minute	Nasal cannulae
• Non-traumatic chest pain/ discomfort	**SpO_2 ≥85–93%** 5–10 litres per minute	Simple face mask
• Implantable cardioverter defibrillator firing • Pregnancy and obstetric emergencies: – birth imminent – haemorrhage during pregnancy – pregnancy induced hypertension – vaginal bleeding. • Abdominal pain • Headache • Hyperventilation syndrome or dysfunctional breathing		
• Most poisonings and drug overdoses (refer to Table 6.7 for **carbon monoxide poisoning** and special cases below for **paraquat or bleomycin** poisoning) • Metabolic and renal disorders • Acute and sub-acute neurological and muscular conditions producing muscle weakness (assess the need for assisted ventilation if **SpO_2 <94%**) • Post convulsion • Gastrointestinal bleeds • Glycaemic emergencies • Heat exhaustion/heat stroke **SPECIAL CASES** • Poisoning with paraquat • Poisoning with bleomycin		

NOTE – patients with **paraquat or bleomycin** poisoning may be harmed by supplemental oxygen so avoid oxygen unless the patient is hypoxaemic. Target saturation 85–88%.

SECTION 6 Drugs

Table 6.11 – Critical illnesses in adults requiring **HIGH** levels of supplemental oxygen

- Cardiac arrest or resuscitation:
  - basic life support
  - advanced life support
  - foreign body airway obstruction
  - traumatic cardiac arrest
  - maternal resuscitation
- Major trauma:
  - abdominal trauma
  - burns and scalds
  - electrocution
  - head trauma
  - limb trauma
  - spinal injury and spinal cord injury
  - pelvic trauma
  - the immersion incident
  - thoracic trauma
  - trauma in pregnancy
- Active convulsion
- Anaphylaxis
- Decompression illness
- Carbon monoxide poisoning
- Hypothermia
- Major pulmonary haemorrhage
- Sepsis (e.g. meningococcal septicaemia)
- Shock

Table 6.12 – Serious illnesses in adults requiring **MODERATE** levels of supplemental oxygen if hypoxaemic

- Acute hypoxaemia
- Deterioration of lung fibrosis or other interstitial lung disease
- Acute asthma
- Acute heart failure
- Pneumonia
- Lung cancer
- Postoperative breathlessness
- Pulmonary embolism
- Pleural effusions
- Pneumothorax
- Severe anaemia
- Sickle cell crisis

Table 6.13 – COPD and other conditions in adults requiring **CONTROLLED OR LOW-DOSE** supplemental oxygen

- Chronic Obstructive Pulmonary Disease (COPD)
- Exacerbation of cystic fibrosis
- Chronic neuromuscular disorders
- Chest wall disorders
- Morbid obesity (body mass index >40 kg/m^2)

Table 6.14 – Conditions in adults **NOT** requiring supplemental oxygen unless the patient is hypoxaemic

- Myocardial infarction and acute coronary syndromes
- Stroke
- Cardiac rhythm disturbance
- Non-traumatic chest pain/discomfort
- Implantable cardioverter defibrillator firing
- Pregnancy and obstetric emergencies:
  - birth imminent
  - haemorrhage during pregnancy
  - pregnancy induced hypertension
  - vaginal bleeding
- Abdominal pain
- Headache
- Hyperventilation syndrome or dysfunctional breathing
- Most poisonings and drug overdoses (except carbon monoxide poisoning)
- Metabolic and renal disorders
- Acute and sub-acute neurological and muscular conditions producing muscle weakness
- Post convulsion
- Gastrointestinal bleeds
- Glycaemic emergencies
- Heat exhaustion/heat stroke

Special cases:

- Paraquat poisoning
- Bleomycin poisoning

Oxygen

Is the patient in CARDIAC and/or RESPIRATORY ARREST or in need of VENTILATORY SUPPORT?

- YES → Administer the maximum dose of oxygen via a bag-valve-mask until the vital signs are normal, then aim for target saturation within the range of **94–98%**
- NO ↓

Do you know or suspect CARBON MONOXIDE poisoning?

- YES → Administer maximum dose of oxygen via a reservoir mask
- NO ↓

Do you know or suspect a critical illness requiring HIGH levels of oxygen? Refer to Table 6.7

- YES → Is SpO_2 ≥94% and are the vital signs normal?
  - NO → Administer 15 l/min of oxygen via a reservoir mask until the vital signs are normal, then aim for target saturation within the range of **94–98%**
  - YES → Monitor SpO_2 and if the saturation falls below **94%** administer oxygen to maintain a saturation within the range of **94–98%**
- NO ↓

Do you know or suspect a condition requiring CONTROLLED OR LOW–DOSE levels of oxygen? Refer to Table 6.9

- YES → Is SpO_2 ≥88%?
  - NO → Administer 4 l/min of oxygen via a 28% Venturi mask or patient's own mask to aim for target saturation within the range of **88–92%**
  - YES → Monitor SpO_2 and if the saturation falls below **88%** administer oxygen to maintain a saturation within the range of **88–92%**
- NO ↓

Do you know or suspect PARAQUAT or BLEOMYCIN poisoning?

- YES → Is SpO_2 ≥85%?
  - NO → SpO_2 <**85%** administer 15 l/min of oxygen via a reservoir mask. SpO_2 **85–87%** administer 2–6 l/m via nasal cannulae or 5–10 l/min of oxygen via a simple face mask. Aim for target saturation within the range of **85–88%**
  - YES → Monitor SpO_2 and if the saturation falls below 85% administer oxygen to maintain a saturation within the range of **85–88%**
- NO ↓

Do you know or suspect a serious illness requiring MODERATE levels oxygen? Refer to Table 6.8

- YES → Is SpO_2 ≥94%?
  - NO → SpO_2 <**85%** administer 10–15 l/min of oxygen via a reservoir mask. SpO_2 **85–93%** administer 2–6 l/m via nasal cannulae or 5–10 l/min of oxygen via a simple face mask. Aim for target saturation within the range of **94–98%**
  - YES → Monitor SpO_2 and if the saturation falls below 94% administer oxygen to maintain a saturation within the range of **94–98%**
- NO ↓

Other conditions NOT requiring oxygen unless hypoxaemic? Refer to Table 6.10

- YES → Is SpO_2 ≥94%?
  - NO → SpO_2 <**85%** administer 10–15 l/min of oxygen via a reservoir mask. SpO_2 **85–93%** administer 2–6 l/m via nasal cannulae or 5–10 l/min of oxygen via a simple face mask. Aim for target saturation within the range of **94–98%**
  - YES → Monitor SpO_2 and if the saturation falls below 94% administer oxygen to maintain a saturation within the range of **94–98%**

Figure 6.1 – Administration of supplemental oxygen algorithm.

Bibliography

1 O'Driscoll BR, Howard LS, Davison AG, on behalf of the British Thoracic Society. BTS guideline for emergency oxygen use in adult patients. *Thorax* 2008, 63(suppl. 6): vi1–vi68.

2 O'Driscoll BR, Howard LS, Earis J, Mak V. BTS guideline for oxgen use in adults in healthcare and emergency settings. *Thorax* 2017, 72: i1–i90.

Paracetamol

Presentation

Both oral and intravenous preparations are available.

Oral

Paracetamol solutions/suspensions:

- **Infant paracetamol suspension** (120 milligrams in 5 ml), used from 3 months to 5 years.
- **Paracetamol 6 plus suspension** (250 milligrams in 5 ml), used from 6 years of age upwards.

Paracetamol tablets

- 500 milligram tablets (tablets may be broken in half).

Intravenous

- Bottle containing paracetamol 1 gram in 100 ml (10 mg/ml) for intravenous infusion for adults, adolescents and children weighing more than 33kg.
- Bottle containing paracetamol 500 milligrams in 50ml (10mg/ml) for intravenous infusion for term newborn, infants, toddlers and children weighing less than 33kg.

Indications

Oral

Relief of mild to moderate pain or high temperature with discomfort (not for high temperature alone).

Intravenous

As part of a balanced analgesic regimen for severe pain paracetamol is effective in reducing opioid requirements while improving analgesic efficacy and is an alternative analgesic when morphine is contraindicated.

Actions

Analgesic (pain relieving) and antipyretic (temperature reducing) drug.

Contra-indications

Known paracetamol allergy.

Do **NOT** give further paracetamol if a paracetamol containing product (e.g. Calpol, co-codamol) has already been given within the last 4 hours (6 hours in patients with renal impairment) or if the maximum cumulative daily dose has already been given.

Cautions

Care must be taken to ensure accurate doses are given to reduce the risk of paracetamol overdose. There are significant risks due to the different preparations and strengths of paracetamol that are available, and potential confusion between millilitres (ml) and milligrams (mg). The intravenous preparations come in different sizes, and due to the small amounts that are recommended for children from birth upwards, and for patients that weigh less than 50kg, extreme vigilance is needed. Refer to local procedure and guidance on how to administer dependant on what preparations are available to you.

Side Effects

Side effects are extremely rare; occasionally intravenous paracetamol may cause hypotension if administered too rapidly.

Additional Information

A febrile child should always be conveyed to hospital except where:

- a full assessment has been carried out,

and

- the child has no apparent serious underlying illness,

and

- the child has a defined clinical pathway for reassessment and follow up, with the full consent of the parent (or carer).

Any IV paracetamol that remains within the giving set can be flushed using 0.9% saline. Take care to ensure that air does not become entrained into the giving set; if there is air in the giving set ensure that it does not run into the patient with further fluids. Ambulance clinicians should strictly adhere to the administration procedure as set out by their Trust to minimise this risk.

Some patients may be at increased risk of experiencing toxicity at therapeutic doses, particularly those with a body weight under 50kg and those with risk factors for hepatotoxicity. Clinical judgement should be used to adjust the dose of oral and intravenous paracetamol in these patients.

Paracetamol is not recommended for patients with cardiac chest pain.

Dosage and Administration

Ensure that:
1. Paracetamol (or an alternative paracetamol-containing product) has not been taken within the previous 4 hours (6 hours in renal impairment).
2. The maximum cumulative daily dose has not already been taken.
3. When administering to children, the correct paracetamol-containing solution/suspension for that patient's age is being used, i.e. 'infant paracetamol suspension' for those aged 0–5 year and 'paracetamol 6 plus suspension' for ages 6 years and over.

Route: Oral – infant paracetamol suspension (i.e. ages 3 months – 5 years).

AGE	INITIAL DOSE	REPEAT DOSE	DOSE INTERVAL	CONCENTRATION	VOLUME	MAXIMUM DOSE
Adult	N/A	N/A	N/A	N/A	N/A	N/A
11 years	N/A	N/A	N/A	N/A	N/A	N/A
10 years	N/A	N/A	N/A	N/A	N/A	N/A
9 years	N/A	N/A	N/A	N/A	N/A	N/A
8 years	N/A	N/A	N/A	N/A	N/A	N/A
7 years	N/A	N/A	N/A	N/A	N/A	N/A
6 years	N/A	N/A	N/A	N/A	N/A	N/A
5 years	240 milligrams	240 milligrams	4–6 hours	120 milligrams in 5 ml	10 ml	960 milligrams in 24 hours
4 years	240 milligrams	240 milligrams	4–6 hours	120 milligrams in 5 ml	10 ml	960 milligrams in 24 hours
3 years	180 milligrams	180 milligrams	4–6 hours	120 milligrams in 5 ml	7.5 ml	720 milligrams in 24 hours
2 years	180 milligrams	180 milligrams	4–6 hours	120 milligrams in 5 ml	7.5 ml	720 milligrams in 24 hours
18 months	120 milligrams	120 milligrams	4–6 hours	120 milligrams in 5 ml	5 ml	480 milligrams in 24 hours
12 months	120 milligrams	120 milligrams	4–6 hours	120 milligrams in 5 ml	5 ml	480 milligrams in 24 hours
9 months	120 milligrams	120 milligrams	4–6 hours	120 milligrams in 5 ml	5 ml	480 milligrams in 24 hours
6 months	120 milligrams	120 milligrams	4–6 hours	120 milligrams in 5 ml	5 ml	480 milligrams in 24 hours
3 months	60 milligrams	60 milligrams	4–6 hours	120 milligrams in 5 ml	2.5 ml	240 milligrams in 24 hours
1 month	N/A	N/A	N/A	N/A	N/A	N/A
Birth	N/A	N/A	N/A	N/A	N/A	N/A

Paracetamol

Ensure that:
1. Paracetamol (or an alternative paracetamol-containing product) has not been taken within the previous 4 hours (6 hours in renal impairment).
2. The maximum cumulative daily dose has not already been taken.
3. When administering to children, the correct paracetamol-containing solution/suspension for that patient's age is being used, i.e. 'infant paracetamol suspension' for those aged 0–5 year and 'paracetamol 6 plus suspension' for ages 6 years and over.

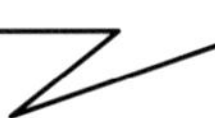

Route: Oral – paracetamol 6 plus suspension (i.e. ages 6 years and over).

AGE	INITIAL DOSE	REPEAT DOSE	DOSE INTERVAL	CONCENTRATION	VOLUME	MAXIMUM DOSE
16 years – Adult AND **over** 50 kg	500 milligrams – 1 gram	500 milligrams – 1 gram	4–6 hours	250 milligrams in 5 ml	10–20 ml	2–4 grams in 24 hours
12 – 15 years OR 50 kg and **under**	500–750 milligrams	500–750 milligrams	4–6 hours	250 milligrams in 5 ml	10–15 ml	2–3 grams in 24 hours
11 years	500 milligrams	500 milligrams	4–6 hours	250 milligrams in 5 ml	10 ml	2 grams in 24 hours
10 years	500 milligrams	500 milligrams	4–6 hours	250 milligrams in 5 ml	10 ml	2 grams in 24 hours
9 years	375 milligrams	375 milligrams	4–6 hours	250 milligrams in 5 ml	7.5 ml	1.5 grams in 24 hours
8 years	375 milligrams	375 milligrams	4–6 hours	250 milligrams in 5 ml	7.5 ml	1.5 grams in 24 hours
7 years	250 milligrams	250 milligrams	4–6 hours	250 milligrams in 5 ml	5 ml	1 gram in 24 hours
6 years	250 milligrams	250 milligrams	4–6 hours	250 milligrams in 5 ml	5 ml	1 gram in 24 hours
5 years	N/A	N/A	N/A	N/A	N/A	N/A
4 years	N/A	N/A	N/A	N/A	N/A	N/A
3 years	N/A	N/A	N/A	N/A	N/A	N/A
2 years	N/A	N/A	N/A	N/A	N/A	N/A
18 months	N/A	N/A	N/A	N/A	N/A	N/A
12 months	N/A	N/A	N/A	N/A	N/A	N/A
9 months	N/A	N/A	N/A	N/A	N/A	N/A
6 months	N/A	N/A	N/A	N/A	N/A	N/A
3 months	N/A	N/A	N/A	N/A	N/A	N/A
1 month	N/A	N/A	N/A	N/A	N/A	N/A
Birth	N/A	N/A	N/A	N/A	N/A	N/A

Paracetamol

> Ensure that:
> 1. Paracetamol (or an alternative paracetamol-containing product) has not been taken within the previous 4 hours (6 hours in renal impairment).
> 2. The maximum cumulative daily dose has not already been taken.

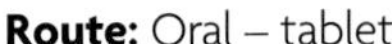

Route: Oral – tablet.

AGE	INITIAL DOSE	REPEAT DOSE	DOSE INTERVAL	CONCENTRATION	VOLUME	MAXIMUM DOSE
16 years – Adult AND **over** 50 kg	500 milligrams – 1 gram	500 milligrams – 1 gram	4–6 hours	500 milligrams per tablet	1–2 tablets	2–4 grams in 24 hours
12 years – 15years OR 50 kg and **under**	500–750 milligrams	500–750 milligrams	4–6 hours	500 milligrams per tablet	1–1.5 tablets	2–3 grams in 24 hours

Paracetamol

Ensure that:
1. Paracetamol (or an alternative paracetamol-containing product) has not been taken within the previous 4 hours (6 hours in renal impairment).
2. The maximum cumulative daily dose has not already been taken.
3. IV paracetamol is only used when managing **severe pain** (use an oral preparation when managing fever with discomfort).

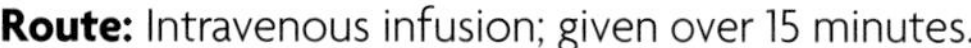

Route: Intravenous infusion; given over 15 minutes.

AGE	INITIAL DOSE	REPEAT DOSE	DOSE INTERVAL	CONCENTRATION	VOLUME	MAXIMUM DOSE
12 years – Adult AND **over** 50 kg	1 gram	1 gram	4–6 hours	10 milligrams in 1 ml	100 ml	4 grams in 24 hours
12 years – Adult AND **under** 50 kg	750 milligrams	750 milligrams	4–6 hours	10 milligrams in 1 ml	75 ml	3 grams in 24 hours
11 years	500 milligrams	500 milligrams	4–6 hours	10 milligrams in 1 ml	50 ml	2 grams in 24 hours
10 years	500 milligrams	500 milligrams	4–6 hours	10 milligrams in 1 ml	50 ml	2 grams in 24 hours
9 years	450 milligrams	450 milligrams	4–6 hours	10 milligrams in 1 ml	45 ml	1.8 grams in 24 hours
8 years	400 milligrams	400 milligrams	4–6 hours	10 milligrams in 1 ml	40 ml	1.6 grams in 24 hours
7 years	350 milligrams	350 milligrams	4–6 hours	10 milligrams in 1 ml	35 ml	1.4 grams in 24 hours
6 years	300 milligrams	300 milligrams	4–6 hours	10 milligrams in 1 ml	30 ml	1.2 grams in 24 hours
5 years	300 milligrams	300 milligrams	4–6 hours	10 milligrams in 1 ml	30 ml	1.2 gram in 24 hours
4 years	250 milligrams	250 milligrams	4–6 hours	10 milligrams in 1 ml	25 ml	1 gram in 24 hours
3 years	200 milligrams	200 milligrams	4–6 hours	10 milligrams in 1 ml	20 ml	800 milligrams in 24 hours
2 years	200 milligrams	200 milligrams	4–6 hours	10 milligrams in 1 ml	20 ml	800 milligrams in 24 hours
18 months	150 milligrams	150 milligrams	4–6 hours	10 milligrams in 1 ml	15 ml	600 milligrams in 24 hours
12 months	150 milligrams	150 milligrams	4–6 hours	10 milligrams in 1 ml	15 ml	600 milligrams in 24 hours
9 months	90 milligrams	90 milligrams	4–6 hours	10 milligrams in 1 ml	9 ml	270 milligrams in 24 hours
6 months	80 milligrams	80 milligrams	4–6 hours	10 milligrams in 1 ml	8 ml	240 milligrams in 24 hours
3 months	60 milligrams	60 milligrams	4–6 hours	10 milligrams in 1 ml	6 ml	180 milligrams in 24 hours
1 month	45 milligrams	45 milligrams	4–6 hours	10 milligrams in 1 ml	4.5 ml	135 milligrams in 24 hours
Birth	35 milligrams	35 milligrams	4–6 hours	10 milligrams in 1 ml	3.5ml	105 milligrams in 24 hours

0.9% Sodium Chloride

Presentation

100 ml, 250 ml, 500 ml and 1,000 ml packs of sodium chloride intravenous infusion 0.9%.

5 ml and 10 ml ampoules for use as flushes.

5 ml and 10 ml pre-loaded syringes for use as flushes.

Indications

Adult fluid therapy

- Medical conditions without haemorrhage.
- Medical conditions with haemorrhage.
- Trauma related haemorrhage.
- Burns.
- Limb crush injury.

Child fluid therapy

- Medical conditions.
- Trauma related haemorrhage.
- Burns.

Flush

- As a flush to confirm patency of an intravenous or intraosseous cannula.
- As a flush following drug administration.

Actions

Increases vascular fluid volume which consequently raises cardiac output and improves perfusion.

Contra-indications

None.

Side Effects

Over-infusion may precipitate pulmonary oedema and cause breathlessness.

Additional Information

Fluid replacement in cases of dehydration should occur over hours; rapid fluid replacement is seldom indicated; refer to **Intravascular Fluid Therapy**.

Dosage and Administration

Route: Intravenous or intraosseous for **ALL** conditions.

FLUSH

AGE	INITIAL DOSE	REPEAT DOSE	DOSE INTERVAL	CONCENTRATION	VOLUME	MAXIMUM DOSE
Adult	2 ml – 5 ml	2 ml – 5 ml	PRN	0.9%	2 – 5 ml	N/A
Adult	10 ml – 20 ml (if infusing glucose)	10 ml – 20 ml (if infusing glucose)	PRN	0.9%	10 – 20 ml	N/A
5 – 11 years	2 ml – 5 ml	2 ml – 5 ml	PRN	0.9%	2 – 5 ml	N/A
5 – 11 years	5 ml – 10 ml (if infusing glucose)	5 ml – 10 ml (if infusing glucose)	PRN	0.9%	5 – 10 ml	N/A
Birth – <5 years	2 ml	2 ml	PRN	0.9%	2 ml	N/A
Birth – <5 years	2 ml – 5 ml (if infusing glucose)	2 ml – 5ml (if infusing glucose)	PRN	0.9%	2 – 5 ml	N/A

0.9% Sodium Chloride

ADULT MEDICAL EMERGENCIES

General medical conditions without haemorrhage: Anaphylaxis, hyperglycaemic ketoacidosis, dehydration[a]

AGE	INITIAL DOSE	REPEAT DOSE	DOSE INTERVAL	CONCENTRATION	VOLUME	MAXIMUM DOSE
Adult	250 ml	250 ml	PRN	0.9%	250 ml	2 litres

Sepsis: Clinical signs of infection **AND** systolic BP<90 mmHg

AGE	INITIAL DOSE	REPEAT DOSE	DOSE INTERVAL	CONCENTRATION	VOLUME	MAXIMUM DOSE
Adult	500 ml	500 ml	15 minutes	0.9%	500 ml	2 litres

Medical conditions with haemorrhage: Systolic BP<90 mmHg and signs of poor perfusion

AGE	INITIAL DOSE	REPEAT DOSE	DOSE INTERVAL	CONCENTRATION	VOLUME	MAXIMUM DOSE
Adult	250 ml	250 ml	PRN	0.9%	250 ml	2 litres

ADULT TRAUMA EMERGENCIES

Blunt trauma, head trauma or penetrating limb trauma: To maintain a palpable central pulse (carotid or femoral)

AGE	INITIAL DOSE	REPEAT DOSE	DOSE INTERVAL	CONCENTRATION	VOLUME	MAXIMUM DOSE
Adult	250 ml	250 ml	PRN	0.9%	250 ml	2 litres

Penetrating torso trauma: To maintain a palpable central pulse (carotid or femoral)

AGE	INITIAL DOSE	REPEAT DOSE	DOSE INTERVAL	CONCENTRATION	VOLUME	MAXIMUM DOSE
Adult	250 ml	250 ml	PRN	0.9%	250 ml	2 litres

Burns:

- Total body surface area (TBSA): between 15% and 25% and time to hospital is greater than 30 minutes
- TBSA: more than 25%

AGE	INITIAL DOSE	REPEAT DOSE	DOSE INTERVAL	CONCENTRATION	VOLUME	MAXIMUM DOSE
Adult	1 litre	NONE	N/A	0.9%	1 litre	1 litre

Limb crush injury

NB Manage crush injury of the torso as per blunt trauma.

AGE	INITIAL DOSE	REPEAT DOSE	DOSE INTERVAL	CONCENTRATION	VOLUME	MAXIMUM DOSE
Adult	2 litres	NONE	N/A	0.9%	2 litres	2 litres

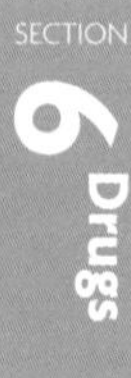

a In cases of dehydration fluid replacement should usually occur over hours.

0.9% Sodium Chloride

MEDICAL EMERGENCIES IN CHILDREN (20 ml/kg)

NB Exceptions: cardiac failure, renal failure, diabetic ketoacidosis (see following).

AGE	INITIAL DOSE	REPEAT DOSE	DOSE INTERVAL	CONCENTRATION	VOLUME	MAXIMUM DOSE
11 years	500 ml	500 ml	PRN	0.9%	500 ml	1,000 ml
10 years	500 ml	500 ml	PRN	0.9%	500 ml	1,000 ml
9 years	500 ml	500 ml	PRN	0.9%	500 ml	1,000 ml
8 years	500 ml	500 ml	PRN	0.9%	500 ml	1,000 ml
7 years	460 ml	460 ml	PRN	0.9%	460 ml	920 ml
6 years	420 ml	420 ml	PRN	0.9%	420 ml	840 ml
5 years	380 ml	380 ml	PRN	0.9%	380 ml	760 ml
4 years	320 ml	320 ml	PRN	0.9%	320 ml	640 ml
3 years	280 ml	280 ml	PRN	0.9%	280 ml	560 ml
2 years	240 ml	240 ml	PRN	0.9%	240 ml	480 ml
18 months	220 ml	220 ml	PRN	0.9%	220 ml	440 ml
12 months	200 ml	200 ml	PRN	0.9%	200 ml	400 ml
9 months	180 ml	180 ml	PRN	0.9%	180 ml	360 ml
6 months	160 ml	160 ml	PRN	0.9%	160 ml	320 ml
3 months	120 ml	120 ml	PRN	0.9%	120 ml	240 ml
1 month	90 ml	90 ml	PRN	0.9%	90 ml	180 ml
Birth	70 ml	70 ml	PRN	0.9%	70 ml	140 ml

MEDICAL EMERGENCIES IN CHILDREN

Heart failure or renal failure (10 ml/kg)

AGE	INITIAL DOSE	REPEAT DOSE	DOSE INTERVAL	CONCENTRATION	VOLUME	MAXIMUM DOSE
11 years	350 ml	350 ml	PRN	0.9%	350 ml	1,000 ml
10 years	320 ml	320 ml	PRN	0.9%	320 ml	1,000 ml
9 years	290 ml	290 ml	PRN	0.9%	290 ml	1,000 ml
8 years	250 ml	250 ml	PRN	0.9%	250 ml	1,000 ml
7 years	230 ml	230 ml	PRN	0.9%	230 ml	920 ml
6 years	210 ml	210 ml	PRN	0.9%	210 ml	840 ml
5 years	190 ml	190 ml	PRN	0.9%	190 ml	760 ml
4 years	160 ml	160 ml	PRN	0.9%	160 ml	640 ml
3 years	140 ml	140 ml	PRN	0.9%	140 ml	560 ml
2 years	120 ml	120 ml	PRN	0.9%	120 ml	480 ml
18 months	110 ml	110 ml	PRN	0.9%	110 ml	440 ml
12 months	100 ml	100 ml	PRN	0.9%	100 ml	400 ml
9 months	90 ml	90 ml	PRN	0.9%	90 ml	360 ml
6 months	80 ml	80 ml	PRN	0.9%	80 ml	320 ml
3 months	60 ml	60 ml	PRN	0.9%	60 ml	240 ml
1 month	45 ml	45 ml	PRN	0.9%	45 ml	180 ml
Birth	35 ml	35 ml	PRN	0.9%	35 ml	140 ml

0.9% Sodium Chloride

MEDICAL EMERGENCIES IN CHILDREN

Diabetic ketoacidosis (10 ml/kg) administer **ONCE** only over 15 minutes.

AGE	INITIAL DOSE	REPEAT DOSE	DOSE INTERVAL	CONCENTRATION	VOLUME	MAXIMUM DOSE
11 years	350 ml	NONE	NA	0.9%	350 ml	350 ml
10 years	320 ml	NONE	NA	0.9%	320 ml	320 ml
9 years	290 ml	NONE	NA	0.9%	290 ml	290 ml
8 years	250 ml	NONE	NA	0.9%	250 ml	250 ml
7 years	230 ml	NONE	NA	0.9%	230 ml	230 ml
6 years	210 ml	NONE	NA	0.9%	210 ml	210 ml
5 years	190 ml	NONE	NA	0.9%	190 ml	190 ml
4 years	160 ml	NONE	NA	0.9%	160 ml	160 ml
3 years	140 ml	NONE	NA	0.9%	140 ml	140 ml
2 years	120 ml	NONE	NA	0.9%	120 ml	120 ml
18 months	110 ml	NONE	NA	0.9%	110 ml	110 ml
12 months	100 ml	NONE	NA	0.9%	100 ml	100 ml
9 months	90 ml	NONE	NA	0.9%	90 ml	90 ml
6 months	80 ml	NONE	NA	0.9%	80 ml	80 ml
3 months	60 ml	NONE	NA	0.9%	60 ml	60 ml
1 month	45 ml	NONE	NA	0.9%	45 ml	45 ml
Birth	35 ml	NONE	NA	0.9%	35 ml	35 ml

TRAUMA EMERGENCIES IN CHILDREN (5 ml/kg)[a]

NB Exceptions: burns.

AGE	INITIAL DOSE	REPEAT DOSE	DOSE INTERVAL	CONCENTRATION	VOLUME	MAXIMUM DOSE
11 years	175 ml	175 ml	PRN	0.9%	175 ml	1,000 ml
10 years	160 ml	160 ml	PRN	0.9%	160 ml	1,000 ml
9 years	145 ml	145 ml	PRN	0.9%	145 ml	1,000 ml
8 years	130 ml	130 ml	PRN	0.9%	130 ml	1,000 ml
7 years	115 ml	115 ml	PRN	0.9%	115 ml	920 ml
6 years	105 ml	105 ml	PRN	0.9%	105 ml	840 ml
5 years	95 ml	95 ml	PRN	0.9%	95 ml	760 ml
4 years	80 ml	80 ml	PRN	0.9%	80 ml	640 ml
3 years	70 ml	70 ml	PRN	0.9%	70 ml	560 ml
2 years	60 ml	60 ml	PRN	0.9%	60 ml	480 ml
18 months	55 ml	55 ml	PRN	0.9%	55 ml	440 ml
12 months	50 ml	50 ml	PRN	0.9%	50 ml	400 ml
9 months	45 ml	45 ml	PRN	0.9%	45 ml	360 ml
6 months	40 ml	40 ml	PRN	0.9%	40 ml	320 ml
3 months	30 ml	30 ml	PRN	0.9%	30 ml	240 ml
1 month	20 ml	20 ml	PRN	0.9%	20 ml	180 ml
Birth	20 ml	20 ml	PRN	0.9%	20 ml	140 ml

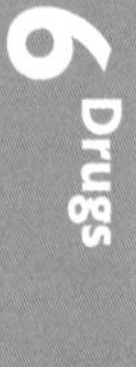

a Seek advice to exceed maximum dose in trauma

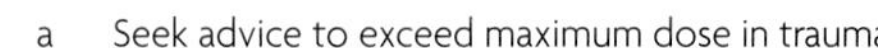

0.9% Sodium Chloride

Burns (10 ml/kg, given over 1 hour):

- TBSA: between 10% and 20% and time to hospital is greater than 30 minutes
- TBSA: more than 20%

AGE	INITIAL DOSE	REPEAT DOSE	DOSE INTERVAL	CONCENTRATION	VOLUME	MAXIMUM DOSE
11 years	350 ml	NONE	N/A	0.9%	350 ml	350 ml
10 years	320 ml	NONE	N/A	0.9%	320 ml	320 ml
9 years	290 ml	NONE	N/A	0.9%	290 ml	290 ml
8 years	250 ml	NONE	N/A	0.9%	250 ml	250 ml
7 years	230 ml	NONE	N/A	0.9%	230 ml	230 ml
6 years	210 ml	NONE	N/A	0.9%	210 ml	210 ml
5 years	190 ml	NONE	N/A	0.9%	190 ml	190 ml
4 years	160 ml	NONE	N/A	0.9%	160 ml	160 ml
3 years	140 ml	NONE	N/A	0.9%	140 ml	140 ml
2 years	120 ml	NONE	N/A	0.9%	120 ml	120 ml
18 months	110 ml	NONE	N/A	0.9%	110 ml	110 ml
12 months	100 ml	NONE	N/A	0.9%	100 ml	100 ml
9 months	90 ml	NONE	N/A	0.9%	90 ml	90 ml
6 months	80 ml	NONE	N/A	0.9%	80 ml	80 ml
3 months	60 ml	NONE	N/A	0.9%	60 ml	60 ml
1 month	45 ml	NONE	N/A	0.9%	45 ml	45 ml
Birth	35 ml	NONE	N/A	0.9%	35 ml	35 ml

Tranexamic Acid

Presentation

Vial containing 500 mg tranexamic acid in 5 ml (100 mg/ml).

Indications

- Patients with **TIME CRITICAL** injury where significant internal/external haemorrhage is suspected.
- Injured patients fulfilling local Step 1 or Step 2 trauma triage protocol – refer to **Appendix in Trauma Emergencies Overview (Adults)**.
- Women suffering from post-partum haemorrhage (PPH). Use TXA alongside uterotonic drugs (drugs that stimulate the uterus to contract) such as syntometrine and misoprostol – refer to **Birth Imminent**.

Actions

Tranexamic acid is an anti-fibrinolytic which reduces the breakdown of blood clot.

Contra-Indications

- Isolated head injury.
- Critical interventions required (if critical interventions leave insufficient time for TXA administration).
- Bleeding now stopped.

Side Effects

Rapid injection might rarely cause hypotension.

Additional Information

- There are good data that this treatment is safe and effective (giving a 9% reduction in the number of deaths in patients in the CRASH-2 trial).
- There is no evidence about whether or not tranexamic acid is effective in patients with head injury; however, there is no evidence of harm.
- High dose regimes have been associated with convulsions; however, in the low dose regime recommended here, the benefit from giving TXA in trauma outweighs the risk of convulsions.
- Refer to local PGD for information on administration procedures. May be given by the intraosseous route as per local procedures, but this route is not currently licensed.

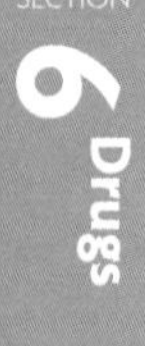

Dosage and Administration

Route: Intravenous only – **administer SLOWLY over 10 minutes – can be given as 10 aliquots administered 1 minute apart.**

AGE	INITIAL DOSE	REPEAT DOSE	DOSE INTERVAL	CONCENTRATION	VOLUME	MAXIMUM DOSE
>12 years – Adult	1 gram	NONE	N/A	100 mg/ml	10 ml	1 gram
11 years	500 mg	NONE	N/A	100 mg/ml	5 ml	500 mg
10 years	500 mg	NONE	N/A	100 mg/ml	5 ml	500 mg
9 years	450 mg	NONE	N/A	100 mg/ml	4.5 ml	450 mg
8 years	400 mg	NONE	N/A	100 mg/ml	4 ml	400 mg
7 years	350 mg	NONE	N/A	100 mg/ml	3.5 ml	350 mg
6 years	300 mg	NONE	N/A	100 mg/ml	3 ml	300 mg
5 years	300 mg	NONE	N/A	100 mg/ml	3 ml	300 mg
4 years	250 mg	NONE	N/A	100 mg/ml	2.5 ml	250 mg
3 years	200 mg	NONE	N/A	100 mg/ml	2 ml	200 mg
2 years	200 mg	NONE	N/A	100 mg/ml	2 ml	200 mg
18 months	150 mg	NONE	N/A	100 mg/ml	1.5 mls	150 mg
12 months	150 mg	NONE	N/A	100 mg/ml	1.5 ml	150 mg
9 months	150 mg	NONE	N/A	100 mg/ml	1.5 ml	150 mg
6 months	100 mg	NONE	N/A	100 mg/ml	1 ml	100 mg
3 months	100 mg	NONE	N/A	100 mg/ml	1 ml	100 mg
1 month	50 mg	NONE	N/A	100 mg/ml	0.5 ml	50 mg
Birth	50 mg	NONE	N/A	100 mg/ml	0.5 ml	50 mg

Bibliography

1 CRASH-2 trial collaborators. Effects of tranexamic acid on death, vascular occlusive events, and blood transfusion in trauma patients with significant haemorrhage (CRASH-2): a randomised, placebo-controlled trial. *The Lancet* 2010, 376(9734): 23–32.

2 CRASH-2 trial collaborators. The importance of early treatment with tranexamic acid in bleeding trauma patients: an exploratory analysis of the CRASH-2 randomised controlled trial. *The Lancet* 2011, 377(9771): 1096–101.e2.

3 Yeguiayan J-M, Rosencher N, Vivien B. Early administration of tranexamic acid in trauma patients. *The Lancet* 2011, 378(9785): 27–8.

4 Cap AP, Baer DG, Orman JA, Aden J, Ryan K, Blackbourne LH. Tranexamic acid for trauma patients: a critical review of the literature. *Journal of Trauma and Acute Care Surgery* 2011, 71(1): S9–14: doi 10.1097/TA.0b013e31822114af.

5 NHS Evidence. *Tranexamic acid.* Available from: http://www.evidence.nhs.uk/formulary/bnf/current/2-cardiovascular-system/211-antifibrinolytic-drugs-and-haemostatics/tranexamic-acid, 2011.

6 World Maternal Antifibrinolytic Trial (The WOMAN Trial). Effect of early tranexamic acid administration on mortality, hysterectomy, and other morbidities in women with post-partum haemorrhage (WOMAN): an international, randomised, double-blind, placebo-controlled trial. *The Lancet 2017*, 389(10084): 2105–2116. Available from: http://thelancet.com/journals/lancet/article/PIIS0140-6736(17)30638-4/fulltext.

Intravascular Fluid Therapy (Adults)

1. Introduction[1, 2, 3, 4, 5, 6, 7, 8]

- Despite a lack of evidence demonstrating any significant beneficial effects, pre-hospital fluid therapy has become an established practice.
- There is, however, a significant body of evidence that indicates that routine pre-hospital intravascular fluid therapy may, in fact, be detrimental.
- Adverse effects may be attributed to prolonged on-scene times delaying time to definitive surgical intervention, thrombus disruption, dilution of clotting factors and other coagulopathies.

2. Pathophysiology[3, 8, 9]

- The objective of fluid therapy is to improve end-organ perfusion and, as a consequence, oxygen delivery.
- By increasing the circulating volume, cardiac output and blood pressure are increased by the Bainbridge Reflex and Frank–Starling Law of the Heart.
- The speed with which a given fluid will produce its effect will largely be determined by how it is distributed throughout the body and how long it remains in the vascular space.

2.1 pH buffering

- Reduced perfusion leads to acidosis as a result of anaerobic metabolism producing lactic acid, phosphoric acids and unoxidised amino acids.
- This acidosis can depress cardiac function (negative inotropic effect) and cause arrhythmias.

2.2 Oxygen transport

- Crystalloid fluids currently used in the pre-hospital environment have no oxygen carrying capacity.
- However, the administration of fluids reduces blood viscosity which in turn may lead to improved peripheral blood flow and hence oxygen delivery.

2.3 Haemostasis

- In general, administration of fluid has a detrimental effect on haemostasis and a tendency to increase bleeding.
- The administration of fluid raises intravascular pressures and usually causes vasodilation, both of which may precipitate disruption of the primary haemostatic thrombus.
- Furthermore, supplemental administration of fluid reduces blood viscosity and dilutes clotting factors both of which can be detrimental to haemostatic mechanisms.
- Finally, in order to minimise hypothermia-induced coagulopathies, the use of cold fluids should be avoided if possible.

3. Haemorrhagic Emergencies[10, 11, 12, 13, 14, 15, 16, 17, 18, 19, 20, 21, 22]

Table 6.15 – EARLY INDICATORS OF IMPAIRED MAJOR ORGAN PERFUSION

SIGNS	CAUSE
Tachypnoea	↑ Metabolic acidosis
Tachycardia	↓ Cardiac output
Hypotension	↓ Vascular volume
↓ Consciousness	↓ Cerebral perfusion

- Haemorrhage may occur as a result of traumatic or medical aetiologies and may be classified as:
  - **apparent** (external) blood loss
  - **concealed** (internal) blood loss.
- Current thinking suggests that fluids should **ONLY** be administered when there are signs of impaired major organ perfusion (refer to Table 6.15).
- Control of external haemorrhage must be achieved before administering fluids.

3.1 Trauma

3.1.1 Penetrating trauma to the trunk

- Penetrating trauma to the trunk carries the risk of significant disruption of major vessels that, due to their location, are not amenable to compression or other methods of haemorrhage control.
- As a consequence of this inability to control further bleeding, the general aim of fluid therapy is to maintain a palpable central pulse (carotid or femoral).

3.1.2 Penetrating trauma to the limbs

- Penetrating trauma to the limbs also carries a risk of significant disruption of major vessels; however, these vessels are both fewer and more amenable to compression or other methods of haemorrhage control.
- As a consequence of this ability to control further bleeding, the general aim of fluid therapy is to maintain a palpable central pulse (carotid or femoral).

3.1.3 Blunt trauma to trunk or limbs

- Blunt trauma to the trunk carries a lower risk of major vessel disruption; consequently, the trigger point for fluid administration is different from penetrating trauma.
- In cases of blunt trauma to the trunk or limbs, the aim of fluid therapy is to maintain a palpable central pulse (carotid or femoral).

3.1.4 Trauma to the head (all types)

- Significant head injury results in raised intracranial pressure (ICP) as cerebral tissues swell within the enclosed skull; to ensure adequate cerebral perfusion pressure (CPP) the body compensates and raises the mean arterial blood pressure (MAP).

CPP = MAP – ICP

- As a result of this compensatory mechanism, significant head injuries are usually associated with hypertension and **NOT** hypotension.
- Hypotension in the setting of significant head injury indicates not only significant blood loss but also **CRITICALLY IMPAIRED CEREBRAL PERFUSION.**
- In order to support cerebral perfusion the administration of fluids may be required.
- In the setting of significant head injury with hypotension, fluid therapy should be titrated to maintain a palpable central pulse (carotid or femoral).
- Hypertensive head injury does not normally require fluid therapy. Research concerning pre-hospital hypertonic saline has yet to demonstrate conclusive evidence of beneficial effect.

3.2 Medical conditions

- Principles of fluid therapy in medically related haemorrhage are fundamentally no different from those of blunt trauma.
- Generally, the aim of fluid therapy is to maintain systolic blood pressure at 90 mmHg.
- Medically related haemorrhage may also be complicated by vascular disease, coagulopathies or the presence of tumours.

3.3 Fluid therapy following haemorrhage

- **DO NOT** delay at scene to obtain vascular access or to commence fluid replacement; wherever possible obtain vascular access and administer fluid **EN-ROUTE TO HOSPITAL.**
- If the clinician determines that there is a definite need for fluid therapy they should obtain vascular access.
- Clinicians should attempt to gain intravenous access in the first instance; however, they may consider intraosseous access where intravenous access fails or is unlikely to be successful.
- Vascular access devices should be flushed with 5 ml of 0.9% sodium chloride for injection to confirm patency prior to administering large volumes of fluid.
- Once patent vascular access is confirmed, administer a single bolus of 250 ml of crystalloid (refer to Table 6.16).
- Where the need for intravascular fluid therapy is less certain, clinicians should still obtain vascular access and flush to confirm patency.
- **Do not connect any fluids to the cannula unless intravascular fluid therapy is indicated.**

NB The slow administration of fluids to keep a vein open (TKO/TKVO) should not be practised to avoid inadvertent excess fluid administration.

Table 6.16 – DOSAGES FOR FLUID THERAPY – HAEMORRHAGIC EMERGENCIES

INITIAL DOSE	REPEAT DOSE	REPEAT INTERVAL	MAXIMUM DOSE
250 ml	250 ml	PRN	2 litres

- Monitor the physiological response; re-assess perfusion, pulse, respiratory rate and blood pressure wherever possible.
- If these observations improve, suspend any further administration.
- If there is no improvement administer further 250 ml boluses, re-assessing for improvement after each fluid bolus (refer to Table 6.16).
- The maximum cumulative fluid dose is usually 2 litres (refer to Table 6.16).
- If the patient remains hypotensive despite repeated 250 ml boluses **OR** the patient is likely to remain on scene for a considerable time (e.g. due to entrapment), request senior clinical support (according to local procedures).

3.4 Exceptions and special circumstances

3.4.1 Crush injury

- A crush injury is caused by direct compressive force on the body. Crush syndrome is the systemic manifestation of muscle cell damage resulting from pressure or crushing.
- The severity of the injury is related to both the magnitude of the compressing force, and the bulk of muscle affected, but not necessarily the duration for which the force has been applied.
- The pathophysiology of crush syndrome results from the leakiness of the cellular membranes as a consequence of pressure or stretching. Sodium, calcium and water leak through the cellular membrane into the muscle cell, trapping extracellular fluid inside the muscle cells. In addition to the influx of these elements into the cell, the cell releases potassium and other toxic substances such as myoglobin, phosphate and uric acid into the circulation.
- The end result of these events is hypotension, hyperkalaemia (which may precipitate cardiac arrest), hypocalcaemia, metabolic acidosis, compartment syndrome (due to swelling), and acute renal failure (ARF).
- If possible, fluid therapy should commence prior to extrication; however, extrication or transport **MUST NOT** be unnecessarily delayed in order to obtain intravenous access or to administer fluid.
- In crush injury of the limbs an initial fluid bolus of 2 litres of 0.9% sodium chloride should be administered (refer to Table 6.17).
- In crush injury of the torso follow blunt trauma fluid therapy practices (see 3.1.3).

- If possible, request senior clinical support to guide further therapy.

Table 6.17 – DOSAGES FOR FLUID THERAPY – CRUSH INJURY OF THE LIMBS

INITIAL DOSE	REPEAT DOSE	REPEAT INTERVAL	MAXIMUM DOSE
2 litres	NONE	N/A	2 litres

3.4.2 Obstetric emergencies

- Clinicians must remember that the gravid uterus may compress the inferior vena cava in a pregnant patient who is supine. Appropriate positioning of the patient, including manual displacement of the gravid uterus (rather than left lateral tilt) must be used to ensure adequate venous return before determining that a pregnant patient is in need of fluid resuscitation.
- Due to their increase in blood volume, the obstetric patient is able to tolerate far greater blood loss, up to 50%, before showing signs of hypovolaemia/shock.
- In obstetric patients, the uterus, and thus the fetus, will often become 'underperfused' **PRIOR** to the pregnant women showing outward signs of shock (i.e. becoming tachycardic or hypotensive).
- Signs of shock appear very late during pregnancy and hypotension is an extremely late sign.
- Clinicians should take frequent clinical observations and be vigilant for subtle changes that may indicate the onset of shock.
- Fluid replacement should aim to maintain a systolic blood pressure of 90 mmHg in obstetric patients who are bleeding.

4. Non-Haemorrhagic Emergencies[23, 24, 15, 16, 17, 18, 19, 20, 25, 26, 27, 28, 29, 30, 31, 32, 33, 34, 35]

4.1 Trauma

- The loss of bodily fluids other than blood, as a result of trauma, is rare. Burn injuries are notable exceptions (see exceptions and special circumstances below).

4.2 Medical conditions

- Patients suffering medical emergencies may experience fluid loss as a result of dehydration (e.g. heat related illness, vomiting or diarrhoea) and/or redistribution of fluid from the vascular compartment (e.g. as a result of anaphylaxis).
- The volume of fluids lost to such processes can easily be underestimated.
- Such patients may be significantly dehydrated resulting in reduced fluid volumes in both the vascular and tissue compartments which has usually taken time to develop and will take time to correct.
- Rapid fluid replacement into the vascular compartment can compromise the cardiovascular system particularly where there is pre-existing cardiovascular disease and in the elderly.
- In cases of dehydration, fluid replacement should be aimed at gradual re-hydration over many hours rather than minutes. Oral electrolyte solutions may be an appropriate consideration in some patients (e.g. heat illness).

4.3 Fluid therapy

- **DO NOT** delay at scene to obtain vascular access or to provide fluid replacement; wherever possible obtain vascular access and administer fluid **EN-ROUTE TO HOSPITAL.**
- If the clinician determines that there is a definite need for fluid therapy, they should obtain vascular access.
- Clinicians should attempt to gain intravenous access in the first instance; however, they may consider intraosseous access where intravenous access fails or is unlikely to be successful.
- Vascular access devices should be flushed with 5 ml of 0.9% sodium chloride for injection to confirm patency prior to administering large volumes of fluid.
- Once patent vascular access is confirmed, administer a single bolus of 250 ml of crystalloid (refer to Table 6.18).
- Where the need for intravascular fluid therapy is less certain, clinicians should still obtain vascular access and flush to confirm patency.
- **Do not connect any fluids to the cannula unless intravascular fluid therapy is indicated.**

NB The slow administration of fluids to keep a vein open (TKO/TKVO) should not be practised to avoid inadvertent excess fluid administration.

Table 6.18 – DOSAGES FOR FLUID THERAPY

INITIAL DOSE	REPEAT DOSE	REPEAT INTERVAL	MAXIMUM DOSE
250 ml	250 ml	PRN	2 litres

- Monitor the physiological response, re-assess perfusion, pulse, respiratory rate and blood pressure wherever possible.
- If these observations improve, suspend any further administration.
- If there is no improvement, administer further 250 ml boluses, reassessing for improvement after each fluid bolus (refer toTable 6.18).
- The maximum cumulative fluid dose is usually 2 litres (refer to Table 6.18).
- If the patient remains hypotensive despite repeated 250 ml boluses OR the patient is likely to remain on scene for a considerable time (e.g. due to extrication difficulties), request senior clinical support (according to local procedures).

Intravascular Fluid Therapy (Adults)

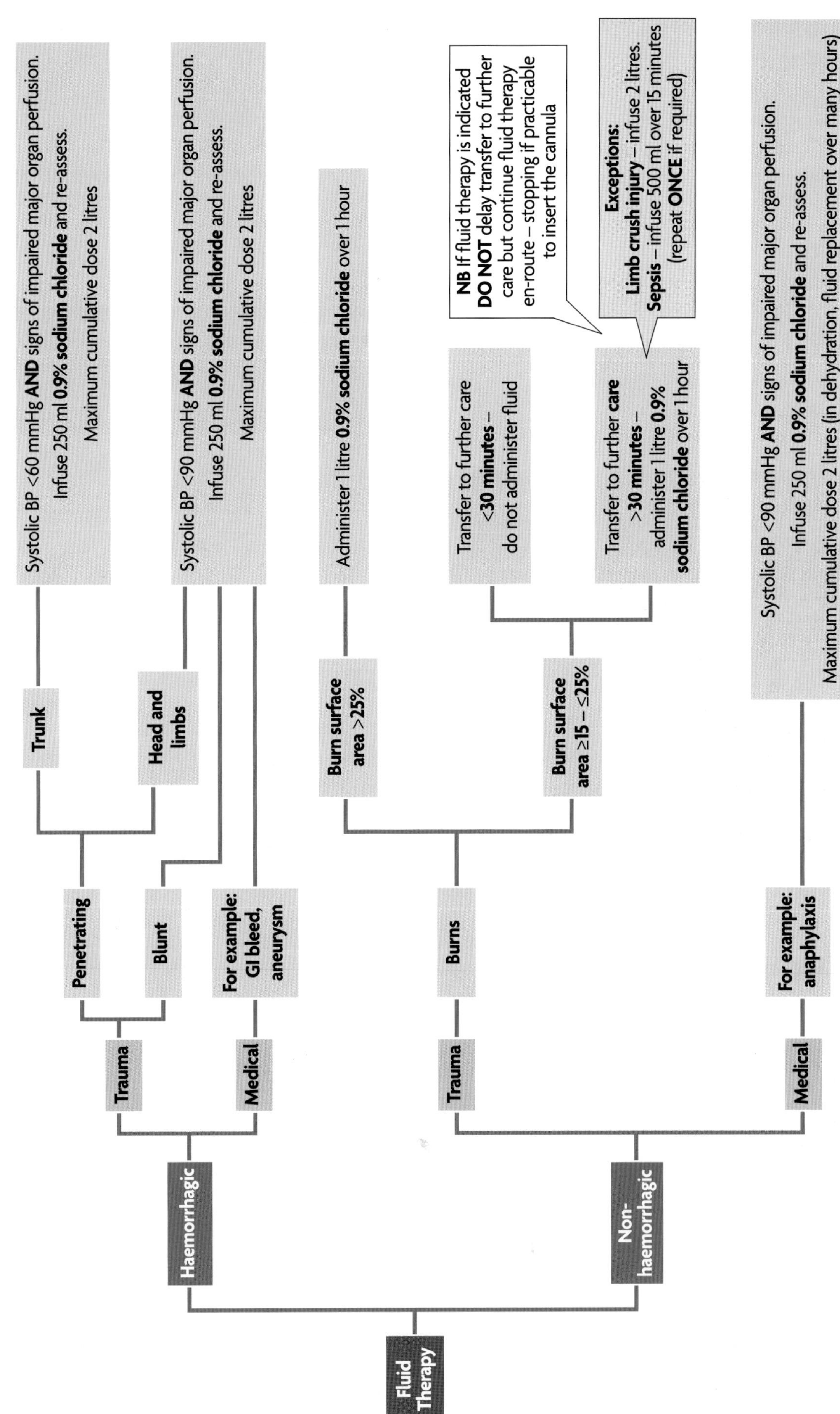

Figure 6.2 – Intravascular fluid therapy algorithm – adults

4.4 Exceptions and special circumstances

4.4.1 Burns

Where burn surface area is:

- <15% do not administer fluid.
- ≥15 – <25% and time to hospital is greater than 30 minutes, then administer 1 litre sodium chloride 0.9% (refer to Table 6.19).
- ≥25% administer 1 litre sodium chloride 0.9% (refer to Table 6.19).

NB If fluid therapy is indicated **DO NOT** delay transfer to further care but continue fluid therapy en-route – stopping if practicable to insert the cannula.

- Care must be taken to ensure that elderly or heart failure patients are not over-infused.
- In order to minimise the risk of hypothermia, the use of cold fluids should be avoided if possible.

Table 6.19 – DOSAGES FOR FLUID THERAPY – BURNS

INITIAL DOSE	REPEAT DOSE	REPEAT INTERVAL	MAXIMUM DOSE
1 litre over 1 hour	NONE[a]	N/A	1 litre

4.4.2 Sepsis

- Sepsis should be suspected in patients who:
  - present with fever/feeling unwell
  - **and** NEWS greater than or equal to 5
  - **and/or** look unwell with history of infection.
- Patients with sepsis will benefit from early fluid therapy and an appropriate hospital alert/information call.
- Intravascular fluid should be administered in cases of suspected sepsis (refer to Table 3.10 and Table 3.11 in **Sepsis**).

Table 6.20 – DOSAGES FOR FLUID THERAPY – SEPSIS

INITIAL DOSE	REPEAT DOSE	REPEAT INTERVAL	MAXIMUM DOSE
500ml over 15 minutes	Repeat ONCE if still hypotensive	PRN	2 litres

KEY POINTS

Intravascular Fluid Therapy (Adults)

- **Current research shows little evidence to support the routine use of IV fluids in adult acute blood loss.**
- **Current thinking is that fluids should only be administered when major organ perfusion is impaired.**
- **DO NOT delay on scene for vascular access or fluid replacement; wherever possible obtain vascular access and administer fluid EN-ROUTE TO HOSPITAL stopping if practicable to insert the cannula.**

Bibliography

1 Revell M, Porter K, Greaves I. Fluid resuscitation in pre-hospital trauma care: a consensus view. *Emergency Medicine Journal* 2002, 19(6): 494–498.

2 Bickell WH, Wall MJJ, Pepe PE, Martin RR, Ginger VF, Allen M K, et al. Immediate versus delayed fluid resuscitation in patients with trauma. *New England Journal of Medicine* 1994, 331: 1105–9.

3 Consensus Working Group on Pre-hospital Fluids. Fluid resuscitation in pre-hospital trauma care: a consensus *view. Journal of the Royal Army Medical Corps* 2001, 147(2): 147–52.

4 Cotton BA, Jerome R, Collier BR, Khetarpal S, Holevar M, Tucker B, et al. Guidelines for pre-hospital fluid resuscitation in the injured patient. *Journal of Trauma* 2009, 67(2): 389–402.

5 Dalton AM. Pre-hospital intravenous fluid replacement in trauma: an outmoded concept? *Journal of the Royal Society of Medicine* 1995, 88(4): 213P–216P.

6 Gausche M, Tadeo RE, Zane MC, Lewis RJ. Out-of-hospital intravenous access: unnecessary procedures and excessive cost. *Academic Emergency Medicine* 1998, 5(9): 878–82.

7 Henderson RA, Thomson DP, Bahrs BA, Norman MP. Unnecessary intravenous access in the emergency setting. *Prehospital Emergency Care* 1998, 2(4): 312–16.

8 Mitra B, Cameron PA, Mori A, Fitzgerald M. Acute coagulopathy and early deaths post major trauma. *Injury* 2012, 43(1): 22–5.

9 Roberts K, Revell M, Youssef H, Bradbury AW, Adam DJ. Hypotensive resuscitation in patients with ruptured abdominal aortic aneurysm. *European Journal of Vascular & Endovascular Surgery* 2005, 31(4): 339–44.

10 Kaweski SM, Sise MJ, Virgilio RW. The effect of pre-hospital fluids on survival in trauma patients. *Journal of Trauma* 1990, 30(10): 1215–18; discussion 1218–19.

11 Spahn D, Cerny V, Coats T, Duranteau J, Fernandez-Mondejar F, Gordini G, et al. Management of bleeding following major trauma: a European guideline. *Critical Care* 2007, 11(1): R17.

12 Eckstein M, Chan L, Schneir A, Palmer R. Effect of pre-hospital advanced life support on outcomes of major trauma patients. *Journal of Trauma* 2000, 48(4): 643–8.

a Seek senior clinical input for prolonged delays

13 Honigman B, Rohweder K, Moore EE, Lowenstein SR, Pons PT. Pre-hospital advanced trauma life support for penetrating cardiac wounds. *Annals of Emergency Medicine* 1990, 19(2): 145–50.

14 National Institute for Clinical Excellence. *Pre-hospital Initiation of Fluid Replacement Therapy in Trauma* (TA74). London: NICE. Available from: https://www.nice.org.uk/guidance/ta74, 2004.

15 Bulger EM, May S, Brasel KJ, Schreiber M, Kerby JD, Tisherman SA, et al. Out-of-hospital hypertonic resuscitation following severe traumatic brain injury: a randomized controlled trial. *Journal of the American Medical Association* 2010, 304(13): 1455–64.

16 Chung KK, Wolf SE, Cancio LC, Alvarado R, Jones JA, McCorcle J, et al. Resuscitation of severely burned military casualties: fluid begets more fluid. *Journal of Trauma* 2009, 67(2): 231–7; discussion 237.

17 Cooper DJ, Myles PS, McDermott FT, Murray LJ, Laidlaw J, Cooper G, et al. Pre-hospital hypertonic saline resuscitation of patients with hypotension and severe traumatic brain injury: a randomized controlled trial. *Journal of the American Medical* Association 2004, 291(11): 1350–7.

18 Holcroft JW, Vassar MJ, Turner JE, Derlet RW, Kramer GC. 3% NaCl and 7.5% NaCl/dextran 70 in the resuscitation of severely injured patients. *Annals of Surgery* 1987, 206(3): 279–88.

19 Maningas PA, Mattox KL, Pepe PE, Jones RL, Feliciano DV, Burch JM. Hypertonic saline-dextran solutions for the pre-hospital management of traumatic hypotension. *American Journal of Surgery* 1989, 157(5): 528–33; discussion 533–4.

20 Thompson R, Greaves I. Hypertonic saline-hydroxyethyl starch in trauma resuscitation. *Journal of the Royal Army Medical Corps* 2006, 152(1): 6–12.

21 Vassar MJ, Perry CA, Gannaway WL, Holcroft JW. 7.5% sodium chloride/dextran for resuscitation of trauma patients undergoing helicopter transport. *Archives of Surgery* 1991, 126(9): 1065–72.

22 Vassar MJ, Perry CA, Holcroft JW. Pre-hospital resuscitation of hypotensive trauma patients with 7.5% NaCl versus 7.5% NaCl with added dextran: a controlled trial. *Journal of Trauma* 1993, 34(5): 622–32; discussion 632–3.

23 Allison K, Porter K. Consensus on the pre-hospital approach to burns patient management. *Emergency Medicine Journal* 2004, 21(1): 112–14.

24 Williams G, Dziewulski P. Intravascular fluid therapy in burns injury. In Group. TJRCALGD, editor, 2011.

25 Greaves I, Porter K, Smith JE. Consensus statement on the early management of crush injury and prevention of crush syndrome. *Journal of the Royal Army Medical Corps* 2003, 149(4): 255–9.

26 Holcomb JB. Fluid resuscitation in modern combat casualty care: lessons learned from Somalia. *Journal of Trauma* 2003, 54(suppl.): S46–51.

27 Treharne LJ, Kay AR. The initial management of acute burns. *Journal of the Royal Army Medical Corps* 2001, 147(2): 198–205.

28 Mattox KL, Maningas PA, Moore EE, Mateer JR, Marx JA, Aprahamian C, et al. Pre-hospital hypertonic saline/dextran infusion for post-traumatic hypotension: the U.S.A. Multicenter Trial. *Annals of Surgery* 1991, 213(5): 482–91.

29 Smith JE, Hall MJ. Hypertonic saline. *Journal of the Royal Army Medical Corps* 2004, 150(4): 239–43.

30 Pons PT, Moore EE, Cusick JM, Brunko M, Antuna B, Owens L. Pre-hospital venous access in an urban paramedic system: a prospective on-scene analysis. *Journal of Trauma* 1988, 28(10): 1460–3.

31 Jones SE, Nesper TP, Alcouloumre E. Pre-hospital intravenous line placement: a prospective study. *Annals of Emergency Medicine* 1989, 18(3): 244–6.

32 Minville V, Pianezza A, Asehnoune K, Cabardis S, Smail N. Pre-hospital intravenous line placement assessment in the French emergency system: a prospective study. *European Journal of Anaesthesia* 2006, 23(7): 594–7.

33 Sampalis JS, Tamim H, Denis R, Boukas S, Ruest SA, Nikolis A, et al. Ineffectiveness of on-site intravenous lines: is pre-hospital time the culprit? *Journal of Trauma* 1997, 43(4): 608–15; discussion 615–17.

34 Daniels R. Surviving Sepsis Campaign: indications for fluid administration in patients with sepsis. Personal communication, 2011.

35 Dellinger RP, Levy MM, Cadet JM, Bion J, Parker MM, Jaeschke R, et al. Surviving Sepsis Campaign: international guidelines for management of severe sepsis and septic shock 2008. *Critical Care Medicine* 2008, 36(1): 296–327: doi 10.1097/01.CCM.0000298158.12101.41.

Index

Below is an index of terms included in these 2017 supplementary guidelines. For a list of topics in the 2016 edition, refer to Contents of the 2016 Edition and 2017 Supplementary Guidelines, which appears at the end of this index.